ALL YOU NEEDLE TO KNOW

All you Needle to Know

By Nita Lemonia McHugh

Published by. Nita Lemonia McHugh

Published in 2025

First Edition

ISBN: 978-0-646-74265-6

Imprint: Published by Lemonia McHugh

Cover Design by hcjart.com.au | stock glove image by freepik

Dedications

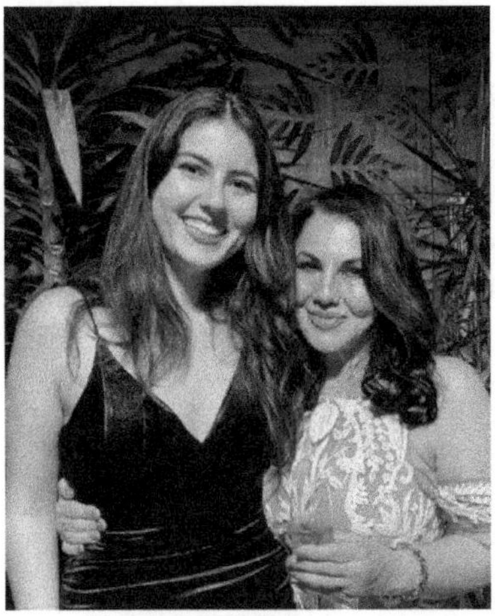

This book is dedicated to my daughter, Antonia, whose patience, curiosity, and sharp wit have been a constant source of inspiration. She spent countless hours in my clinic's waiting room, diligently doing her homework, chatting with clients, and even turning school show-and-tell into a lesson on the differences between fillers and Botox. Her keen eye and clever mind gave this book its perfect title, All You NEEDLE to Know.

Antonia, thank you for growing up alongside my passion and for always believing in the work I do. This book, in many ways, is as much yours as it is mine.

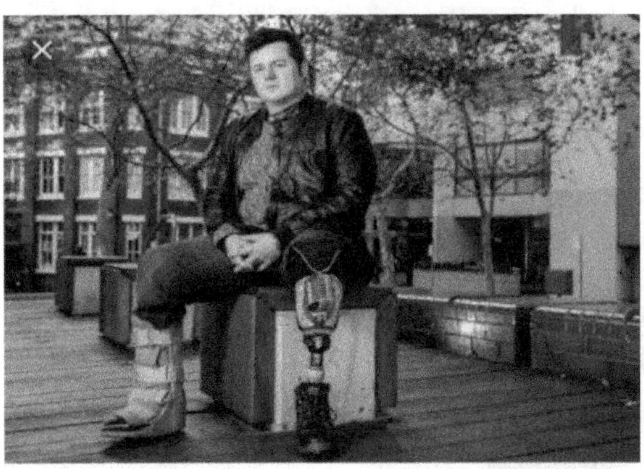

Daily Telegraph

"To my son, Mathew whose courage and determination inspire me daily. Your strength in overcoming adversity is a testament to the human spirit."

To Dr. Soo-Keat Lim, Your unwavering support and belief in my abilities have been instrumental in shaping my journey. Your mentorship has not only enhanced my professional growth but has also profoundly influenced my personal development. I am deeply grateful for your guidance, which has been a cornerstone in my achievements.

Thank you for believing in me and guiding me at the very beginning of my aesthetic journey. Together, we founded Rejuven8 Cosmetic Clinic—one of the first of its kind in Western Sydney—and your unwavering support, kindness, and faith in my abilities made all the difference.

A true gentleman, a pioneer in liposculpture, and a past president of the ACCS, your generosity with knowledge and your humility in treating every patient equally—no matter their walk of life—continues to inspire me.

With deepest appreciation,

Nita Lemonia McHugh

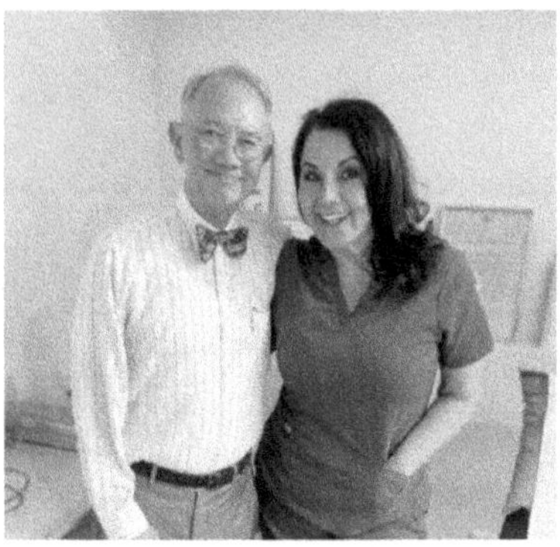

Esteemed Cosmetic Physician , former President of the ACCS. Dr Soo-Keat Lim . Working together since 1998. We often joke that our working relationship has lasted more than most marriages!

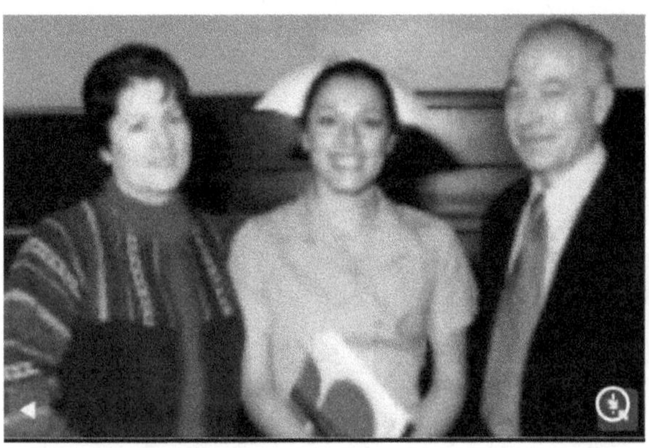

To my dear departed parents. Hope I have made you proud. Here I am as a registered nurse in 1974 receiving the Superintendent Proficiency award , with my parents.

About the Author

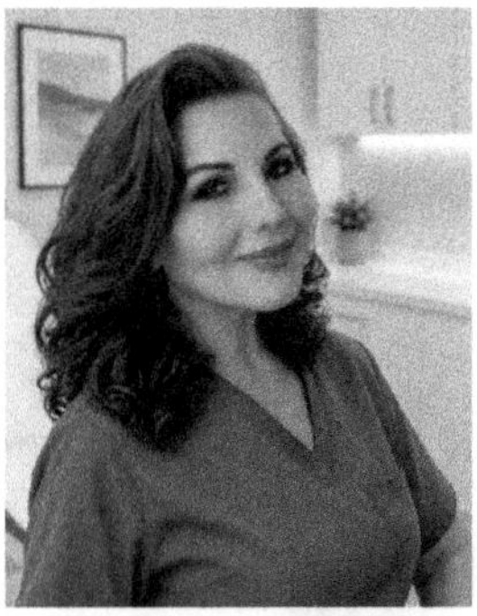

Welcome to *All You NEEDLE to Know.*

This book is the culmination of a lifetime spent caring for people, learning from experts, and witnessing the extraordinary impact that confidence and self-esteem can have on a person's life.

I have been a Registered Nurse for over five decades and have dedicated more than thirty years to the field of aesthetic medicine. During that time, I have attended hundreds of conferences, workshops, anatomy masterclasses, and training programs throughout Australia and internationally. I have been privileged to learn from some of the most respected practitioners in the world and to work alongside outstanding mentors, colleagues, and educators.

Yet some of my greatest lessons have not come from textbooks or conferences. They have come from my patients.

Over the years, I have shared in countless life journeys. I have celebrated engagements, weddings, new babies, career achievements, and personal transformations. I have also supported people through loss, illness, divorce, grief, menopause, ageing, and changes in confidence. Through these experiences, I have learned that aesthetic medicine is never simply about skin, wrinkles, lips, or volume. It is about identity, self-expression, confidence, and feeling comfortable in your own skin.

This book is not intended to replace medical advice, nor is it a technical textbook. Rather, it is a practical guide written from the perspective of an experienced nurse who believes that informed patients make the best decisions. My goal is to help you understand the treatments available, ask better questions, recognise quality care, and appreciate both the possibilities and limitations of aesthetic medicine.

Throughout these pages, I share not only clinical knowledge but also the wisdom gained from decades of experience, observation, and continuous learning. You will find information about facial ageing, cosmetic injectables, regenerative medicine, skin treatments, anatomy, safety, and treatment planning, along with many of the pearls I have collected throughout my career.

My philosophy has always been simple: enhance, don't change. The best aesthetic treatments should respect individuality, preserve character, and help people look refreshed rather than different.

Whether you are considering your first treatment, have been enjoying aesthetic treatments for years, or are a practitioner beginning your own journey, I hope this book provides valuable insights, practical guidance, and reassurance.

Most of all, I hope it reminds you that beauty is never about perfection. True beauty comes from confidence, authenticity, vitality, and embracing who you are at every stage of life.

Thank you for allowing me to share this journey with you.

With gratitude,

Nita McHugh

Registered Nurse • Aesthetic Educator • Cosmetic Injector

Instagram: @nitamchugh_rn   Website: www.nitamchugh.com.au

Email: cosmeticnurse@outlook.com.

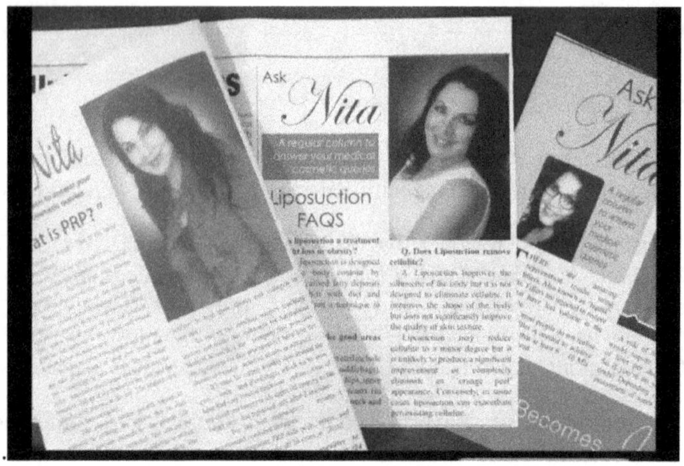

For years, Nita was a regular columnist for Nepean News, writing the popular "Ask Nita" editorial. Through this platform, she educated the Nepean district of Western Sydney about cosmetic injectable procedures and products, helping readers make informed decisions about aesthetic treatments

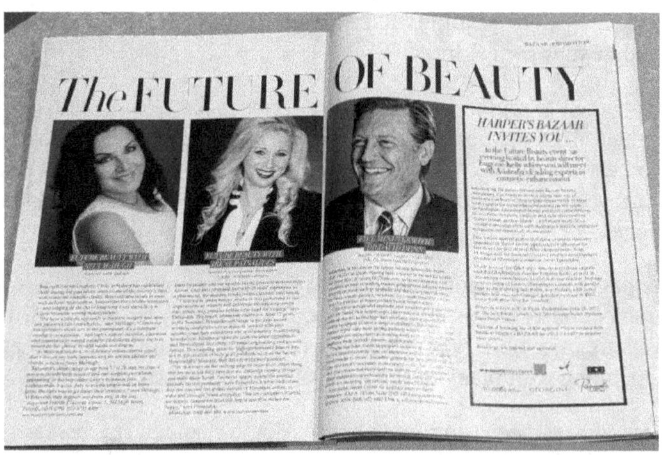

Nita McHugh featured in Harper's Bazaar Magazine July 2012.

ALL YOU NEEDLE TO KNOW

Table of Contents

COLLEAGUES AND FRIENDS ALONG THE JOURNEY

CONFERENCE AND TRAINING COLLEAGUES

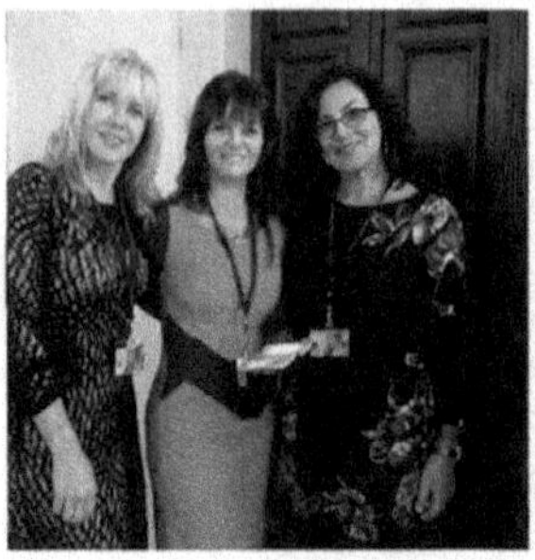
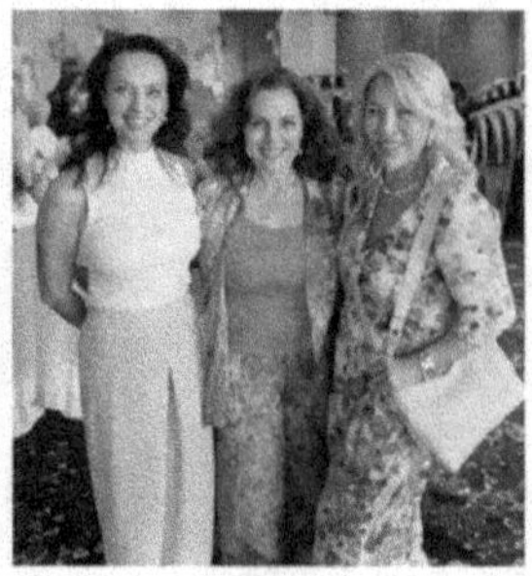
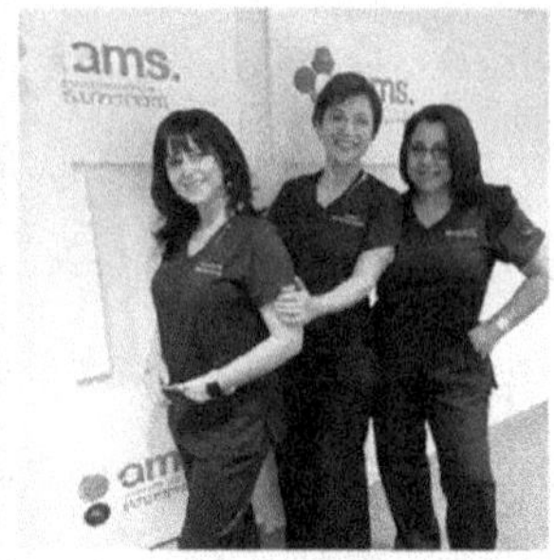

INDUSTRY MENTORS AND EDUCATORS

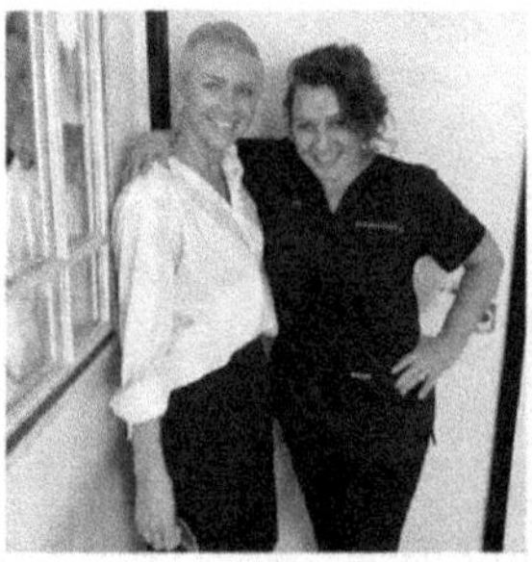
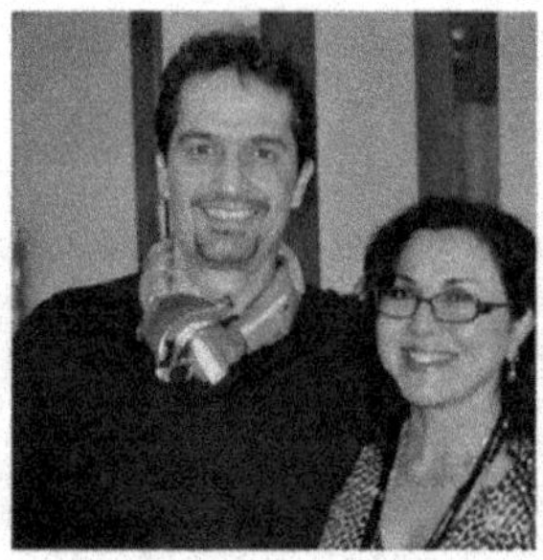
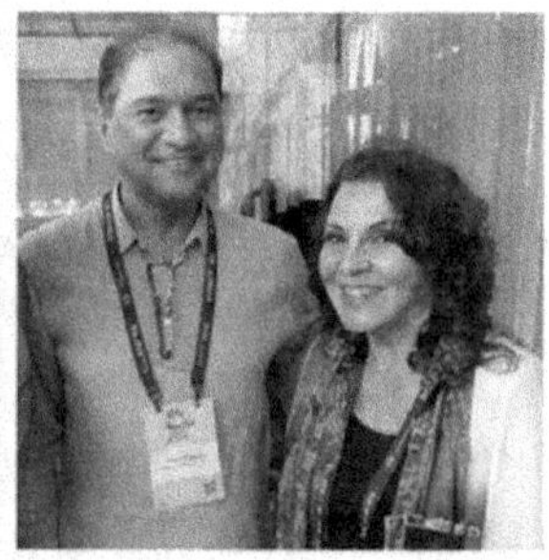

SOCIAL EVENTS AND GATHERINGS

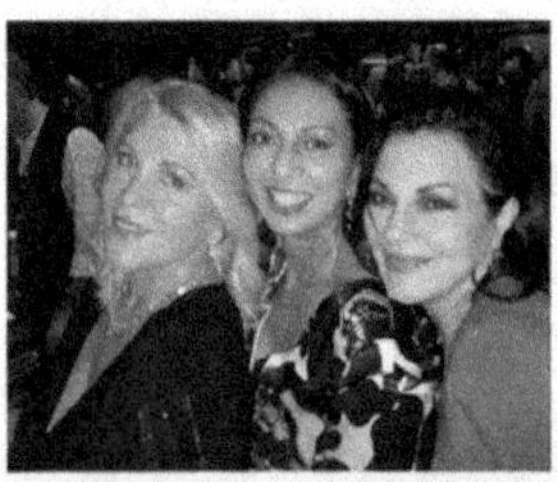
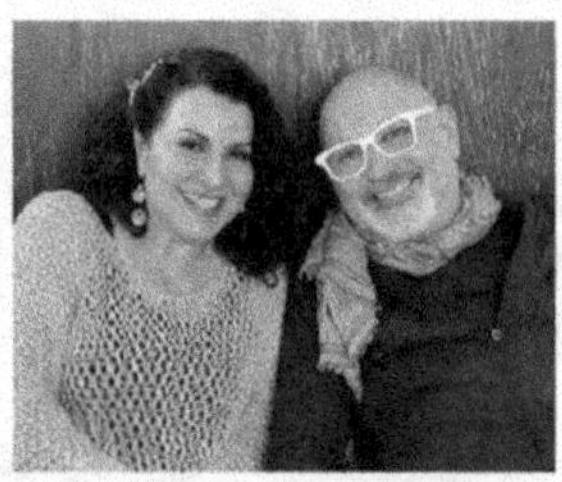
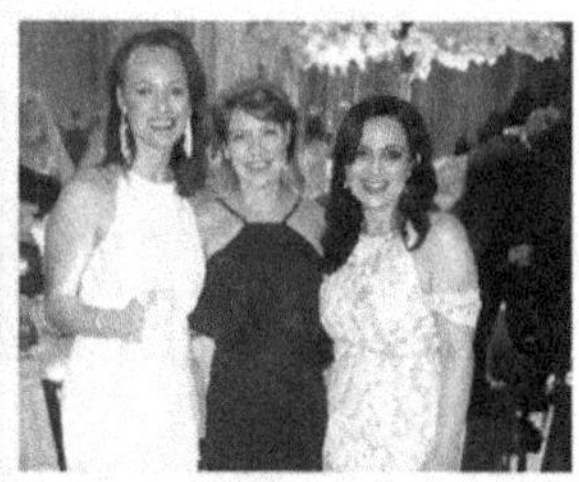
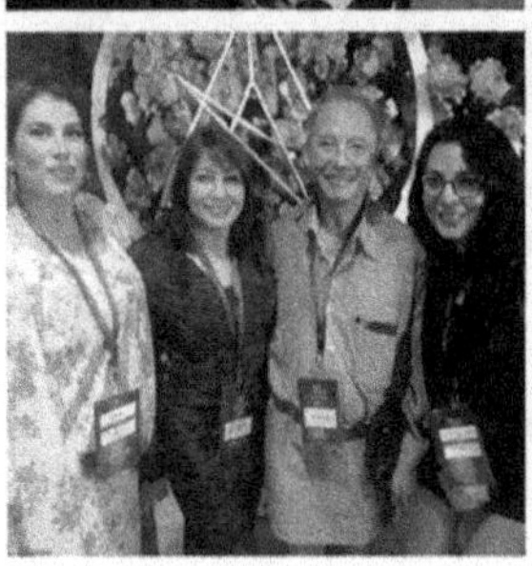
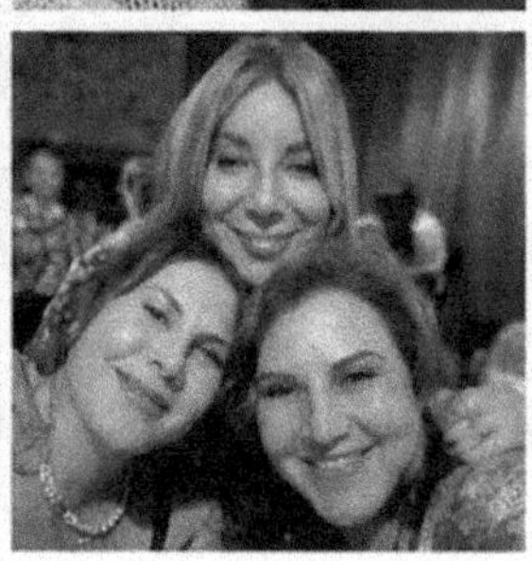
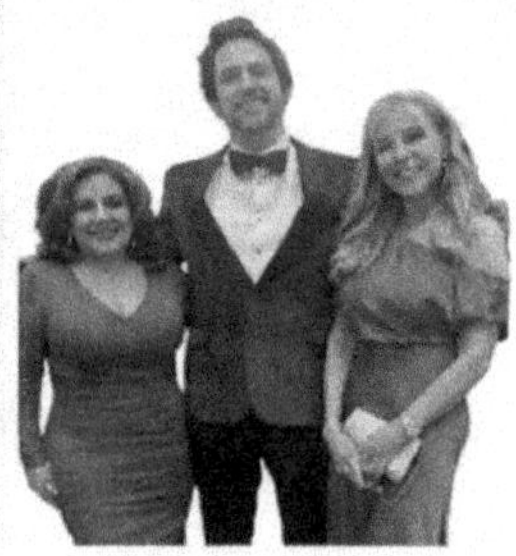

To my colleagues—pictured and not pictured—thank you for the laughter, friendship, mentorship and support that enriched my aesthetic career.

To my colleagues—pictured and not—thank you for the laughter and support you brought to my aesthetic career.

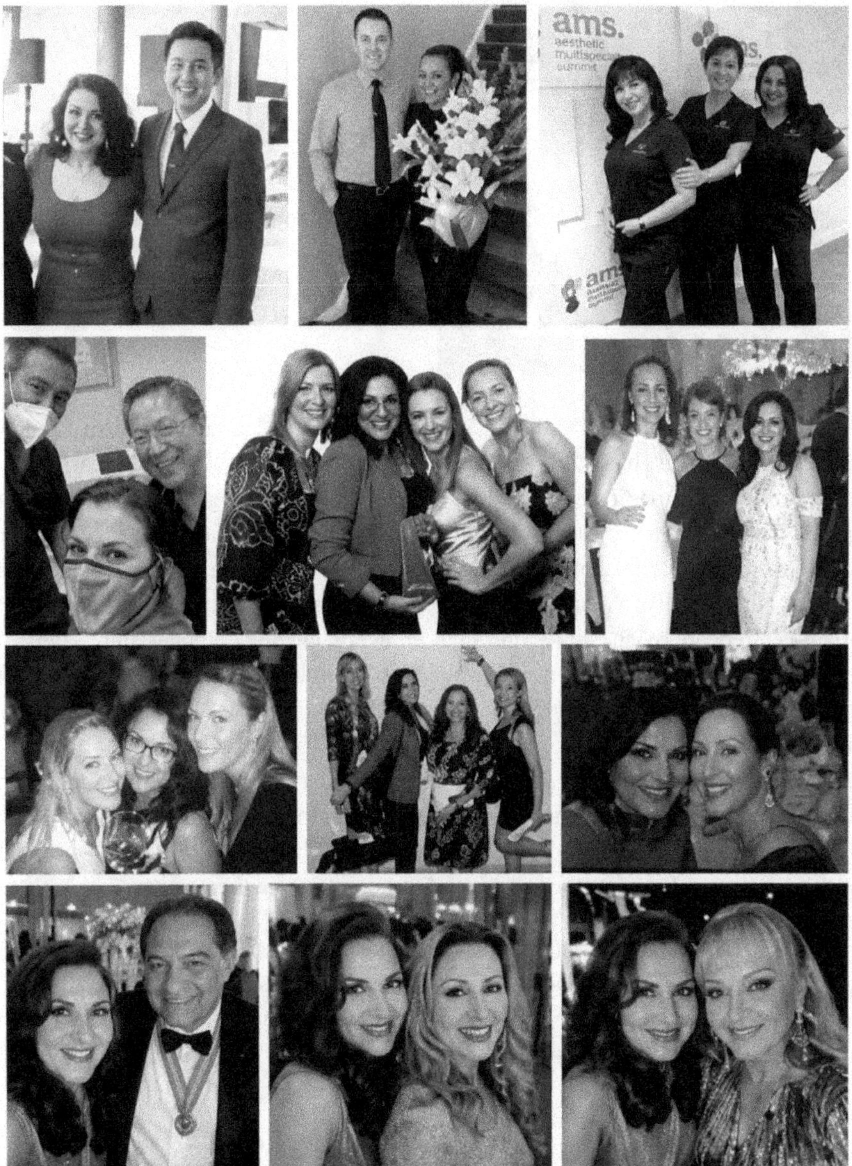

Foreward from A/Prof. Tim Papadopoulos

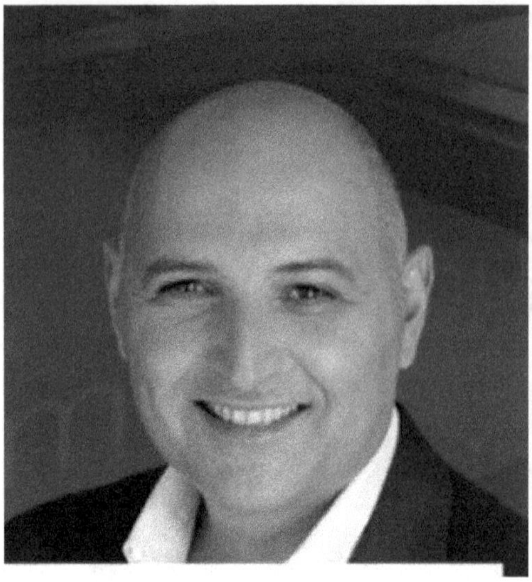

With great pleasure, I introduce "All You NEEDLE to Know," a comprehensive guide to the world of aesthetic injectables written by Nita McHugh, RN. With 50 years of nursing experience and 30 years dedicated to aesthetic medicine, Nita brings unparalleled expertise to this subject. Throughout these pages, she seamlessly blends scientific knowledge with practical wisdom, offering valuable insights for both practitioners and patients. What makes this book exceptional is Nita's ability to demystify complex concepts while maintaining clinical accuracy. Her patient-centred approach shines through in every chapter, emphasising safety, natural results, and ethical practice. From the science of botulinum toxin and dermal fillers to regenerative treatments and emerging technologies, Nita covers the full spectrum of injectable aesthetics with clarity and depth. I have witnessed Nita's dedication to excellence and continuous learning throughout her career. I can attest to her commitment to advancing the field of aesthetic medicine. Her focus on evidence-based practices and holistic patient care exemplifies the highest standards of our profession. This book represents her extensive knowledge and passion for educating others and improving patient outcomes.

"All You NEEDLE to Know" will be an invaluable resource for healthcare professionals seeking to enhance their understanding of aesthetic injectables and patients wanting to make informed treatment decisions. It is a testament to Nita's legacy as a skilled practitioner and a generous educator.

A/Prof. Tim Papadopoulos

BSc, MBBS, MBA, FRACS (Gen), FRACS (Plast), GAICD

Foreward from Dr Bonnie Hawthorne

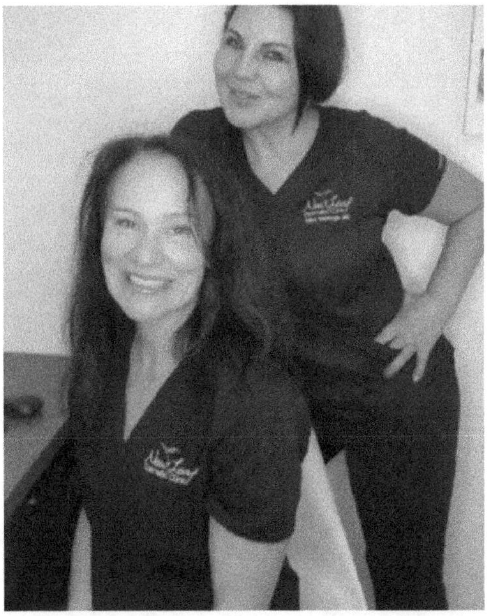

It is an honor to introduce this book, written by someone with a profound understanding of cosmetic injectables and the true essence of beauty. I have been privileged to learn from Nita McHugh, a master of her craft and, in my opinion, a true artist with decades of experience.

Nita possesses a rare gift—the ability to empower individuals to feel confident in their own skin. Her knowledge, skill, and passion shine through in every aspect of her work, and she has successfully shared that wisdom within these pages.

On a personal note, I want to express just how much Nita means to me. She is more than a mentor; she is my teacher, my guide, and my Mama No. 2. Her honesty, talent, and unwavering dedication to her craft are truly inspiring. Every time I watch her work, I am in awe of her unique approach, her meticulous attention to detail, and the care she brings to every procedure. Nita, you are one of a kind—a compassionate healer, a gifted educator, and a guardian angel to those lucky enough to know you. I am incredibly grateful to have you in my life, and I know that readers of this book will gain invaluable insight from your expertise.

Dr. Bonnie Hawthorne

MD MRCS(ENG) DFSRH FRAC GP

Cosmetic Physician

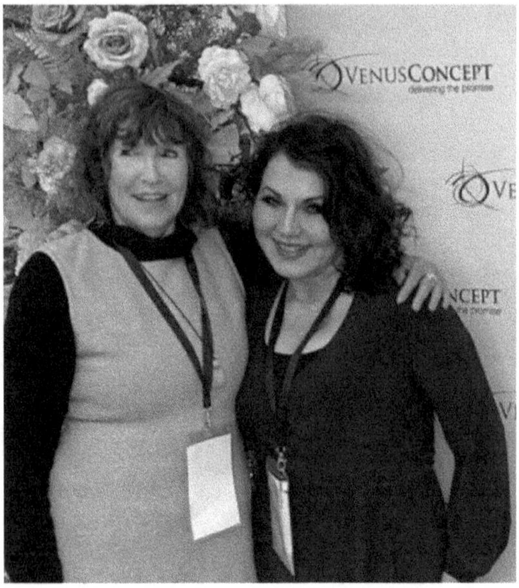

I first met Nita when she attended one of my Paramedical training courses. I was impressed from day one with her professionalism and her desire to work at a high standard, in the cosmetic enhancement industry. Nita, over the years, has made sure that she attended every training available and that her standard of care was always the highest possible.

Her patient interactions were always based on that extremely high knowledge base as well as her desire to do the right thing from a knowledge sharing basis for all who worked for her as well. I feel that Nita's contribution to the cosmetic enhancement industry has been great and will continue to be so for many years to come. This book is another way for Nita to give to the industry she so loves.

Ricky Allen
Beauty Editor Vogue Magazine
Nurse Educator

Introduction

Welcome to ALL YOU NEEDLE TO KNOW—your essential guide to the world of cosmetic injectables. If you've ever considered an aesthetic treatment but felt overwhelmed by the vast array of options, confusing terminology, or conflicting information, you're not alone. This book is here to simplify the process, answer your questions, and empower you with knowledge so that you can make informed decisions about your skin and overall appearance.

I'm Nita McHugh, a registered nurse since 1978 and an aesthetic nurse for over 30 years. My personal journey into cosmetic injectables began with my own desire to correct my skin and smooth out frown lines. I initially started with medical skin treatments before incorporating injectables into my practice. Having started Botox treatments at age 38, I understand firsthand both the curiosity and concerns that come with aesthetic enhancements. Over the years, I have worked with countless clients who, like you, want to look refreshed and natural—not "overdone" or unrecognisable.

Cosmetic injectables have come a long way from the early days of Botox and dermal fillers. Today, the industry offers a wide range of treatments designed not only to smooth wrinkles but also to enhance facial contours, restore lost volume, and even improve skin quality. However, with more choices comes more confusion. Should you opt for Botox or a filler? What's the difference between hyaluronic acid and biostimulatory injectables? How do you ensure that your treatment results are both safe and effective?

This book will break down everything you need to know, from the science behind injectables to the practicalities of choosing a qualified practitioner. Based in Sydney, Australia, I have witnessed the evolution of this industry and the growing demand for natural, rejuvenating treatments. My goal is to cut through the marketing hype and provide clear, factual, and professional insights, ensuring that you decide with the confidence, to make the best choices for yourself.

Whether you're completely new to the world of injectables or looking to refine your knowledge, ALL YOU NEEDLE TO KNOW will serve as your trusted companion in navigating this exciting and ever-advancing field.

Let's get started on your journey to informed and confident beauty choices!

Why This Book Exists

After more than 30 years in aesthetics, I've come to a simple realisation:

People don't need more treatments.

They need better understanding.

When I first entered this industry, things were far simpler. We had Botox and collagen, and that was enough. There weren't endless choices, constant trends, or the pressure to keep chasing the next new thing.

Today, aesthetics has evolved into a far more complex world — fillers, biostimulants, skin boosters, devices, regenerative medicine, and social media influences everywhere you look.

With that evolution has come incredible opportunity, but also confusion.

Patients are overwhelmed.

Trends change constantly.

Social media has blurred the line between what is real and what is not.

And somewhere along the way, many people lost sight of what truly matters:

Natural results.

Good judgement.

Understanding the face.

Over the years, I've seen beautiful work that restores confidence and helps people feel refreshed and empowered. But I've also seen the other side — faces overfilled, treatments performed without a long-term plan, and patients chasing perfection instead of balance.

This book was written to bring things back to centre.

Not to sell treatments.

Not to follow trends.

But to help you understand what is being done — and why.

Because when you understand your face, your ageing process, and your options, you make better decisions.

And better decisions almost always lead to better outcomes.

How to Use This Book

This is not a book you need to read from beginning to end.

It has been written so you can move through it in a way that feels right for you.

You may read a chapter, put it down, and return to it later. You may jump straight to a topic that relates to your own concerns, or gradually work through the book as your understanding grows.

If you are new to aesthetics, I suggest starting with the earlier chapters — understanding the face, the consultation process, and the foundations of treatment.

If you've already had treatments, you may find yourself naturally drawn to the sections on planning, treatment combinations, ageing patterns, and long-term maintenance.

There is no perfect way to read this book.

What matters is that you take something valuable from it.

Some chapters may challenge what you've previously heard or believed, and that is okay. Aesthetics is constantly evolving, and part of growth is being willing to rethink old ideas and approaches.

My intention is not to overwhelm you with information, but to guide you with clarity.

To help you ask better questions.

To help you understand your choices.

And to help you feel more confident navigating an industry that can often feel confusing and noisy.

Take your time with it.

Come back to it whenever you need to.

Because the more you understand, the more empowered you become in making decisions about your own face, ageing journey, and sense of self.

After more than thirty years as a cosmetic nurse, I've learned one simple truth: what people think they need is often very different from what they actually need.

Throughout my career, I have sat across from thousands of faces. Beautiful faces that have laughed, cried, loved, worried, celebrated, and endured life's challenges. Every face tells a story. Yet despite their uniqueness, many people arrive asking for the same things—more filler, bigger lips, higher cheeks, a sharper jawline, or a more youthful appearance.

Over the years, I noticed a pattern. The issue was often not what patients believed it to be. Many of the best outcomes I've achieved came not from doing more, but from doing less.

Less volume. Less chasing trends.

Less comparison to social media filters.

Less trying to recreate a face that was never meant to be theirs.

Somewhere along the way, aesthetics lost its direction. What began as a specialty focused on subtle enhancement gradually became an industry obsessed with transformation. We moved from helping people look refreshed to helping them look altered. Natural beauty gave way to trends, and in some cases, beautiful faces became unrecognisable versions of themselves.

The most concerning part is how gradually it happens. A little filler here, a little more there, another tweak, another syringe. Before long, the face no longer reflects the person in the mirror.

Many patients arrive with photographs of celebrities, filtered images, or edited versions of themselves and ask me to recreate what they see on a screen. The problem is that these images often don't exist in real life. They are carefully curated illusions that create unrealistic expectations and can pull people further from their natural beauty.

The truth is that your face is not a trend. It is not something to be moulded into whatever happens to be fashionable this year. Your face is part of your identity. It reflects your heritage, personality, emotions, and life experiences. The way you smile, the crinkle around your eyes when you laugh, and the subtle characteristics that make you recognisable to those who love you are not flaws that need correcting.

When we treat the face like a construction project—adding volume, freezing movement, and lifting tissue without understanding the underlying causes of ageing—we risk losing something far more important than a wrinkle.

We risk losing authenticity.

That is why I wrote this book.

Not to persuade you to have cosmetic treatments.

And certainly not to persuade you against them.

I wrote it to help you understand them.

My goal is to give you the information I wish every patient had before sitting in an injector's chair. I want you to understand what treatments do and don't do, what is worth your money, and when it may be wiser to walk away.

Throughout my career, I have seen remarkable results achieved with the lightest touch. I have watched faces become fresher, healthier, and more balanced without anyone noticing treatment had been performed. I have also seen faces changed by over-treatment—sometimes to the point where they appear older rather than younger.

Because despite what advertising may suggest, more filler is not always the answer. Sometimes the very thing people believe will make them look younger is the thing that ages them most.

Fortunately, I believe the industry is beginning to shift. Patients are becoming more educated, and practitioners are focusing less on volume and more on skin quality, tissue health, collagen stimulation, and regeneration. The conversation is moving away from creating different faces and back toward supporting the face you already have.

That is where this book belongs.

Not in trends. Not in hype. Not in unrealistic promises.

But in honest aesthetics.

In the chapters ahead, I will guide you through the world of cosmetic medicine—from injectables and lasers to skin treatments and regenerative therapies. More importantly, I will teach you how to look at your own face with greater understanding and confidence.

Because when you understand what is really happening beneath the skin, you stop chasing treatments and start making informed decisions.

And when that happens, something wonderful occurs.

You stop trying to become someone else.

You simply become the best version of yourself.

And in my experience, that is where true beauty begins.

My Personal Aesthetic Journey

At 35, I became aware of something I could no longer ignore — my frown lines. I frowned while driving, thinking, and even sleeping. It had become such a habit that I once tried placing a Band-Aid across my forehead at night to stop the movement. Unfortunately, it only deepened the creases rather than smoothing them.

Then I discovered Botox, and it was a revelation. Relaxing the muscles responsible for my frown lines softened not only my expression, but in many ways, my confidence too. Now, more than 35 years later, my frown lines have largely disappeared — not just because of Botox, but because my brain eventually learned that constant frowning was unnecessary. Today, I rarely require treatment in that area.

Botox became my introduction to the world of aesthetics, but over the years I explored many other treatments in the pursuit of natural, balanced rejuvenation.

I have had filler placed in my lips and cheeks to restore contour and volume. However, because I naturally have a fuller face, I discovered that too much filler could sometimes make me appear puffy rather than refreshed. That experience taught me an important lesson: more is not always better.

As I aged, I also noticed heaviness developing around my eyes. I eventually underwent upper and lower blepharoplasty — one of the best decisions I made. The surgery refreshed my eyes without changing my natural expression and restored brightness to my face.

In recent years, my focus has shifted more toward regenerative aesthetics. Rather than simply adding volume, I became interested in stimulating collagen and improving skin quality for longer-lasting, more authentic results.

Sculptra has become one of my favourite treatments because it gradually rebuilds collagen and creates subtle structure without looking obvious. For jawline definition, I have found Radiesse incredibly effective, providing both contour and collagen stimulation over time.

I also strongly believe in annual PRP (Platelet-Rich Plasma) treatments for both skin and hair rejuvenation. I regularly treat my face, neck, and scalp to support collagen, texture, and hair thickness.

Not every treatment suited me. I tried thread lifting, but personally found the discomfort and temporary results were not worth it for my face type. Threads can work beautifully in the right candidate, but I believe heavier faces require careful assessment.

Beyond injectables, skin quality has always been a priority for me. I maintain my skin with regular treatments including chemical peels, Dermapen microneedling, MOXI laser, and Ultherapy to stimulate collagen, improve texture, and maintain firmness.

Now approaching 70, I see myself as an example of ageing with intention rather than chasing trends. My philosophy has never been about looking younger than I am, but about looking healthy, rested, and natural.

Aesthetic medicine has evolved enormously over the decades, and I have evolved with it. These experiences have shaped not only how I treat myself, but how I guide my patients.

Because true rejuvenation is not about fighting ageing.

It is about ageing well — gracefully, naturally, and confidently.

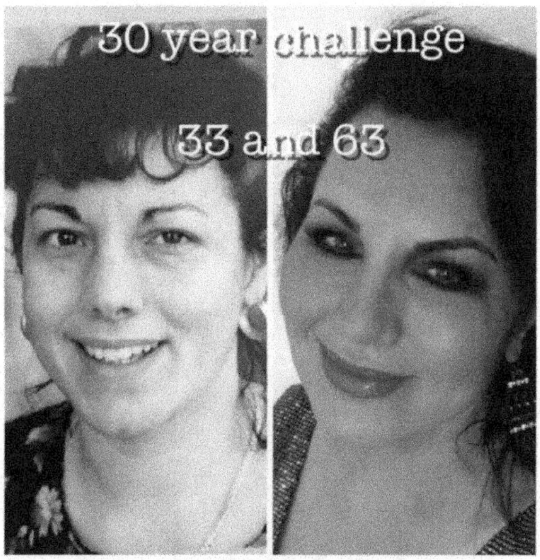

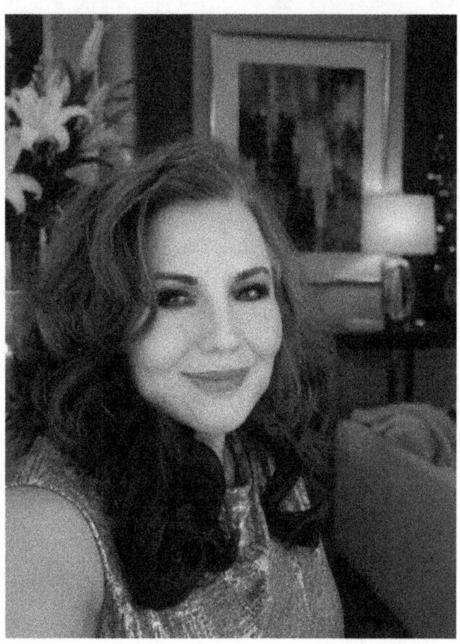

Nita at 70

PART 1 - THE HUMAN SIDE OF AESTHETICS

Chapter 1: The Psychology Behind Cosmetic Treatments

Treating the Person, Not Just the Face

Cosmetic medicine is often discussed in terms of muscles, collagen, volume loss, and skin quality. But after more than 30 years in the treatment room, I can tell you this:

People rarely come in because of a wrinkle alone. They come in because of how that wrinkle makes them feel.

Behind every request for Botox, filler, skin tightening, or rejuvenation is usually a deeper story. Sometimes it is about confidence. Sometimes it follows stress, divorce, menopause, illness, grief, burnout, or simply the shock of looking in the mirror one day and not recognising yourself anymore. Understanding the psychology behind cosmetic treatments is just as important as understanding facial anatomy.

Most patients do not walk into a clinic saying, "I want my corrugator muscles weakened." Instead, they say things like:

"I look tired all the time."

"I look angry even when I'm not."

"I don't feel like myself anymore."

"I just want to look fresher."

Cosmetic treatments are rarely about vanity alone. More often, they are connected to confidence, identity, and emotional wellbeing. Many patients seek treatment during major life transitions — menopause, retirement, divorce, career changes, illness, or when children leave home. At the same time life is shifting emotionally, the face is also changing physically.

That combination can feel confronting.

The Mirror and the Mind

The face is deeply connected to our sense of self. It is how we recognise ourselves, how others respond to us, and how we communicate emotion without speaking.

When people begin to notice sagging skin, deepening lines, hollow eyes, or a permanently tired expression, it can affect far more than appearance. It can influence confidence, mood, social behaviour, and even relationships.

Over the years, I have heard patients quietly confess:

"I stopped going out."

"I hate photos now."

"I feel invisible."

Small, subtle treatments can sometimes create a surprisingly emotional response. Not because the person suddenly looks like someone else, but because they begin to look like themselves again.

That moment is powerful.

Healthy Motivation vs Unrealistic Expectations

There is a significant difference between healthy cosmetic motivation and unhealthy psychological drivers.

Patients with healthy expectations usually want to look fresher, softer, or less tired. They understand ageing is normal and are looking for subtle support rather than perfection. These patients are generally calm, realistic, and open to professional advice.

On the other hand, some patients arrive chasing perfection, wanting to look filtered, celebrity-like, or dramatically different from their natural appearance. They are often dissatisfied no matter how much treatment they have had. They may move from injector to injector searching for an impossible outcome.

This is where psychology becomes critical in aesthetic medicine.

Body Dysmorphic Disorder (BDD) is a real psychological condition where a person becomes fixated on perceived flaws that others may barely notice. These patients may constantly check mirrors, obsess over one area of the face, repeatedly seek treatments without satisfaction, and hold unrealistic expectations about what cosmetic procedures can achieve.

No amount of filler or Botox can heal a psychological wound.

An ethical injector must sometimes say:

"I don't think treatment is the right solution for you right now."

That conversation can be uncomfortable, but it is often the most responsible and caring decision.

The Emotional Consultation

A good consultation is never just about the face.

It is about listening carefully, observing body language, understanding emotional state, and recognising what may sit underneath the request for treatment.

Sometimes the real issue is not the wrinkle itself — it is what the wrinkle represents.

A patient may say she hates the lines around her mouth, but as the consultation unfolds, you discover she has recently gone through a divorce, feels unattractive, or has not dated in years. The treatment becomes more than a cosmetic procedure. It becomes part of rebuilding confidence and reconnecting with herself.

This is why empathy matters so much in aesthetics.

The Influence of Social Media and Filters

We now live in a world dominated by filters, editing apps, AI-enhanced images, and unrealistic beauty standards. Many patients bring heavily filtered photos into consultations and ask to look exactly like the image on the screen.

The problem is that these images are not real.

They erase pores, soften texture, alter proportions, remove movement, and create impossible standards. This creates a dangerous gap between reality and expectation.

An experienced injector helps patients understand not only what is achievable, but also what is appropriate for their own unique face.

Good aesthetics should enhance individuality — not erase it.

The Role of the Injector

A good injector is not simply a technician.

They are part clinician, part artist, part listener, and part guide.

Their role is not to inject everything a patient asks for, but to educate, set realistic expectations, and sometimes recommend less treatment — or no treatment at all.

One of the most important skills in aesthetic medicine is knowing when not to treat.

Ethical practice is not about selling syringes.

It is about protecting the patient.

Midlife, Hormones, and Identity

Many cosmetic patients are women navigating midlife. This stage often includes hormonal changes, menopause, career transitions, relationship shifts, ageing parents, or children leaving home.

At the exact same time life is changing emotionally, the face is changing physically.

This can create feelings of loss — loss of youth, identity, femininity, confidence, or attractiveness.

When done well, cosmetic treatments can gently support someone through this stage of life. They can restore confidence, improve self-image, and help patients feel more aligned with how they feel inside.

Some of the most emotional moments in my career have not come from dramatic transformations, but from subtle ones.

A patient looks in the mirror after treatment and quietly says:

"Oh… I look like me again."

That moment is not about vanity.

It is about recognition, relief, and confidence.

Cosmetic Treatments and Self-Worth

Cosmetic treatments should never be used as a substitute for self-esteem, emotional healing, relationship repair, or mental health support.

They can enhance confidence, improve appearance, and support self-image — but they are not a cure for deeper emotional pain.

Before having cosmetic treatment, I believe every patient should ask themselves:

Am I doing this for me, or for someone else?

Do I want to look fresher, or completely different?

Are my expectations realistic?

Would subtle improvement be enough?

The best cosmetic treatments are usually the ones where people simply say:

"You look well."

"You look rested."

"You look happy."

Not:

"What have you had done?"

Because the true goal of aesthetics is not to change who you are.

It is to help you feel comfortable in your own skin.

Chapter 2: Emotional Anatomy of The Face

In aesthetic medicine, we are trained to study anatomy in extraordinary detail. We learn about muscles, ligaments, fat pads, septa, blood vessels, and bone structure. We are taught where to inject, how deep to place product, how many units or millilitres to use, and how the face changes as we age.

But after more than thirty years in the treatment room, I have come to realise there is another anatomy equally as important as the physical one.

Every face has an emotional anatomy.

Behind every wrinkle, hollow, clenched jaw, or request for Botox or filler, there is often a feeling, a story, or a life transition. People rarely walk into a clinic talking about collagen loss or muscle activity. They come because of how their face makes them feel. More importantly, they come because of how they think the world sees them.

If you truly want to understand cosmetic medicine, you must understand not only the physical anatomy of the face, but the emotional anatomy as well.

The face reflects our lives in ways most people never consciously realise. Over time, stress, grief, anxiety, exhaustion, sadness, anger, and even resilience become etched into our expressions. The face remembers repeated emotions. The muscles contract in familiar ways, the skin folds along certain lines, tension settles into the jaw, and slowly those temporary expressions can become permanent.

Sometimes people no longer feel angry, yet their face still communicates anger. Others may feel vibrant and energetic, but hollowing beneath the eyes makes them appear permanently exhausted. Many patients sit in my chair and say the same things.

"I look tired all the time."

"People keep asking if I'm upset."

"I look sad in photos."

"I don't feel like myself anymore."

What they are noticing is not simply ageing. They are noticing changes in their emotional anatomy.

The forehead and frown area are often the first places where emotional tension becomes visible. Deep lines between the brows can create a constant expression of worry, irritation, seriousness, or stress. Many people spend years unconsciously frowning while concentrating, working, parenting, caregiving, or simply navigating difficult periods of life. Eventually those lines remain, even when the face is at rest.

I often hear patients say, "I'm not angry, but everyone thinks I am."

Softening this area carefully with toxin can create a more relaxed and approachable appearance without removing natural expression. The goal should never be a frozen face. A beautiful result is not about paralysis; it is about softness, balance, and harmony.

The eyes reveal emotion perhaps more than any other area of the face. Hollowing beneath the eyes can create shadows that make a person appear tired, stressed, sad, or unwell, even when they are healthy and sleeping well. As volume loss occurs around the eyes, the face can lose brightness and vitality.

Patients often tell me, "No matter how much I sleep, I still look exhausted."

When treated conservatively and correctly, restoring support around the eyes can refresh the entire face. The person does not necessarily look younger; they simply look more rested and more like themselves again.

The midface and cheeks are closely linked to youthfulness, vitality, and positive emotional expression. Full cheeks reflect light beautifully and create an appearance of energy and health. As we age, the cheeks gradually flatten and descend. Support is lost through the midface, and the lower face often begins to appear heavier or sadder.

What fascinates me is how interconnected the face truly is. A small amount of support placed correctly in the cheeks can indirectly soften the lower face, improve facial balance, and subtly change emotional expression. Sometimes restoring the cheeks restores far more than volume. It restores vitality.

The mouth and lower face carry enormous emotional significance. Downturned mouth corners, marionette lines, and loss of support around the lips can unintentionally create an expression of sadness, disappointment, bitterness, or ageing. Patients frequently say, "I look miserable in photographs," even though they feel perfectly content.

Sometimes only millimetres separate a sad-looking face from a refreshed and harmonious one. Tiny changes in this area can dramatically soften expression without making someone look artificial.

The jawline and lower face tell another emotional story altogether. This area is associated with structure, confidence, strength, and vitality, but it is also where many people physically carry emotional stress.

One of the most common patterns I see in clinic is enlargement of the masseter muscles due to chronic clenching and grinding of the teeth. Many patients are completely unaware they are doing it. During periods of anxiety, emotional overwhelm, stress, or poor sleep, people often tighten their jaw unconsciously throughout the day and especially at night.

The body stores stress in different places, and for many people, it settles in the jaw.

Over time, chronic clenching enlarges the masseter muscles, creating a heavier, squarer lower face. It may also contribute to headaches, jaw pain, TMJ symptoms, dental wear, facial tension, and even neck discomfort. Emotionally anxious people often carry this tension constantly without realising it.

When appropriate, relaxing the masseters with toxin can do far more than slim the lower face aesthetically. Many patients describe a sense of relief afterward, as though their entire face feels softer and lighter. The treatment often reduces pain, headaches, and muscular tension while also creating a gentler facial shape.

This is where aesthetics and emotional wellbeing quietly intersect.

As the jawline and neck lose definition with age, the lower face can also begin to appear heavier or more fatigued. Careful structural treatments can restore support, improve facial harmony, and create a fresher and more confident profile.

What I have learned over the years is that patients rarely seek treatment because of a specific anatomical concern. They do not walk in asking for correction of a nasolabial fold or a millimetre of volume loss. What they are really saying is far more personal.

"I don't feel like myself anymore."

"I want to look fresher."

"I want the outside to match how I feel inside."

Cosmetic treatments are often about identity as much as appearance. Many people seek treatment during periods of significant transition — menopause, divorce, illness, grief, retirement, career changes, or emotional exhaustion. When the face changes at the same time life is changing, it can feel deeply confronting. People look into the mirror and no longer recognise themselves.

The face is intimately tied to self-image. It is how we recognise ourselves, how we communicate emotion, and how the world responds to us. When someone constantly sees heaviness, sagging, deep lines, or exhaustion reflected back at them, it can affect confidence, mood, social interactions, and professional presence.

Sometimes a very subtle treatment creates an unexpectedly profound emotional shift, not because the person looks dramatically different, but because they feel like themselves again.

That is very different from chasing perfection.

Not all cosmetic motivations are healthy, and this is something every ethical injector must understand. There is a difference between wanting to look fresher and becoming obsessed with flaws. There is a difference between healthy self-care and chasing filtered perfection.

Some patients arrive wanting subtle support and realistic improvement. Others remain chronically dissatisfied no matter how much treatment they receive. Some become fixated on tiny imperfections invisible to everyone else. These patients may not need more filler. They may need emotional support, reassurance, or deeper healing.

A skilled injector is not simply a technician. They are also a listener, an observer, and a guide. A good consultation involves far more than analysing anatomy. We must assess emotional readiness, expectations, motivation, and psychological wellbeing alongside the physical face sitting in front of us.

Sometimes the most professional thing an injector can say is, "I don't think treatment is right for you at this time."

That takes integrity.

Some of the most meaningful moments in aesthetic medicine come from the smallest changes. A patient looks into the mirror and quietly says, "I look like me again."

That moment is never really about vanity.

It is about recognition, confidence, relief, and emotional restoration.

The best cosmetic treatments are usually the ones people cannot identify. Instead of saying, "What have you had done?" people simply say:

"You look well."

"You look rested."

"You look happy."

Because the true goal of aesthetics should never be to change who someone is. The goal is to help the outer face reflect the inner self once again.

That is the true art of understanding both the physical anatomy and the emotional anatomy of the face.

Chapter 3: Reasons why people seeking cosmetic enhancements

There are many reasons why both women and men seek cosmetic enhancements — and contrary to outdated perceptions, it rarely has anything to do with vanity. More often, it comes down to self-care, confidence, and a quiet desire to feel like yourself again. The motivations are as varied as the people who walk through my door, but a few themes come up again and again.

1. Career & Professional Image

The reality of today's workplace is that appearance still carries weight. Many professionals feel pressure to look youthful and energetic, particularly in industries that favour younger candidates. Whether it's preparing for a job interview, going for a promotion, or simply maintaining a polished presence in a client-facing role — a refreshed, confident appearance can make a genuine difference. Those working in sales, hospitality, real estate, and media know this better than most.

2. Social & Personal Confidence

Life changes can shake us to our core. A divorce or the end of a long relationship often brings with it a loss of confidence and self-worth, and many clients come to me during exactly these moments — not to transform themselves for someone else, but to reclaim themselves for their own sake. When you feel good in your skin, it shows. And for those stepping back into the world — including the dating scene — that renewed sense of self can be everything.

3. Milestone Events

Weddings, significant birthdays, reunions, cultural celebrations — these occasions have a wonderful way of inspiring people to put their best face forward. It's not just brides either. Parents of the couple, lifelong friends, and guests all want to show up feeling their absolute best and looking it too.

4. Everyday Self-Care

Not every client arrives with a dramatic turning point. Sometimes it's simply a matter of the mirror not reflecting how you actually feel. Work stress, poor sleep, and the natural ageing process can leave people looking far more tired and worn than they truly are. Treatments like Botox or dermal fillers can gently restore that well-rested, refreshed look. I also see a great many teachers, nurses, and public speakers — professionals whose work involves constant facial expression — who develop deep frown lines over time, leaving them looking stern or fatigued when they're anything but.

5. Post-Health Challenges

For those who have been through significant weight loss, illness, or prolonged stress, aesthetic treatments can play a meaningful role in feeling whole again. Losing a large amount of weight, for example, can leave the skin needing support that the body can't provide alone. Similarly, medical treatment or chronic illness can take a visible toll — and restoring the face can help restore a sense of normalcy and confidence alongside it.

6. Men Are Increasingly Seeking Treatments Too

More and more men are finding their way to aesthetic clinics, and it makes complete sense. They face the same professional pressures women do, and social expectations around grooming and appearance are evolving quickly. Men tend to prefer subtle treatments — what the industry calls "tweakments" — enough to look refreshed and vital without it being obvious. With careers lasting longer and dating apps changing how we meet people, men are quietly but confidently embracing aesthetic care as part of looking and feeling their best.

Ultimately, cosmetic enhancement is about self-care, confidence, and feeling good in your own skin. Whether it's about staying competitive professionally, marking a new chapter personally, or simply wanting your reflection to match how you feel inside — the decision is always deeply personal, and always valid.

I am forever grateful to every client who has trusted me — not only with their appearance, but with their story.

All my clients have a story. To be trusted with someone's life as well as their looks is a privilege I never take lightly. Over the years I have come to think of myself as an accidental counsellor — someone people open up to, perhaps because the treatment room offers a rare kind of quiet honesty. To help a client rebuild their confidence, to witness the chapters of their life, and to play even a small part in helping them move forward — that is what makes this work so deeply rewarding.

One particular client has never left my memory.

She came in for a consultation, and as I was taking her before photographs, I noticed it immediately — an unmistakable sadness behind her eyes. Her face was gaunt, her hair cut into a simple bob. She was thin, her skin crinkled, her lips pressed tightly together as though she were holding something fragile just beneath the surface.

When she finally spoke, her voice was barely steady.

"My husband left me for a younger woman."

She was utterly devastated.

But she was also determined. She committed to a course of treatments — Sculptra to restore volume to her face, fillers to bring life back to her lips, and Botox to soften the lines that time and heartbreak had deepened. Gradually, visit by visit, something shifted. Her smile returned. Her posture changed. And as her appearance was lovingly restored, something far more beautiful began to emerge from within — her own quiet radiance.

Then, as it so often does, karma arrived in its own time.

Eight years later, the younger woman her ex-husband had left her for had become overweight and deeply unhappy. Meanwhile, my client had transformed entirely — poised, graceful, her hair now long and flowing, her whole presence carrying an effortless confidence that no treatment alone could create. That came entirely from her.

At their son's wedding, her ex-husband could not take his eyes off her. His marriage had long since unravelled, and the regret, by all accounts, has never left him.

She, on the other hand, continues to visit me every three months — not out of insecurity, but out of genuine self-care and the joy of feeling her very best.

He lives with regret. She lives with freedom, beauty, and confidence.

And that, more than anything, is what this work is truly about.

Real Stories from the Treatment Room

What the Needle Has Taught Me

After more than three decades in aesthetic medicine, I've come to understand one thing with absolute certainty — cosmetic treatments are never just about the face. They are about people. About emotions, life stages, confidence, heartbreak, and reinvention. Sometimes, yes, pure vanity too. But far more often, something much deeper.

The treatment room is a quiet confessional.

Over the years, I've sat with women through marriages and divorces, new relationships and painful endings, illness and recovery, career changes, motherhood, menopause, and the remarkable reinventions that so often happen in the fifties, sixties, and beyond. Some of my clients have been with me for decades. I've watched them grow, change, struggle, and flourish. The needle, in those moments, becomes a small but meaningful part of a much bigger life story.

These are some of the moments that have stayed with me.

The Tiny Red Dot

A woman in her fifties walked into the clinic one afternoon. From across the room I could already see it — sun-damaged skin, deep frown lines, hollow eyes, dry and weathered texture. In my mind, I was quietly mapping out a treatment plan: skin rejuvenation, Botox, perhaps some structural support.

When she sat down, I asked her what concerned her most.
She pointed to a tiny red dot on her cheek.

"That," she said simply.

It was a small cherry angioma — something easily treated with hyfrecation in a matter of minutes. She had walked in worried about a speck, while I had been looking at her entire face.

It was a powerful reminder that we don't always see ourselves the way others see us. And as practitioners, we must always listen before we treat. Our job is to address what matters to the person in front of us — not what we notice first.

The Loyal Clients

Some clients don't just pass through your career — they become woven into it.
Over the years I've had women come to me before their weddings, return after their divorces, find new love, start new careers, and become grandmothers. I've watched them grow older, wiser, and so often more comfortable in their own skin. We've shared laughter, tears, and more conversations than I could count.

For many of them, the clinic becomes something beyond a place of treatment. It becomes a safe space — a moment carved out of a busy life that belongs entirely to them. That trust is something I hold with great care.

The Overfilled Lips

A young woman came in with very large, heavily filled lips, obvious breast implants, and a petite frame. She sat down and told me she wanted more filler in her lips.

I looked at her carefully and said, honestly, that I felt her lips were already overfilled — and that I would actually recommend dissolving some of the existing filler to restore a more natural result.
She shook her head without hesitation.
"No. I love the attention they get from men."

In that moment, I understood. Her lips weren't really about aesthetics at all. They were about validation — about the attention they drew and what that meant to her. It wasn't my place to judge that. But it was my place to be honest. I declined to add more, explained my reasoning clearly, and left the decision with her.

Sometimes what a client wants and what is genuinely best for them are two different things. Navigating that with honesty and compassion is one of the most important skills in this profession.

Beauty as a Tool

Another woman came in requesting lip filler and, as we talked, she told me quite openly that she was a sex worker. Her lips, she explained, were part of her professional image — part of how she made her living.
"My lips are my tools," she said, matter-of-factly.

There was no apology in it, and none was needed. It was simply her reality. That conversation reminded me, as so many have over the years, that cosmetic treatments carry entirely different meanings for different people. For some it is confidence. For others, identity. For others still, livelihood. My role is not to filter those motivations — it is to listen, advise honestly, and treat with skill.

The Sixty-Year-Old Gentleman

A man in his sixties arrived at the clinic one day — a little nervous, but quietly determined. He had recently separated from his partner and wanted to start dating again. The problem, he said, was that he felt old and tired compared to the women he was meeting.

We discussed a gentle, considered approach: softening his frown lines, improving his skin quality, a little structural support where it was needed. Nothing dramatic — just enough to help him look as vital as he felt.
A few months later he returned looking relaxed and confident, and he smiled as he said:

"I feel like I've got a second chance."

That, to me, is exactly what this work can do at its best.

The Divorced Woman Who Reclaimed Herself

A woman came to see me in the aftermath of a difficult divorce. She looked exhausted and defeated — hollow cheeks, deep lines, the corners of her mouth pulled downward as though weighted by everything she had been through.

We began with a gentle, staged approach: Botox, structural filler, skin boosters. Over time, something remarkable happened. Her face softened — but more than that, her whole energy shifted. She became brighter, more social, more confident. She started going out again, building her independence, reconnecting with the life she still had ahead of her.

The treatments hadn't simply changed her face. They had helped her reclaim herself.

The Cleft Palate Patient

A young woman came in, visibly shy and self-conscious about her lips. She had a repaired cleft palate and had spent years feeling uncomfortable with the asymmetry it left behind.

With careful, conservative filler, we gently balanced her lip shape and softened the unevenness. When she looked in the mirror, her eyes filled with tears.
"I've never liked my lips before," she said quietly.

That moment had nothing to do with trends or aesthetics in the conventional sense. It was about a young woman finally feeling at ease in her own face. Those are the appointments that remind you why this work matters.

The Woman with Bell's Palsy

A woman who had experienced Bell's palsy came to me with a noticeably uneven smile — one side of her face significantly stronger than the other. Using carefully placed Botox, we relaxed the stronger side and brought better balance to her facial movement.

When she saw the result, she looked at herself for a long moment and said:
"I feel normal again."

The Girl with No Top Lip

A young woman came in feeling deeply self-conscious about her upper lip, which was almost entirely absent. She avoided photographs and struggled with her confidence in social settings.

With a small, subtle amount of filler, we created a gentle shape and restored proportion. The change was not dramatic — but to her, it was everything. She stood taller walking out than she had walking in.

The Teacher with the Scary Frown

A schoolteacher arrived at the clinic with a concern that made me smile inwardly. Her students, she said, thought she was always angry. She had developed a deep, permanent frown from years of concentration and expression, and it gave her a stern resting face that didn't reflect who she was at all.

We treated the area with Botox, and when she came back for her review she laughed and said:
"The kids keep asking me why I look so nice lately."

It's a small thing — and yet it changed how an entire classroom of children experienced their teacher every day.

The Receded Chin and the Wedding Photos

An Asian bride-to-be came in ahead of her wedding, concerned about her profile in photographs. She had a noticeably receded chin that she felt threw her features off balance.

With a small amount of chin filler, we improved her profile and brought better proportion to her face overall. When she saw the result she smiled and said:
"Now I feel ready for my wedding photos."

The Resting Expression

One patient came to me frustrated by what she described, with good humour, as her "resting bitch face." Her mouth corners naturally turned downward, giving her an expression of displeasure even when she felt perfectly content — and people read it that way constantly.

With careful treatment to soften the depressor muscles and gently support the corners of the mouth, her expression became noticeably warmer and more approachable. She told me afterwards:

"People smile at me more now."

It Takes All Kinds

A woman with six children came in regularly. Her husband always paid for her treatments and, she told me with great delight, would take her out for a beautiful dinner afterwards. Following one particularly thorough full-face rejuvenation session, she laughed and winked as she was leaving:

"I suppose I'll have to give my husband a special thank-you on the way home."

Moments like that remind you — people come from all walks of life, with all kinds of relationships and motivations. In this profession, you truly do see everything. And if you approach it all without judgment and with genuine warmth, you are privileged for it.

The Tricky Waiting Room

One of the more delicate situations I have ever navigated involved a married couple and their company secretary.

The wife came to see me and, in the course of conversation, shared that her husband had been having an affair with the secretary — a woman she described as manipulative and calculating. Not long afterwards, the secretary herself became a client. She had an entirely different version of events, telling me the wife was demanding and difficult, and that the husband had since moved in with her.

I treated both women professionally and with equal care.

The real skill, however, lay in ensuring they were never in the waiting room at the same time.

In aesthetics, discretion is not optional. It is everything.

What These Stories Have Taught Me

After decades in this profession, I have learned that cosmetic treatments are rarely straightforward — they are layered with emotion, meaning, and personal history. People come for many different reasons, and not every request should simply be granted. Listening, always, is more important than injecting.

Confidence, when it is genuinely restored, can change the entire trajectory of a person's life.

But the most important lesson of all is this: the needle is never just about the face. It is about the person behind it. And when it is used with skill, honesty, and genuine compassion, it can do far more than smooth a line or restore a contour.

It can help someone feel like themselves again.

And there is no greater privilege than that.

When to Do Aesthetic Treatments, How Often, and How to Plan for Special Occasions

Aesthetic treatments deliver their best results when they are timed thoughtfully and planned well in advance. While many procedures are described as having little to no downtime, the skin and underlying tissues still need time to settle, heal, and truly look their best. Rushing the process rarely ends well — and when there is a special occasion involved, the stakes feel even higher.

This section walks you through when to have each treatment, how frequently to repeat it, and how far ahead you should be planning before any important event.

Planning Around Special Occasions
Whether you are preparing for a wedding, a milestone birthday, a professional event, a holiday, or a photo shoot, timing is everything. Even with the most skilled technique, injectables can cause temporary swelling, bruising, tenderness, or mild asymmetry while the product settles. These are normal and expected — but they need time to resolve before you walk into a room wanting to look your absolute best.

As a general guide: allow at least three weeks before any special occasion for injectable treatments. If it is your first time having a particular treatment, or you are combining multiple treatments, give yourself four to six weeks minimum.

Last-minute injectables increase stress and reduce control over outcomes. Plan ahead — always.

Botox & Anti-Wrinkle Treatments
Botox works by gradually relaxing the muscles responsible for expression lines. The results are not immediate — the treatment takes time to fully develop, and any unevenness can only be assessed and corrected once it has settled.

Botox can be used preventatively in younger patients or to soften established lines in those with deeper concerns. Either way, patience is part of the process.

How often: Every three to four months.

Before a special occasion: Have your Botox done at least two to three weeks beforehand. This gives the treatment time to reach its full effect and allows for a review appointment if needed.

Botox performed too close to an event may not yet have reached its full effect — and there is nothing to be done but wait.

Skin Treatments (Non-Injectable)
Skin treatments — including facials, peels, microneedling, laser, LED, and radiofrequency — improve texture, clarity, and radiance, and work beautifully alongside injectable treatments. The key variable is downtime, which ranges from minimal to significant depending on the intensity of the treatment.

How often: Light treatments can be performed monthly. More corrective treatments are typically delivered in a course of three to six sessions.

Before a special occasion:
Light facials and LED therapy: three to seven days before
Peels, microneedling, laser, and radiofrequency: three to six weeks before, depending on the strength of the treatment
For any important event, skin should look calm and settled — not as though it has just been worked on.

Lip Fillers
The lips are one of the most expressive and sensitive areas of the face, and filler here can cause noticeable swelling and bruising in the first week, particularly for first-time patients. Lips may also appear slightly uneven while the product integrates — this is entirely normal, but it does require time.

How often: Every nine to eighteen months.

Before a special occasion: Allow at least three to four weeks. For first-time lip filler, allow a full six weeks — the initial result will look more pronounced than the final outcome, and you want to see how your lips settle before the big day.

Lips need time to soften and integrate. Last-minute lip filler is rarely subtle — and subtle is almost always the goal.

Facial Fillers (Cheeks, Jawline, Chin)
Structural fillers in areas such as the cheeks, jawline, and chin take time to fully settle into the tissues. Swelling can be present for several days, and the final contour often refines itself over two to four weeks. These treatments should never be rushed.

How often: Every twelve to twenty-four months.

Before a special occasion: Plan facial fillers four to six weeks in advance. This allows any bruising to fully resolve and gives the face time to find its natural balance with the new structure.

The face needs time to "find itself" after structural filler. What you see immediately after treatment is not the final result.

Biostimulants and Bio-Fillers
Biostimulants such as Sculptra and Radiesse work differently from traditional fillers. Rather than producing an immediate volumising effect, their benefit comes from stimulating the body's own collagen production over a period of weeks and months. The results are gradual, natural, and long-lasting — but they cannot be rushed.

How often: An initial course of one to three treatments, followed by maintenance every twelve to twenty-four months.

Before a special occasion: These treatments should be planned months in advance, not weeks. They are not designed to deliver a result for a specific date — they are an investment in long-term skin health and quality.

Biostimulants are for the long game, not last-minute preparation.

PRP for Face and Neck

Platelet-Rich Plasma therapy uses your own growth factors to improve skin quality, tone, and radiance from within. Initial redness, swelling, and mild bruising are common, and the skin's improvement builds gradually over several weeks as collagen remodelling takes place.

How often: Three initial sessions, followed by maintenance every six to twelve months.

Before a special occasion: Allow at least four weeks after your final PRP session before the event.

PRP enhances your natural glow over time — it is not a quick fix, and it should never be treated as one.

Hands — Radiesse® or Bio-Fillers

The hands are often overlooked in aesthetic planning, yet they are almost always visible in photographs and can betray age when the face has been beautifully maintained. Filler in the hands can cause bruising and swelling that may actually be more pronounced than in the face, and adequate settling time is essential.

How often: Every twelve to twenty-four months.

Before a special occasion: Allow four to six weeks — particularly if your hands will be prominently featured in photographs, such as at a wedding.

Hands show bruising easily and settle in their own time. Factor this into your planning from the start.

When Combining Multiple Treatments

When planning a course of treatments ahead of a special occasion, the golden rule is to work from longest-acting to shortest-acting, and from deepest to most superficial. Layering treatments in the wrong order — or too close together — can compromise results and increase recovery time unnecessarily.

A sensible sequence might look like this:

1. Biostimulants — well in advance (months before)
2. Structural facial fillers and hand treatments
3. PRP
4. Botox
5. Skin treatments such as peels or microneedling
6. Light facials and LED — closest to the event

Good outcomes are planned, not rushed. The more important the occasion, the earlier the planning should begin.

The Bottom Line

Aesthetic treatments are not a last-minute solution. They are part of a considered, ongoing approach to ageing well — one that requires forethought, patience, and a realistic understanding of how the body heals and responds.

If something matters enough to celebrate, it matters enough to plan properly.

When treatments are timed correctly and given the space to settle, the results look exactly as they should — natural, relaxed, and entirely effortless. As though you simply woke up that way.

And that, ultimately, is the art of it.

Chapter 4: The Face We Inherit

Before we discuss ageing, wrinkles, fillers, skin boosters, or surgery, we need to talk about something far more important.

Genetics

Long before your first wrinkle appears, your face has already been shaped by generations that came before you.

The colour of your eyes, the thickness of your skin, the shape of your nose, the fullness of your lips, the prominence of your cheekbones, and even how you age are all influenced by the DNA you inherited from your ancestors.

As cosmetic practitioners, we often compare one patient to another, but the truth is that no two faces begin from the same starting point.

The face you see in the mirror today is the result of thousands of years of genetic history.

Your Face Is Your Family Tree

Have you ever looked at old family photographs and recognised your own features staring back at you?

Perhaps you inherited your father's jawline, your mother's eyes, your grandmother's cheeks, or your grandfather's nose.

Certain facial characteristics tend to run strongly through families.

These may include:

Deep-set eyes, Prominent noses, Thin lips, Full lips, Strong chins, Heavy eyelids, Round faces, High cheekbones, Large ears, Dimples

Even the way we age often follows family patterns.

Patients frequently tell me:

"My mother developed jowls at this age."

"Everyone in my family gets eye bags."

"My father always had a strong jawline."

Often they are right.

Genetics plays a major role in determining not only how we look but how we age.

Thick Skin Versus Thin Skin

One of the most important genetic differences is skin thickness.

Not all skin is created equal.

Some people are born with naturally thick, robust skin that contains more collagen and stronger support structures.

Others inherit delicate, thinner skin that shows ageing earlier.

Thin skin tends to: Show wrinkles earlier, Develop crepey texture, Reveal blood vessels more easily, Bruise more readily, Display volume loss sooner

Thick skin tends to: Age more slowly, Develop fewer fine lines, Maintain support longer, Hide underlying structures, Remain firmer for longer

However, thick skin is not always an advantage.

Patients with thicker skin may develop heavier lower faces, more pronounced jowls, and deeper folds later in life.

Thin skin often wrinkles first. Thick skin often sags first.

Ethnicity and Facial Ageing

One of the most fascinating aspects of aesthetic medicine is observing how different ethnic groups age.

While every individual is unique, certain characteristics are commonly seen within different populations.

Anglo-Saxon and Northern European Skin

Fair-skinned individuals often have thinner skin and lower levels of protective melanin.

As a result they tend to: Develop wrinkles earlier, Experience more sun damage, Show redness and broken capillaries, Develop skin cancers more frequently, Lose collagen at a faster visible rate

Many of these patients present with fine lines and texture changes before significant facial sagging occurs.

Mediterranean and Southern European Skin

Greek, Italian, Spanish, and Middle Eastern populations often inherit thicker skin and stronger facial structure.

Common characteristics include: Olive complexions, Higher melanin levels, Stronger bone structure, More pronounced noses, Better resistance to sun-induced wrinkling

These patients often maintain youthful skin quality for longer but may later develop heavier lower-face ageing and deeper folds.

As a Greek woman myself, I often see these characteristics reflected in both my family and many of my patients.

Asian Skin

Many Asian populations possess thicker dermal layers and higher collagen density.

Common features include: Smoother skin texture, Less early wrinkling, Broader midface support, Flatter nasal bridges, Stronger resistance to visible ageing

These patients often maintain youthful skin appearance well into later decades but may experience volume changes and skin laxity as ageing progresses.

Indian and South Asian Skin

South Asian skin typically contains higher levels of melanin and often demonstrates excellent resistance to premature wrinkling.

Common characteristics include: Strong pigmentation, Good collagen support, Fuller facial proportions, Delayed wrinkle formation, Greater tendency toward pigmentation disorders

The challenge is often managing uneven pigmentation rather than wrinkles.

African Skin

African skin contains the highest levels of natural melanin protection.

Common characteristics include: Exceptional resistance to photoageing, Delayed wrinkle formation, Thicker dermis, Excellent collagen preservation, Later onset of visible ageing

Many patients retain remarkably youthful skin for decades, although volume loss and tissue descent still occur with age.

Bone Structure Matters

Much of what we perceive as beauty comes from the underlying skeleton.

A person may have beautiful skin but still inherit a weaker chin, flatter cheeks, or a recessed jaw.

Others are naturally gifted with strong facial architecture.

Facial bones determine: Facial width, Projection, Symmetry, Jawline shape, Chin position, Cheek prominence, Eye support, Nasal structure

Many aesthetic treatments aim to restore or mimic the support that strong bone structure naturally provides.

Fat Pads Are Genetic Too

The face contains multiple fat compartments that contribute to youthful contours.

Some people inherit naturally fuller faces.

Others are genetically lean.

Patients who have always had fuller faces may dislike their cheeks in their twenties but often appreciate them in their sixties.

Those born with lean faces often enjoy defined features when young but may experience earlier hollowing as they age.

The face that frustrated you at twenty may become the face you appreciate most at sixty.

The Genetics of Beauty

Modern society often promotes a single beauty ideal. Yet beauty exists in countless forms.

The high cheekbones of Eastern Europe.

The olive skin of the Mediterranean.

The almond eyes of Asia.

The rich skin tones of Africa.

The strong bone structure of Northern Europe.

The full lips of many Middle Eastern and African populations.

Beauty has never belonged to one ethnicity. Every face carries the story of its ancestry.

As practitioners, our role is not to erase those characteristics. It is to respect them.

Working With Nature, Not Against It

The best cosmetic outcomes occur when we enhance what nature has already provided.

A successful treatment should not make a Greek woman look Scandinavian.

It should not make an Asian patient look European.

It should not erase ethnic identity.

Instead, it should restore, refresh, and celebrate the unique features that make each face individual.

Understanding genetics allows us to create treatment plans that are realistic, respectful, and natural.

Because the goal of aesthetic medicine is not to change who you are.

It is to help you become the best version of the face you inherited.

Chapter 5: What is Dysmorphia

What is Body Dysmorphic Disorder?

Body Dysmorphic Disorder — commonly referred to as BDD or dysmorphia — is a psychological condition in which a person becomes excessively and persistently preoccupied with a perceived flaw in their appearance. That flaw may be minor, barely noticeable to others, or in some cases entirely imagined. But to the person experiencing it, the concern feels very real, deeply distressing, and almost impossible to set aside.

It is important to distinguish BDD from ordinary self-consciousness. Most of us have features we would change if we could — that is entirely human. BDD is something quite different. It is an obsessive, consuming preoccupation that begins to interfere with daily life, relationships, work, and emotional wellbeing. It is not vanity. It is not superficiality. It is a recognised mental health condition that deserves to be taken seriously.

How Do You Know If You Might Be Experiencing BDD?

If you find yourself frequently preoccupied with your appearance, it is worth asking honestly: is this concern proportionate, or is it beginning to take over my thoughts and affect how I live?

The following are signs that what you are experiencing may go beyond ordinary self-criticism.

You are fixated on a specific feature. You spend significant time each day thinking about a particular aspect of your appearance. You check mirrors repeatedly — or avoid them altogether. You photograph yourself frequently, zooming in to scrutinise the feature that concerns you, and find it difficult to move past what you see.

Your sense of self-worth is closely tied to how you look. Your mood, confidence, and ability to engage with the world fluctuates depending on how you feel you look on any given day. A perceived bad appearance day can spiral into anxiety, low mood, or social withdrawal.

You constantly compare yourself to others. Scrolling through images of influencers or celebrities leaves you feeling inadequate. You rely heavily on filters or editing tools to create a version of yourself you feel more comfortable sharing, and the unedited image feels unacceptable.

Reassurance never feels like enough. You frequently seek confirmation from others that the flaw you see isn't visible — but even when people reassure you, you cannot fully believe them. The relief, if it comes at all, is fleeting.

You have had repeated cosmetic treatments without lasting satisfaction. You have pursued multiple procedures but continue to feel dissatisfied. Each treatment brings temporary relief, but the anxiety quickly returns — sometimes shifting to an entirely different feature. You continue searching for a fix that never quite arrives, even when practitioners advise you that further treatment is not appropriate.

Your daily life is being affected. You avoid social situations because of self-consciousness about your appearance. You spend considerable time, energy, or money on makeup, skincare, or cosmetic treatments in an attempt to manage the anxiety. Thoughts about your appearance cause you genuine distress.

If several of these resonate with you, it may be worth speaking to someone — not because anything is wrong with you, but because you deserve support.

What Can Be Done?

BDD is a treatable condition. Recognising that your thoughts about your appearance may not be an accurate reflection of reality is a significant and courageous first step. From there, there is real help available.

Seek professional support. A psychologist or therapist with experience in body image and OCD-spectrum conditions can make an enormous difference. Cognitive Behavioural Therapy — CBT — is considered the gold standard treatment for BDD. It works by helping individuals identify, challenge, and gradually reframe the distorted thought patterns that are driving their distress.

Reduce mirror-checking and social media exposure. Limiting time spent scrutinising your reflection, taking selfies, or consuming social media content that promotes unrealistic beauty standards can help break the cycle of comparison and rumination. Small, consistent changes here can have a meaningful impact over time.

Step back from cosmetic procedures. If you have had multiple treatments and still feel deeply unsatisfied, further procedures are very unlikely to resolve what you are experiencing. Reputable aesthetic practitioners have an ethical responsibility to recognise the signs of BDD and to decline treatment when it is clearly not in a client's best interest. A good practitioner will always refer you to appropriate support rather than simply accommodating every request.

Reconnect with what your body can do. Shifting focus from how you look to how you feel — and what your body is capable of — can be genuinely therapeutic. Movement that brings joy, whether that is exercise, yoga, swimming, or dance, can help rebuild a more compassionate relationship with yourself.

Practice self-compassion. Perfection does not exist. Beauty is subjective, changeable, and far less fixed than social media would have us believe. Learning to speak to yourself with the same kindness you would offer a close friend is not a small thing — it is, in many ways, the most important work of all.

Consider medication where appropriate. In more severe cases, SSRIs — a class of antidepressant medication — can help reduce the intensity of obsessive thoughts. This is always a conversation to have with a qualified mental health professional, who can assess whether medication is appropriate as part of a broader treatment plan.

A Final Word

Aesthetic treatments, at their best, should enhance confidence and help people feel more like themselves. They should never be a way of feeding an insecurity that no procedure could ever truly resolve.

If concerns about your appearance are beginning to dominate your thoughts, affect your relationships, or limit how fully you are able to live your life — please consider that it may be more than dissatisfaction. It may be dysmorphia. And dysmorphia is not something any needle can fix.

Seeking help is not about giving up on looking good. It is about building a healthier, kinder relationship with yourself — one that no treatment, however skilfully administered, can create on your behalf.

True confidence is not found in the mirror. It is found within.

Chapter 6: How to Choose the Right Injector

The Most Important Decision You Will Make

When it comes to cosmetic injectables, people often ask about products — which brand of filler, which formulation of toxin, which the latest innovation is. And while product quality does matter, it is not the most important factor in your outcome.

The injector is.

Botulinum toxin, dermal fillers, and biostimulants are tools. Extraordinary tools, when used correctly — but tools nonetheless. In the right hands, they produce results that are subtle, beautiful, and entirely natural. In the wrong hands, they can lead to poor outcomes, avoidable complications, and in some cases, long-term damage that is both physically and emotionally costly to address.

Choosing your injector is the single most important decision in your entire aesthetic journey. Everything else follows from that.

Why the Injector Matters More Than the Product

It is very common for patients to ask which brand of filler a clinic uses. It is a far less common — but far more important — question to ask who will actually be holding the syringe.

A skilled injector brings a deep understanding of facial anatomy, how faces age, the principles of proportion and balance, and crucially, how to recognise and manage complications if they arise. They also bring something that cannot be taught in a weekend course — an aesthetic eye. An intuitive sense of what a face needs, and equally, what it does not.

The same product, placed by two different practitioners, can produce results that are worlds apart. One face looks refreshed, harmonious, entirely natural. Another looks overdone, distorted, and somehow less like the person it belongs to. The difference is never the syringe. It is always the artist behind it.

Who Can Perform Injectable Treatments?

In Australia and many other countries, cosmetic injectables may legally be performed by doctors, registered nurses, nurse practitioners, and in some contexts, dentists. Each of these professions is capable of producing excellent results — but professional title alone tells you very little about the quality of work you can expect.

A nurse with fifteen years of dedicated aesthetic experience will, in most cases, be considerably more skilled than a doctor who completed a weekend introductory course last month. What matters far more than the letters after someone's name is their experience, their commitment to ongoing education, their safety knowledge, and the quality of their aesthetic judgment.

The Experience Factor

Cosmetic injecting is both a science and an art, and it takes years to truly master. When you are considering an injector, it is entirely reasonable — and genuinely important — to ask how long they have been practising, whether they inject full time or only occasionally, and how regularly they attend professional training and industry conferences.

Experience teaches things that simply cannot be learned from a textbook. It teaches how different faces age, how products behave in different tissue types, how to anticipate and avoid complications, and how to respond swiftly and calmly when something unexpected occurs. An injector who has treated thousands of faces will notice things in a consultation that a less experienced practitioner may overlook entirely.

What to Look for in a Good Injector

A natural aesthetic. Before committing to any practitioner, look carefully at their work. Do their patients look like refreshed, improved versions of themselves — or do they look overfilled, frozen, or oddly similar to one another? A skilled injector always aims for balance, subtlety, and age-appropriate harmony. If a clinic's social media is full of identical pillow cheeks, overfilled lips, and expressionless foreheads, that tells you a great deal about their aesthetic philosophy — and it may not align with yours.

A thorough consultation. A professional injector will take time before any treatment to ask about your medical history, listen carefully to your concerns, examine your face from multiple angles, walk you through your options, and set realistic expectations. They will treat the consultation as an essential part of the process — not an inconvenience to rush through on the way to picking up a syringe.

A clear red flag: if an injector asks how many syringes you want before they have even properly looked at your face, that is not a practitioner who is assessing your needs. That is a practitioner who is taking your order.

The ability to say no. This is, in my view, one of the most telling signs of a genuinely skilled and ethical injector. A responsible practitioner will decline requests they feel are unrealistic, unsafe, or simply not in your best interest. They will offer honest alternatives and explain their reasoning clearly. An injector who will do anything, to anyone, at any time, simply because the client has asked — that is not competent practice. That is a liability.

An honest conversation about risks. Before any treatment, your injector should discuss possible side effects and complications openly, provide written aftercare instructions, and offer a follow-up appointment to review your results. They should also be able to tell you clearly what they would do if something went wrong. Ask whether they carry hyaluronidase — the reversal agent for hyaluronic acid fillers — and ask about their emergency protocol. A confident, experienced injector will answer these questions without hesitation. If the question makes them uncomfortable, that is important information.

A clean, professional environment. The clinic or treatment room should be visibly clean, well-organised, and operating to proper medical standards — sterile single-use needles, appropriate medical supplies, and a professional atmosphere throughout. If a treatment is being offered at a beauty party, a pop-up event, or somewhere that feels makeshift or informal, think very carefully before proceeding. The setting in which you are treated matters enormously.

Red Flags to Watch For

Approach with caution if you encounter any of the following: extremely low prices or constant discount promotions; pressure to purchase packages before you have had a proper consultation; no discussion of risks or aftercare; no follow-up offered; or treatments being performed in non-clinical settings.

In aesthetics, pricing generally reflects experience, product quality, consultation time, clinic standards, and safety protocols. When the price seems too good to be true, it usually is — and the cost of correcting poor work, both financially and emotionally, is almost always far greater than the cost of doing it properly the first time.

Social Media Is Not a Substitute for Experience

In the current landscape, many practitioners are judged — and chosen — on the basis of their Instagram following, their TikTok presence, and the volume of before-and-after photographs they post. Social media can be a useful window into a practitioner's aesthetic style, but it does not tell you about their long-term results, their complication management, or the depth of their clinical knowledge.

Some of the most skilled injectors I know have modest social media profiles. They do not need a large following because their work speaks for itself, and their patients return year after year and recommend them to everyone they know. Word of mouth built over years of consistent, honest, high-quality work is a far more reliable measure of excellence than follower count.

Questions Worth Asking Before You Commit

You have every right to ask your injector the following before treatment begins:

- How many years have you been performing injectable treatments?
- What training have you completed, and how recently?
- Do you carry hyaluronidase, and are you trained in its use?
- What is your protocol if a complication occurs?
- Do you offer follow-up review appointments?

These are not rude or difficult questions. They are responsible ones. Any practitioner worth choosing will welcome them.

The Value of a Thoughtful Treatment Plan

A skilled injector does not simply treat a single line or isolated area in response to whatever a patient points at in the mirror. They assess the face as a whole — its proportions, its structure, the way it has aged and how it is likely to continue ageing — and they plan accordingly. They may recommend staged treatments over time rather than attempting to address everything at once, which almost always produces more refined, natural, and lasting results.

A well-considered treatment plan leads to better outcomes, fewer complications, and genuinely better value over time. It reflects a practitioner who is thinking about your long-term result, not just today's appointment.

The Bottom Line

In aesthetics, the cheapest option is rarely the best value. Good work, performed safely by an experienced and ethical practitioner, will serve you far better — and far longer — than a bargain that needs correcting.

When choosing your injector, trust experience over hype, skill over price, and natural results over whatever trend is currently dominating social media. Trust your instincts in the consultation room too. The right practitioner will make you feel genuinely heard, respected, and safe.

And when the work is done well, nobody will ask who did your lips or comment on your cheeks. They will simply look at you and say: "You look fantastic."

That is the true mark of a great injector — and it is exactly what you deserve.

Chapter 7: What to Expect at the Initial Consultation

The initial consultation is one of the most important parts of any aesthetic journey. Before any treatment is performed, a thorough assessment is essential to ensure safety, suitability, and realistic expectations.

A good consultation is not simply about deciding where to place filler or how many units of anti-wrinkle treatment are required. It is about understanding the whole person — their concerns, facial structure, medical history, lifestyle, and treatment goals — so that a personalised and appropriate plan can be created.

Every face ages differently. Skin, muscle, fat, ligaments, and bone all change over time, and these changes interact with one another. For this reason, aesthetic medicine should never focus only on isolated lines or individual features. The consultation is where the underlying cause of concerns is identified.

Medical History and Lifestyle Assessment

The consultation begins with a detailed medical history. Previous cosmetic treatments are discussed, including injectables, lasers, skin treatments, and any prior complications or adverse reactions.

Medical conditions are also important, particularly autoimmune disorders, inflammatory skin conditions, bleeding disorders, or any condition that may affect healing and collagen response.

Medications and supplements are carefully reviewed, especially blood thinners, anti-inflammatory medications, steroids, immunosuppressants, and herbal supplements that may increase bruising or interfere with healing.

Lifestyle factors also play a significant role in treatment outcomes. Smoking, alcohol consumption, sun exposure, stress, sleep quality, and skincare habits can all affect skin health, collagen production, healing, and longevity of results.

Understanding Bruising and Healing Risks

Some patients are naturally more prone to bruising or swelling than others. Blood-thinning medications, impaired platelet function, low iron levels, and certain medical conditions may increase the likelihood of bruising and prolong recovery time.

Aesthetic treatments must always be tailored to the individual, with consideration given to healing capacity, inflammation, and skin integrity.

Understanding the Patient's Goals

An important part of the consultation is understanding what the patient is hoping to achieve.

Some patients are concerned about volume loss, facial sagging, wrinkles, pigmentation, or skin quality. Others simply want to look fresher or less tired.

It is also important to clarify expectations. Some treatments provide immediate improvement, while others work gradually by stimulating collagen and improving skin quality over time.

Event planning is another important consideration. Certain procedures may involve swelling, bruising, or downtime, so timing treatments appropriately is essential.

Clinical Assessment of the Face

The facial examination is comprehensive and focuses on identifying the true cause of ageing changes rather than simply treating what is visible on the surface.

Assessment includes:

- Bone structure and facial framework
- Deep and superficial fat compartments
- Muscle movement and facial expression
- Ligament support and facial sagging
- Skin quality, elasticity, and hydration
- Facial symmetry and proportions

The face is assessed as a whole, not as isolated parts.

For example, nasolabial folds are often not caused by the fold itself. They are frequently the result of volume loss and structural change in the cheeks and surrounding support structures. Treating the fold alone can create heaviness and unnatural results, whereas restoring support in the midface often softens the fold more naturally.

This holistic approach creates better facial harmony and more balanced outcomes.

Skin and Vascular Assessment

Skin quality and vascular health are also evaluated carefully before treatment.

Thin, fragile, sun-damaged, or highly vascular skin may require a more conservative approach. Patients with a history of herpes simplex infections around the lips may require preventative antiviral medication before lip treatments to reduce the risk of an outbreak.

Safety is always the priority.

Before Treatment Proceeds

Before any treatment is performed, the treatment plan is discussed in detail, including expected outcomes, risks, possible side effects, recovery, and aftercare instructions.

Informed consent must always be obtained, and in Australia, cosmetic injectable treatments require medical oversight, including prescription approval by a doctor for the treating cosmetic nurse.

A thorough consultation forms the foundation of safe, ethical, and effective aesthetic practice.

My Philosophy When Consulting

Over the years, I have learnt that the best aesthetic outcomes do not come from doing more treatment. They come from understanding the face properly before treating anything at all.

Many patients arrive requesting a specific procedure.

"I want filler here."

"I need Botox there."

But what a patient asks for is not always what they truly need.

Rather than focusing immediately on the requested treatment, I focus on understanding the reason behind the concern. If you treat only the symptom and not the cause, you simply create a cycle of ongoing correction.

The face does not age in isolated parts. Skin, fat pads, ligaments, muscle, and bone all change together. This is why a proper consultation matters far more than simply choosing a product or procedure.

When I assess a face, I look at structure, volume, movement, skin quality, and how these elements interact with one another.

A line may not actually be a skin problem. It may be caused by volume loss, muscle movement, ligament laxity, or structural change.

Over time, I developed a simple framework for consultations:

Look — assess the entire face and how it moves.

Listen — understand the patient's concerns and expectations.

Locate — identify the true cause of the issue.

Then:

Educate — explain what is happening anatomically.

Encourage — guide the patient toward appropriate treatment options.

Ensure — confirm understanding, safety, and comfort with the plan.

I believe strongly in treating the cause, not simply the complaint.

A patient may focus on their lips when the real issue is loss of support through the midface. Another may worry about lines when skin quality is the primary concern.

When the underlying cause is treated properly, results appear softer, fresher, and more natural.

A Natural Approach

My goal has never been to change faces. It is to refine, support, and restore them while preserving individuality and movement.

Natural results come from restraint, balance, and respecting the face as a whole.

Over-treatment often creates heaviness, distortion, and loss of expression. In contrast, subtle, well-planned treatments allow patients to look refreshed without looking altered.

Modern aesthetics has also shifted away from excessive volume and toward skin quality, regeneration, and collagen stimulation. Healthy skin will always look more youthful and natural than an overfilled face.

Natural results should never erase personality or facial character. The aim is not perfection. It is recognition.

The best compliment a patient can receive is not:

"You look like you've had work done."

It is:

"You look well."

"You look refreshed."

"You still look like yourself."

That is the essence of good aesthetic medicine.

Because ultimately, the quality of the consultation will determine the quality of the result.

How I Assess the face

The 3 Ls and 3 Es

After more than 30 years in aesthetics, I have learnt that good results do not begin with the syringe. They begin with observation.

Over time, I developed a simple framework that guides the way I assess every patient who sits in front of me.

I call it: The 3 Ls and 3 Es.

It keeps the consultation focused, structured, and patient-centred, while helping me understand not only the anatomy of the face, but the person behind it.

The First Step — Understanding

Look

The first thing I do is look at the face as a whole.

Not just the line, wrinkle, or feature the patient is concerned about, but how everything works together.

I assess:

- Facial structure, Volume distribution, Skin quality
- Symmetry, Movement and expression

I observe the face both at rest and in motion. A face tells a completely different story when someone smiles, laughs, talks, or frowns.

Movement often reveals where ageing is occurring, where support has been lost, and where muscles are overcompensating.

For example, strong masseter muscles may reflect years of clenching or grinding from stress and anxiety. Forehead lines may tell the story of chronic expression, tension, or compensating for heavy brows. Sometimes the face carries emotional patterns just as much as anatomical ones.

I also pay close attention to how patients present themselves when they walk into the room.

Body language reveals far more than most people realise.

I notice:

- Posture, Eye contact
- Facial expression, Confidence or hesitation
- Whether they appear relaxed, anxious, guarded, or self-conscious

Some patients avoid mirrors. Some continually apologise for ageing. Others focus obsessively on one tiny feature that nobody else notices.

These observations matter because aesthetic medicine is never just about anatomy. Often, there is emotion sitting quietly underneath the concern.

Listen

Listening is one of the most important parts of the consultation.

Patients will usually tell you what bothers them physically, but if you listen carefully, they will also tell you how those changes are affecting them emotionally.

I listen to:

- Their concerns, Their expectations
- The language they use, Their emotional tone

Sometimes a patient asking for "filler everywhere" is actually saying: "I look tired."

"I don't feel confident anymore."

"I don't recognise myself."

Others may come in wanting dramatic change when what they really need is subtle support and reassurance.

Listening allows me to understand whether expectations are realistic and whether the requested treatment aligns with what will actually look balanced and natural.

Locate

Once I have observed and listened, the next step is locating the true cause of the concern.

This is where clinical assessment becomes critical.

A line is not always caused by the skin itself. It may be related to:

- Volume loss, Muscle activity
- Bone resorption, Ligament laxity
- Skin thinning, Repetitive facial movement

Similarly, a hollow or fold may not need direct filling at all. Sometimes the issue originates from loss of support in another area of the face.

If you do not identify the cause correctly, you risk treating symptoms rather than creating meaningful improvement.

The Second Step — Guiding

Educate

Once I understand what is happening anatomically, I explain it clearly to the patient.

I believe patients should understand:

- Why changes are occurring, What treatment options exist
- What results are realistic, What limitations may exist

Education creates confidence and helps patients make informed decisions instead of emotional ones.

Encourage

Encouragement is not about convincing someone to have treatment.

It is about guiding them toward the most appropriate and balanced approach.

Sometimes that means:

- Starting conservatively, Improving skin quality first
- Staging treatments gradually, Choosing less treatment rather than more

Patients often feel relieved when they realise they do not need to dramatically change their face to look fresher.

Ensure

Before any treatment proceeds, I ensure the patient:

- Understands the plan, Feels comfortable
- Has realistic expectations, Understands risks, downtime, and aftercare

This is where trust is built.

A patient should never feel rushed, pressured, or confused during a consultation.

The consultation itself should leave them feeling informed, reassured, and confident in their decisions.

Why This Framework Matters

Without a structured approach, it becomes easy to over-treat, miss the true cause of a concern, or create imbalance in the face.

The 3 Ls and 3 Es help create: Better assessment, Better communication, Better treatment planning, Better long-term outcomes

Most practitioners treat what they see.

The best practitioners look deeper and treat what is causing it.

Look. Listen. Locate.

Educate. Encourage. Ensure.

Chapter 8: Understanding Consent- What Every Patient Should Know Before Treatment

Why Consent Matters

Consent is far more than signing a piece of paper.

True informed consent means you understand:

- What treatment is being performed
- Why it is being recommended
- The expected benefits
- Alternative treatments available
- Potential risks and complications
- Expected recovery time
- Cost implications
- What to do if complications occur

A consent form should never be signed under pressure. Patients should have sufficient time to ask questions and make an informed decision.

Botulinum Toxin Type A Consent

What Is It?

Botulinum toxin is a prescription medicine used to temporarily relax targeted muscles responsible for dynamic wrinkles.

Common treatment areas include:

- Frown lines, Forehead lines, Crow's feet, Bunny lines
- Chin dimpling, Neck bands, Jaw slimming, Excessive sweating

Expected Benefits

- Softer facial lines, Prevention of wrinkle formation, Improved facial balance, Reduced muscle activity

Possible Side Effects

Common:

- Redness, Swelling, Bruising, Tenderness

Less Common:

- Headache, Flu-like symptoms, Temporary asymmetry, Eyelid droop (ptosis), Brow heaviness

Rare:

- Allergic reaction, Difficulty swallowing, Vision disturbances

Alternatives

- No treatment, Skincare, Laser treatments, Surgery

Hyaluronic Acid Dermal Filler Consent

What Are Dermal Fillers?

Hyaluronic acid fillers are injectable gels used to restore volume, improve contours and support facial structures.

Areas Commonly Treated

- Lips, Cheeks, Chin, Jawline, Temples, Tear troughs, Nasolabial folds, Marionette lines

Expected Benefits

- Volume restoration, Facial balancing, Improved contours, Hydration

Common Side Effects

- Swelling, Bruising, Tenderness, Temporary lumpiness

Significant Risks

- Infection, Delayed inflammatory reactions, Nodules, Filler migration

Serious Vascular Complications

Although rare, filler can enter or compress a blood vessel causing: Skin necrosis, Scarring, Blindness, Stroke

Patients should immediately report: Severe pain, Blanching, Mottled skin, Vision changes

Alternatives

- Skin boosters, Biostimulators, Surgery, No treatment

Biostimulator Consent

Sculptra (PLLA) and Calcium Hydroxyapatite (CaHA)

What Are Biostimulators?

Biostimulators work by encouraging your body to produce collagen rather than simply adding volume.

Examples include: Sculptra (PLLA), Radiesse (CaHA)

Expected Benefits

- Improved skin quality, Increased collagen production, Firmer skin, Gradual rejuvenation

Treatment Expectations

Results develop gradually over:

- 6–12 weeks, Often require multiple sessions

Common Side Effects

- Swelling, Bruising, Tenderness

Specific Risks

PLLA:

- Papules, Nodules, Granulomas

CaHA:

- Nodules, Unevenness, Vascular occlusion

Alternatives

- Dermal fillers, PRP, Skin boosters, Surgery

Skin Booster Consent

What Are Skin Boosters?

Skin boosters are injectable products designed primarily to improve hydration and skin quality rather than create volume.

Examples include:

- Profhilo, Skinvive, Restylane Skinboosters, Redensity 1, Neauvia Hydro Deluxe, Sunekos

Expected Benefits

- Increased hydration, Improved skin texture, Improved elasticity, Skin luminosity

Common Side Effects

- Injection bumps, Bruising, Swelling, Tenderness

Rare Risks

- Infection, Allergic reaction, Vascular compromise

PRP Consent

Platelet Rich Plasma

What Is PRP?

PRP uses your own blood. A sample is collected, processed and concentrated platelets are re-injected or microneedled into the treatment area.

Common Treatment Areas

- Face, Neck, Décolletage, Hair restoration

Expected Benefits

- Improved skin quality, Enhanced healing, Improved hair growth, Increased collagen production

Risks

- Bruising, Swelling, Infection, Discomfort

Limitations

Results vary between individuals and cannot be guaranteed.

PRP Biofiller Consent

What Is Biofiller?

Biofiller is created by heating and processing platelet-rich plasma into a gel-like substance that can provide temporary volume.

Benefits

- Uses your own tissue, Natural appearance, Regenerative effects, Improved skin quality

Risks

- Bruising, Swelling, Lump formation, Uneven correction, Infection

Limitations

Biofiller generally lasts less time than commercial fillers.

Chemical Peel Consent

What Is a Chemical Peel?

A chemical peel uses acids to remove damaged skin cells and stimulate skin renewal.

Benefits

- Improved pigmentation, Smoother texture, Reduced acne, Improved skin brightness

Common Reactions

- Redness, Peeling, Dryness, Tightness

Potential Risks

- Hyperpigmentation, Hypopigmentation, Infection, Scarring, Cold sore activation

Post Treatment Responsibilities

Patients must: Wear sunscreen daily, Avoid picking peeling skin, Follow aftercare instructions carefully

Final Patient Declaration

Before proceeding, patients should acknowledge:

✓ I understand the treatment.

✓ I understand the potential risks and benefits.

✓ I have had the opportunity to ask questions.

✓ No guarantee of results has been made.

✓ I understand that complications can occur despite appropriate treatment.

✓ I consent voluntarily to proceed.

Medical Legal aspect of consent

Legal Importance of Signing Consent Forms: A signed consent form is an important legal document that provides evidence the patient was informed about the proposed treatment, its benefits, risks, possible complications, alternatives, and expected outcomes before proceeding.

While a signature alone does not prove informed consent was obtained, it supports the clinician's documentation that a consent discussion occurred and that the patient voluntarily agreed to treatment.

In the event of a complaint, regulatory investigation, or legal claim, a properly completed and signed consent form, together with detailed clinical notes, can be critical in demonstrating that the practitioner met their professional and legal obligations to obtain informed consent.

Chapter 9: Facial Assessing and Marking

Beauty Assessments- Understanding Facial Proportions

One of the most common questions I hear from patients is: "What makes a face attractive?"

The answer is surprisingly complex.

Beauty is influenced by culture, ethnicity, personality, expression, confidence, and individual features. There is no single perfect face, nor should there be.

However, throughout history artists, sculptors, architects, and aesthetic practitioners have recognised certain facial proportions that tend to create balance and harmony.

These measurements are not rigid rules. They are assessment tools that help us understand facial structure and guide treatment planning.

In aesthetics, we are not trying to make every face identical. We are simply looking for balance.

Facial Thirds

One of the most basic methods of facial assessment is dividing the face into thirds. Ideally, the face can be divided into three approximately equal horizontal sections.

Diagram: Facial Thirds

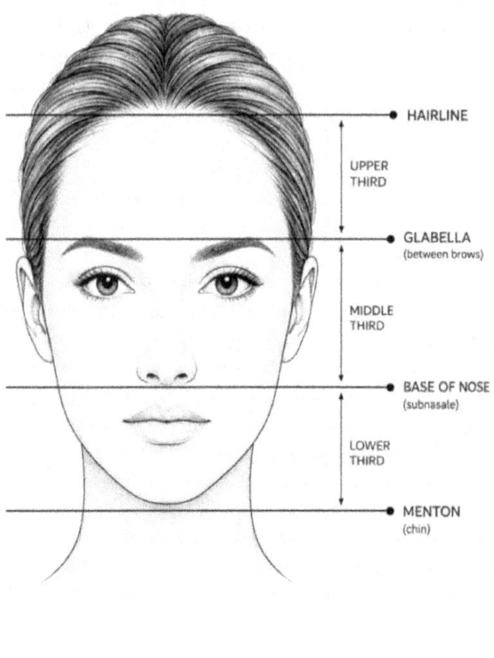

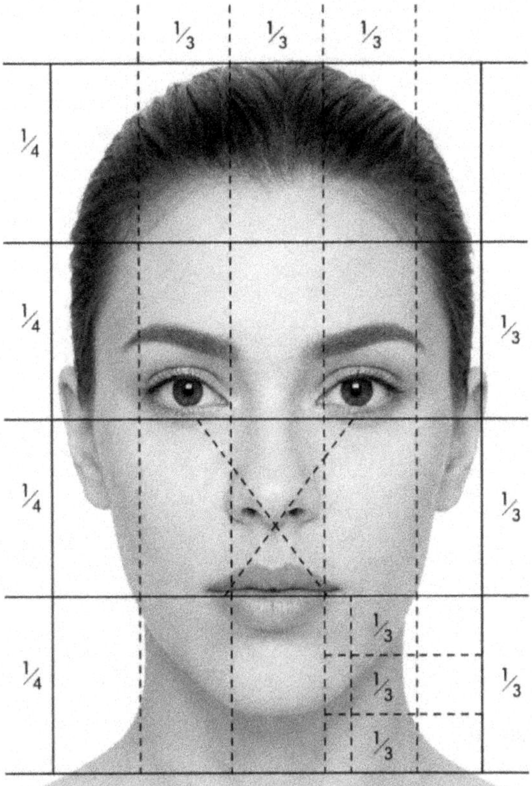

Fig. 9

Fig. 9 (a) The head is divided into four equal parts: i.e. from top of head to normal hairline; hairline to brows; brows to base of nose; bottom of nose to base of chin.

(b) The face is divided into three equal sections: normal hairline to brows; brows to bottom of nose; base of nose to base of chin.

(c) The ear measures one-third of the facial length, its top rim being on an imaginary line with the brows and its lobe on a line with base of chin.

(d) The mouth closure line is approximately one-third of the distance from base of nose to base of chin. Its width is approximately one-third of the facial width. (An imaginary diagonal line from the inner corner of the eye to the outer corner of the mouth traverses the outer part of the nostril.)

(e) The space between the eyes measures the width of one eye. Pupil to pupil equals one-third of the facial length.

The Upper Third extends from the hairline to the eyebrows.

The Mid Third extends from the eyebrows to the base of the nose.

The Lower Third extends from the base of the nose to the bottom of the chin.

When assessing patients, we often identify disproportions such as:

A long lower third, A short chin A recessed jaw, A long midface, A shortened upper face

Understanding these proportions helps guide treatments involving the chin, jawline, cheeks, and temples.

Facial Fifths

The face can also be divided vertically into five equal sections.

This assessment helps determine balance across the width of the face.

Diagram: Facial Fifths

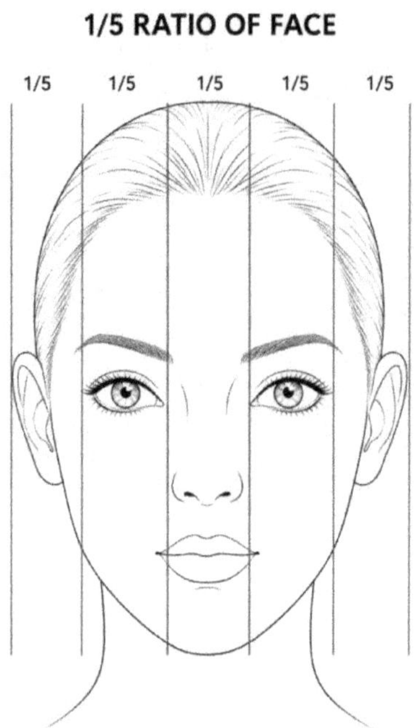

Each fifth should be approximately equal.

Typically:

F1 = outer face to outer eye

F2 = width of one eye

F3 = width between the eyes

F4 = width of one eye

F5 = outer eye to outer face

A useful rule is:

"The distance between the eyes should roughly equal the width of one eye."

When assessing patients, facial fifths help identify:

Eye spacing, Facial asymmetry, Midface width, Orbital proportions, Nasal width

This assessment is particularly useful when planning facial balancing treatments.

The Golden Ratio

For centuries artists and mathematicians have been fascinated by a number known as the Golden Ratio.

Approximately: 1 : 1.618

This proportion appears repeatedly throughout nature.

It can be seen in: Flower petals, Seashells, Tree growth, The human body And facial proportions

Diagram: Golden Ratio

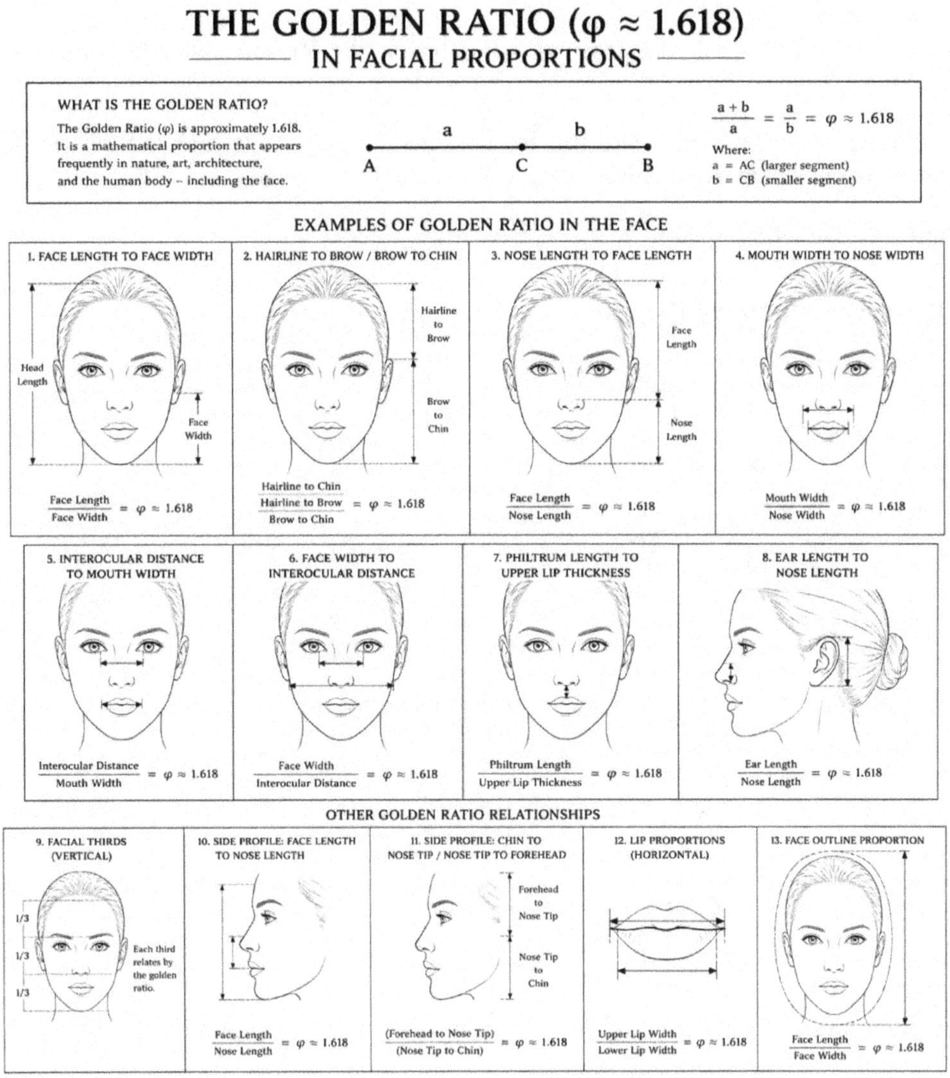

Face Length

Face Width

≈ 1.618

The Golden Ratio should never be considered a beauty rule.

Many beautiful people do not conform to it.

However, it provides an interesting framework for understanding harmony and proportion.

In modern aesthetics it is used as one of many assessment tools rather than a fixed standard.

Ricketts E-Line

One of the most useful tools for assessing lips is the Ricketts Esthetic Line, often called the E-Line.

Developed by orthodontist Dr. Robert Ricketts, it helps evaluate the relationship between the nose, lips, and chin.

Diagram: Ricketts E-Line

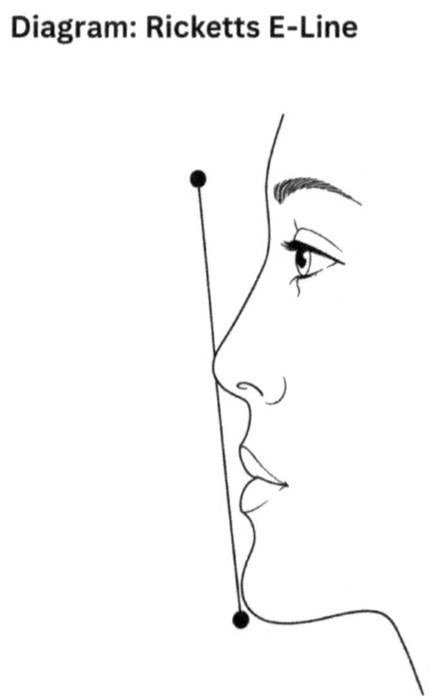

The line is drawn from the tip of the nose to the most prominent point of the chin.

Traditionally:

The upper lip sits approximately 4 mm behind the line.

The lower lip sits approximately 2 mm behind the line.

However, these measurements were developed primarily using Caucasian populations.

Different ethnic groups naturally have different lip positions.

Many Mediterranean, African, Middle Eastern, and Asian faces may have lips that project beyond the traditional E-Line and still appear completely natural and attractive.

This highlights an important principle:

Assessment tools should guide treatment, not dictate treatment.

Female Cheek Assessment

The female cheek apex is typically higher and more lateral, creating the classic "heart-shaped" or inverted triangle appearance.

Markings:

1. Draw a line from the lateral canthus (outer corner of eye) to the corner of the mouth.
2. Draw a second line from the alar base (side of nose) to the tragus.
3. The intersection approximates the female cheek apex.

The ideal projection point is usually:

- Over the zygomatic eminence
- Slightly lateral to the pupil
- High on the cheekbone

Male Cheek Assessment

Men generally require a flatter, broader cheek.

The apex is: More medial, Slightly lower, Less projected

The goal is strength rather than roundness.

Markings:

1. Draw a vertical line through the lateral limbus (outer iris).
2. Draw a horizontal line from the alar base.
3. The intersection indicates the male cheek projection point.

MD Codes Reference

For filler placement:

Female

- Ck1: High lateral cheek, Ck2: Zygomatic arch, Ck3: Anterior cheek

Emphasis is usually on Ck1 and Ck2.

Male

- Ck1: More conservative
- Greater emphasis on Ck3 and lateral support
- Avoid excessive anterior projection

Simple Rule

Female

- High, Lateral, Curved, Heart-shaped

Male

- Flatter, Wider, Stronger, Square appearance

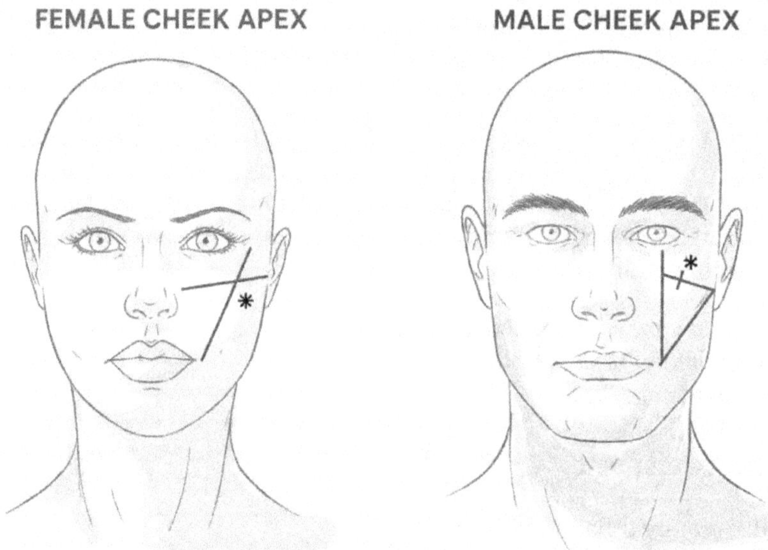

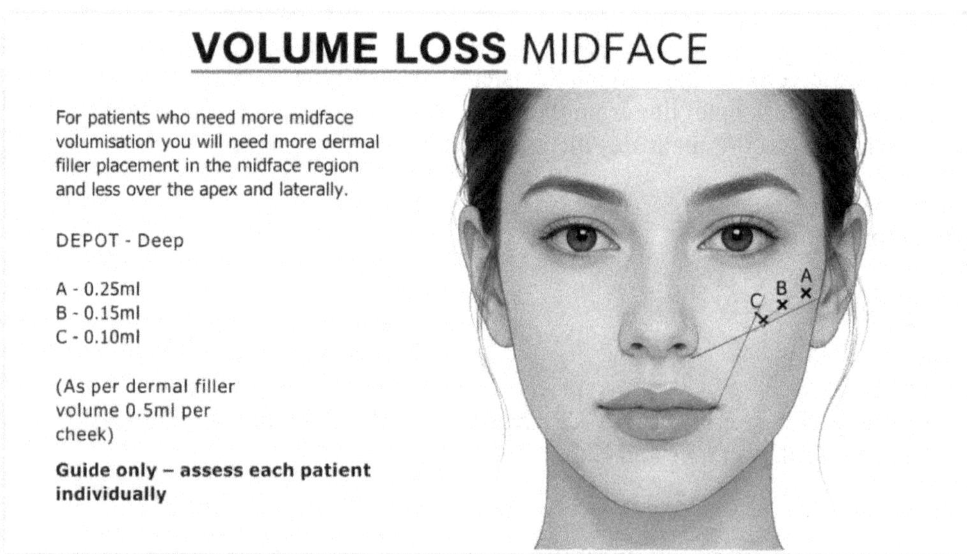

SHAPE AND **CONTOUR**

For patients who request cheek beautification or cheek bone enhancement, dermal filler placement should be more focused on the apex and laterally over the cheek.

DEPOT – Deep

A – 0.10 ml
B – 0.25 ml
C – 0.15 ml

(As per dermal filler volume 0.5ml per cheek)

Guide only – assess each patient individually

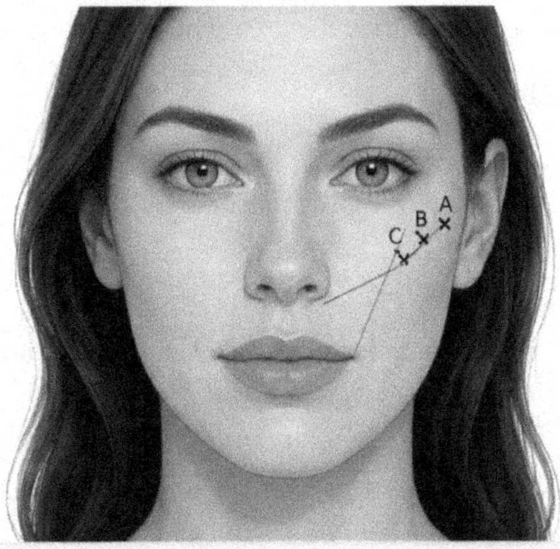

3 Ways to Approach Injecting Cheeks

Before the popularity of MD Codes®, injectors commonly used anatomical guide lines to help determine the ideal location for cheek augmentation. These assessment tools are still useful today, particularly for beginners learning facial proportions and structural support.

The purpose of all three methods is the same:

- Identify the point of maximum cheek projection, Restore lost volume, Create lift and support, Improve facial harmony.

A – Hinderer's Method

Hinderer's lines are created by drawing:

1. A line from the corner of the mouth to the upper ear (tragus).
2. A second line from the outer corner of the eye to the corner of the mouth.

Where the lines intersect identifies the ideal malar prominence (cheek apex).

Best Used For:

- Younger patients with flat cheeks, Patients requiring cheek projection.
- Female patients seeking a softer, heart-shaped appearance, Creating a defined cheek highlight.

Treatment Goal:

Restore projection at the cheek apex and recreate youthful contour.

B – Wilkinson's Method

Wilkinson's approach focuses on the vertical alignment of the lateral cheek.

The line is drawn vertically down from the lateral canthus (outer eye corner) toward the mandibular border.

This technique identifies the area where structural support can be restored to create lift.

Best Used For:

- Mid-face ageing, Mild cheek descent.
- Patients developing nasolabial folds, Patients requiring support rather than projection.

Treatment Goal:

Lift and support the mid-face while maintaining a natural appearance.

C – Powell's Method

Powell's method uses a horizontal line from the nasal bridge combined with an oblique line extending toward the zygomatic arch.

The intersection identifies the area of greatest cheek enhancement.

Best Used For:

- Patients with flattened cheek contours, Facial balancing procedures.
- Patients requiring lateral cheek enhancement., Creating a more sculpted appearance.

Treatment Goal:

Increase cheek width and contour while improving facial proportions.

Which Method Should You Use?

In reality, experienced injectors rarely rely on a single assessment system.

Modern cheek assessment combines: Facial anatomy, Ageing patterns, Fat pad changes, Bone resorption, Individual beauty goals

These classic approaches simply provide landmarks that help guide treatment planning.

As I often tell my students:

"Treat the face in front of you, not the diagram."

The best cheek enhancement is one that restores balance, not one that follows a formula.

3 WAYS TO APPROACH INJECTING CHEEKS

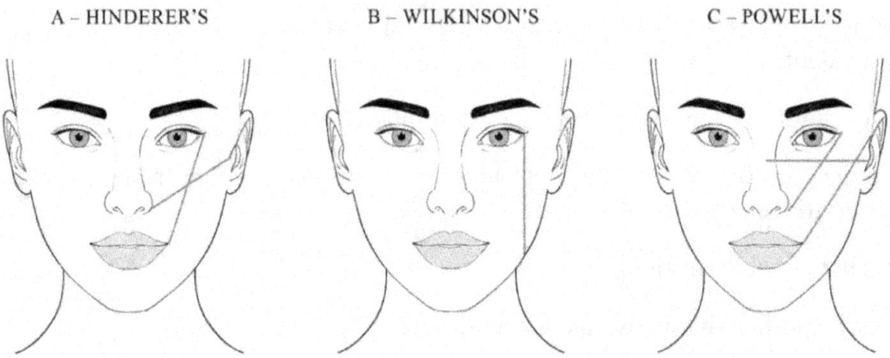

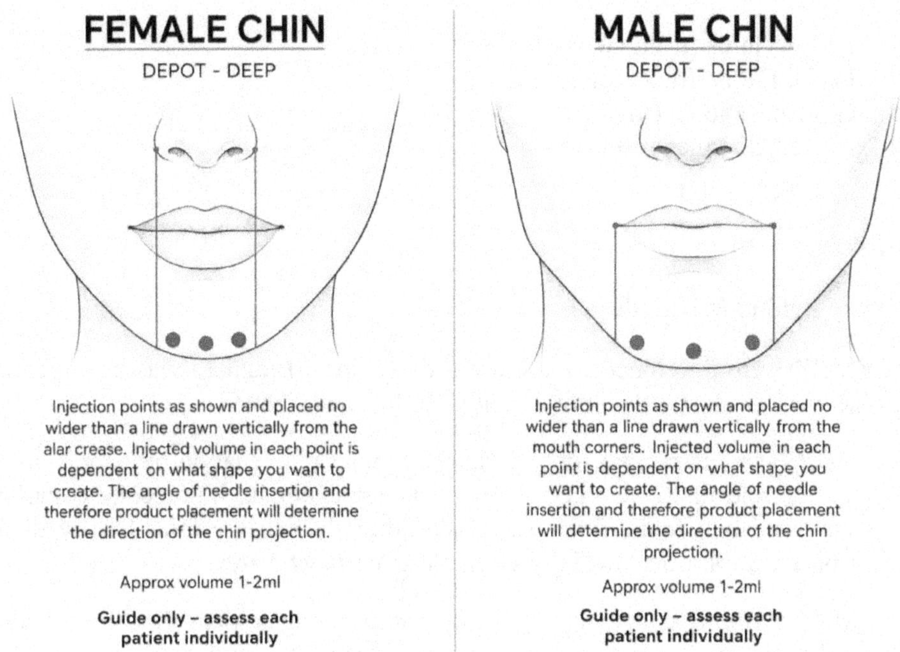

Beauty Is Not Mathematics

While proportions and measurements are valuable, they do not define beauty.

Some of the world's most recognisable faces would fail one or more of these measurements.

What often makes a face attractive is not perfection but character.

A strong nose. A distinctive chin. A unique smile. Expressive eyes.

These features create individuality.

As aesthetic practitioners, our goal is not to force every patient into a mathematical formula.

Our goal is to understand balance, identify areas of concern, and create harmony while preserving identity.

The most beautiful results are rarely the most dramatic.

They are the ones that allow patients to look like themselves—only fresher, healthier, and more confident.

Beauty is not about perfection.

It is about proportion, harmony, and authenticity.

For the published book, I would place four professional black-and-white diagrams alongside this chapter:

1. Facial Thirds (front view)
2. Facial Fifths (front view)
3. Golden Ratio face overlay
4. Ricketts E-Line profile

.

Mapping

The Story Behind MD Codes™

MD Codes™ were developed by Mauricio de Maio, a Brazilian plastic surgeon and one of the world's most influential educators in facial aesthetics.

Before MD Codes, many injectors approached facial rejuvenation by simply treating the wrinkle or fold that concerned the patient. For example, if someone complained about their nasolabial folds, filler was placed directly into the fold. If they disliked their marionette lines, filler was injected into the marionette area.

Dr. de Maio recognised that ageing is far more complex than this. Facial ageing involves changes in bone, ligaments, fat compartments, skin quality, and muscle activity. A fold is often the result of volume loss somewhere else in the face.

To address this, he created the MD Codes system — a structured facial assessment and treatment framework that identifies specific anatomical points where filler can be strategically placed to restore support, volume, shape, and facial balance.

The system allows injectors to:

- Assess the face systematically
- Develop a treatment plan based on facial structure
- Improve communication between practitioners
- Standardise teaching and training
- Focus on facial harmony rather than individual wrinkles

- Achieve more predictable outcomes

Each area of the face is assigned a code.

Examples include:

- CK = Cheek
- T = Tear Trough
- Tm = Temple
- LP = Lips
- C = Chin
- Jw = Jawline
- NLF = Nasolabial Fold
- M = Marionette

Each number identifies a specific injection point within that region.

For example:

- CK1 = Zygomatic Arch
- CK2 = Zygomatic Eminence
- CK3 = Anterior Cheek

Rather than saying "place filler in the upper lateral cheek," an injector can simply refer to CK1 or CK2.

Allergan and MD Codes™

The MD Codes system was later adopted by Allergan Aesthetics as part of its global training programs for the Juvederm range of dermal fillers.

Through extensive education programs, workshops, publications, and anatomical training, Allergan helped introduce MD Codes to thousands of injectors worldwide. Today, the system is recognised as one of the most widely taught facial assessment frameworks in aesthetic medicine.

An Important Point

While MD Codes provide an excellent guide, they should never replace a thorough facial assessment.

Every face is unique.

Bone structure, ethnicity, gender, age, facial shape, and aesthetic goals vary significantly between patients. MD Codes are best viewed as a roadmap rather than a recipe.

As Dr. de Maio often teaches, successful treatment is not about filling lines. It is about understanding the emotional messages conveyed by the face and restoring support, structure, and harmony.

For beginner injectors, MD Codes provide a valuable framework for learning facial anatomy and treatment planning. For experienced injectors, they serve as a common language that helps standardise communication and improve consistency in patient outcomes.

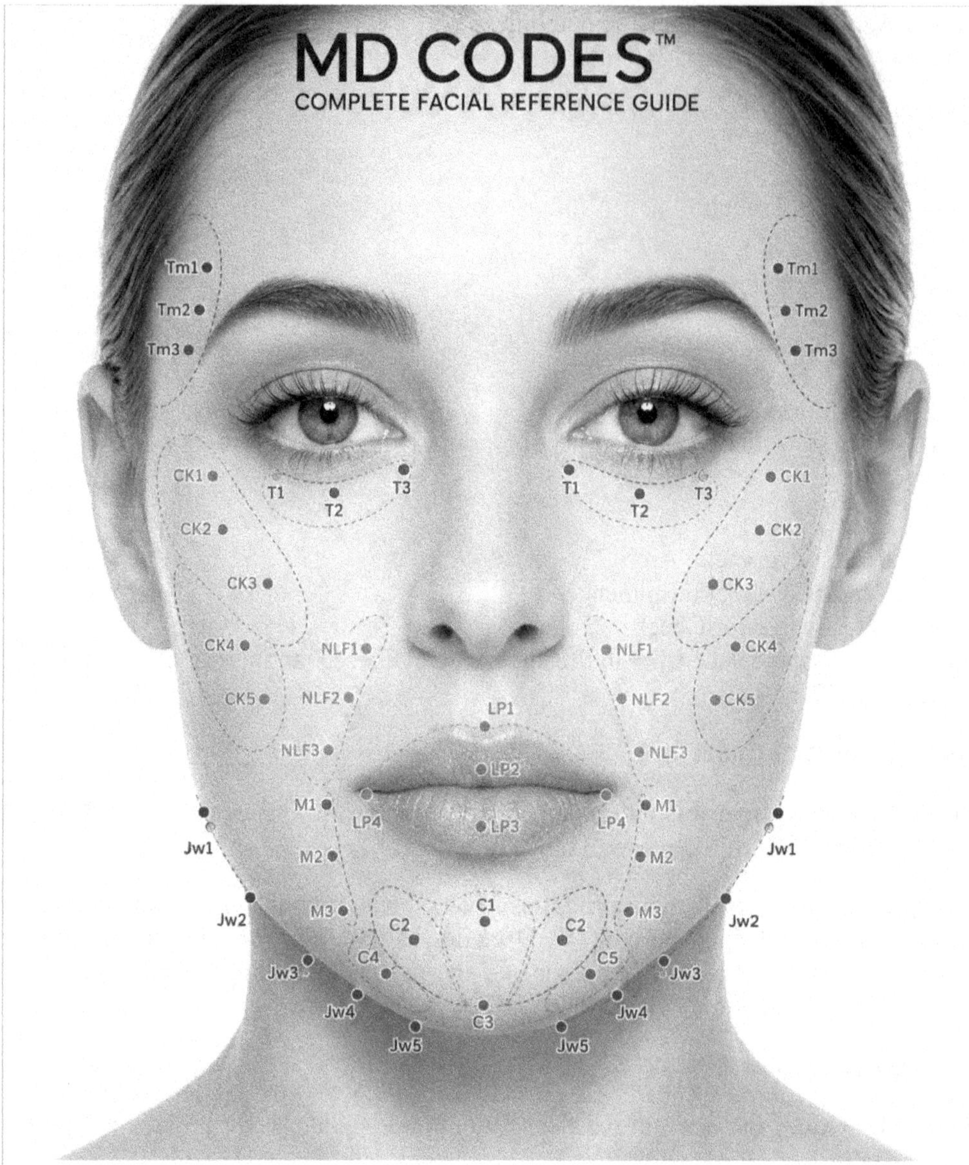

1. CHEEK (CK1–CK5)

- CK1 Zygomatic Arch
- CK2 Zygomatic Eminence
- CK3 Anterior Cheek
- CK4 Lateral Lower Cheek
- CK5 Submalar Region

2. TEMPLE (Tm1–Tm3)

- Tm1 Anterior Temple
- Tm2 Central Temple
- Tm3 Posterior Temple

3. TEAR TROUGH (T1–T3)

- T1 Medial Tear Trough
- T2 Central Tear Trough
- T3 Lateral Tear Trough

4. LIP (LP1–LP4)

- LP1 Cupid's Bow
- LP2 Upper Vermilion
- LP3 Lower Vermilion
- LP4 Oral Commissure

5. NASOLABIAL FOLD (NLF1–NLF3)

- NLF1 Upper Fold
- NLF2 Mid Fold
- NLF3 Lower Fold

6. MARIONETTE (M1–M3)

- M1 Upper Marionette
- M2 Middle Marionette
- M3 Lower Marionette

7. CHIN (C1–C5)

- C1 Central Chin
- C2 Lateral Chin
- C3 Anterior Projection
- C4 Mental Crease Support
- C5 Pre-Jowl Support

8. JAWLINE (Jw1–Jw5)

- Jw1 Mandibular Angle
- Jw2 Posterior Jawline
- Jw3 Mid-Jawline
- Jw4 Pre-Jowl
- Jw5 Anterior Jawline

Chapter 10: Before and After Photos – The Truth is in the Technique

In aesthetic medicine, a photograph is worth far more than a thousand words. Before-and-after images allow practitioners and patients to objectively assess results, track progress, and document treatment outcomes. They provide a visual record that can reveal subtle improvements that may otherwise go unnoticed.

However, photographs can also be misleading if they are not taken correctly.

As both an injector and trainer, I have seen excellent treatments appear disappointing because the photographs were poorly taken. Equally, I have seen average results appear dramatic simply because the lighting, angle, or expression changed between photos.

For photographs to have clinical value, they must be standardised.

The goal is not to make the after photo look better. The goal is to make both photographs identical except for the treatment result.

Why Clinical Photography Matters

Good photography allows the practitioner to:

- Assess treatment outcomes objectively
- Monitor changes over time, Educate patients
- Track ageing progression, Document medical records
- Demonstrate treatment efficacy, Protect both practitioner and patient legally

Many patients forget how they looked before treatment. Months later they may feel little has changed until they compare their original photographs with their current appearance.

The camera often sees what the mirror misses.

The Most Common Photography Mistakes

The biggest mistake is changing the lighting.

Light can dramatically alter the appearance of wrinkles, skin texture, pigmentation, shadows, eye bags, and facial contours.

A patient photographed under harsh overhead lighting may appear tired and aged. The same patient photographed under soft front-facing lighting may look years younger without any treatment at all.

Other common mistakes include: Different camera angles, Different facial expressions, Different hairstyles, Different makeup, Different camera distances, Different backgrounds, Different zoom settings, Different head positions

When these variables change, the comparison becomes unreliable.

The Gold Standard for Before and After Photography

Every clinic should aim to create a dedicated photography area.

Ideally photographs should be taken:

Against a plain neutral background, With consistent lighting

At the same distance from the camera, Using the same camera settings

Using the same focal length, With the patient's hair pulled away from the face

Without glasses, Without smiling unless specifically documenting a dynamic expression

The patient's head should remain in a neutral position with eyes looking directly at the camera.

The Five Essential Views

Every facial assessment should include:

Front view, Right oblique view (45 degrees), Left oblique view (45 degrees)

Right profile, Left profile

These views allow assessment of: Facial symmetry, Volume loss, Jawline definition, Nasal profile, Chin projection, Cheek projection, Neck and jowl changes

For full-face rejuvenation cases, these five views provide the most comprehensive record.

Consistency Is Everything

The most important word in clinical photography is consistency.

If the before photo was taken standing, the after photo should be taken standing.

If the patient wore no makeup before treatment, they should ideally wear no makeup after treatment.

If the camera was positioned one metre away initially, it should remain one metre away at follow-up.

Even subtle changes can influence the final image.

The less variation between photographs, the more trustworthy the results.

Beware the Smile

One of the easiest ways to create a misleading before-and-after image is through facial expression.

A patient who appears serious in the before photograph and smiling in the after photograph will automatically appear happier, younger, and more attractive.

The treatment may have had little to do with the apparent improvement.

For accurate documentation, neutral facial expressions should always be used.

Additional smiling photographs can be taken separately if desired.

Dynamic Photographs

Not all photographs need to be static.

For toxin treatments, dynamic photographs are extremely useful.

Patients can be asked to: Raise their eyebrows, Frown, Squint, Smile, Purse their lips

These images allow practitioners to document muscle activity before and after treatment and demonstrate the effects of neuromodulators such as Botox.

Modern Photography Systems

Many clinics now use dedicated imaging systems that standardise positioning and lighting automatically.

Some systems even provide:

3D imaging, Volume analysis, Skin texture analysis, Pigmentation mapping, Vascular assessment, Ageing simulations

While these technologies are helpful, even a smartphone can produce excellent clinical photographs when consistency is maintained.

Good technique matters more than expensive equipment.

The Ethical Use of Before and After Photos

Photographs should never be manipulated.

No filters. No retouching. No skin smoothing. No digital reshaping.

Patients trust us to present honest results.

Authentic photographs build credibility. Altered photographs destroy it.

In an industry often criticised for unrealistic expectations, honest photography is one of the most powerful ways to educate and protect patients.

A good before-and-after photograph should not exaggerate results.

It should reveal the truth. Because in aesthetic medicine, trust is every bit as important as technique.

Chapter 11: When Not to Treat

Knowing when to pause is part of good practice

One of the most important decisions I make in clinic is not what to treat but **when not to treat**

Aesthetic medicine is not just about skill. It is about judgment

There are times when treatment is not appropriate and recognising this protects both the patient and the outcome

Unrealistic expectations

This is one of the most important red flags

If a patient: Wants to look like someone else, Is chasing perfection, Is never satisfied with previous results, Focuses on very minor "flaws"

Then treatment will not solve the issue

In some cases, this may reflect: Body dysmorphia, Emotional distress, External pressure

No treatment will meet unrealistic expectations and continuing to treat can do harm

When something doesn't feel right

Sometimes there is no obvious reason to say no but something feels off

Over time, I have learnt to trust that instinct

If a patient: Feels rushed, Is unsure, Is emotionally unsettled

It is often better to: Pause, Rebook, Allow time for clarity

Active infections

You should not treat over or near an active infection

This includes: Skin infections, Inflamed acne, Open wounds

Injecting into compromised skin increases the risk of: Spreading infection, Poor healing, Complications

Treatment should be delayed until the skin has fully settled

Cold sores (Herpes Simplex)

If a patient has an active cold sore: Do not treat the area

Injectables, needling, or laser can: Trigger a flare, Spread the virus

In patients prone to cold sores: Preventative antiviral medication may be considered prior to treatment

Pregnancy

Aesthetic treatments are not recommended during pregnancy

This includes: Injectables, Most in-clinic procedures

Not because we know they are harmful but because: There is insufficient safety data, The priority is always caution

Treatment can wait

Breastfeeding

Most practitioners take a cautious approach during breastfeeding

While some treatments may be low risk

There is: Limited evidence, Ongoing debate

In most cases, it is best to: Delay non-essential treatments, Focus on skincare and gentle options if needed

Chemotherapy and active cancer treatment

Patients undergoing chemotherapy or active cancer treatment require careful consideration

Concerns include: Compromised immune system, Poor healing, Increased risk of infection

Treatment should only proceed: With medical clearance And careful planning

Often, it is best to wait until treatment is completed

Roaccutane (Isotretinoin)

Roaccutane affects the skin in several ways: Thins the skin, Reduces oil production, Increases sensitivity, Slows healing.

This increases the risk of: Irritation, Scarring, Poor recovery from procedures

Traditionally, many treatments were avoided during and shortly after Roaccutane use

While guidelines are evolving, caution is still important

I generally: Avoid aggressive treatments, Delay energy-based procedures, Assess the skin carefully before proceeding

Medications and contraindications

Certain medications may increase risk

These include: Blood thinners (increased bruising and bleeding), Immunosuppressants, Some antibiotics or medications affecting healing

This does not always mean treatment cannot be done but it requires: Careful assessment, Adjusted expectations, Informed consent

Before an important event

Timing matters

Bruising, swelling, or delayed results can affect outcomes

Before an important event such as: A wedding, A holiday, A special occasion

I may advise: Delaying treatment or choosing a more conservative approach

Because even the best treatment can have temporary side effects

The importance of timing

Sometimes the issue is not the treatment but the timing

It may be better to: Wait for the skin to settle, Complete another treatment first, Space procedures appropriately.

Good results depend on: **when you treat, not just what you treat**

Saying no is part of good care

It can be difficult to turn a patient away

But saying no when appropriate: Builds trust, Prevents complications, Protects the patient

A practitioner who says yes to everything is not always acting in the patient's best interest

A final thought

Not every concern needs treatment, Not every patient is ready, Not every moment is the right time.

The most important decision you can make is, knowing when to pause because good outcomes are not just about what you do

They are also about what you choose not to do

The right treatment, at the right time, for the right reason

Chapter 12: Treatment Timing and Sequencing

Combining In-Clinic Treatments and Injectables

Why Timing Matters

One of the most important — and often overlooked — aspects of aesthetic medicine is timing.

Modern cosmetic treatments are rarely performed in isolation. Patients commonly combine lasers, radiofrequency, skin treatments, regenerative therapies, biostimulants, fillers, and anti-wrinkle injections as part of an overall treatment plan.

When treatments are timed correctly, they complement and enhance one another beautifully.
When timed poorly, however, they can increase inflammation, compromise healing, affect product placement, and ultimately impact results.

Understanding when to combine treatments is just as important as understanding which treatment to choose.

General Principles of Treatment Layering

In my experience, successful treatment planning follows a few key principles:

- Treat skin quality before adding structure
- Avoid stacking excessive inflammation into the tissue
- Allow tissue time to heal and settle
- Work progressively from regeneration to structural support and then maintenance

Healthy skin will always provide a better foundation for any injectable treatment.

Timing Treatments After Laser Procedures

Laser treatments work by creating controlled injury within the skin to stimulate repair and collagen remodelling. The more aggressive the treatment, the greater the inflammatory response and recovery time.

Light Laser Treatments

Examples may include gentle pigment correction or low-level resurfacing procedures with minimal downtime.

Following lighter laser treatments, the skin generally recovers relatively quickly.

Typical treatment timing may include:

- Skin boosters: approximately 3–5 days
- Polynucleotides: approximately 5–7 days
- Anti-wrinkle injections: often performed on the same day or within several days
- Dermal filler: usually after 1–2 weeks

Medium to Deep Laser Resurfacing

More intensive resurfacing procedures, such as fractional resurfacing, CO2 laser, or erbium laser treatments, create significantly more inflammation and tissue remodelling.

Because the skin barrier and deeper tissues require longer recovery, treatment timing becomes more important.

Typical recovery intervals may include:

- Skin boosters: 2–3 weeks
- Polynucleotides: 2–3 weeks
- Biostimulants: 3–4 weeks
- Dermal filler: 3–4 weeks
- Anti-wrinkle injections: approximately 1–2 weeks

Injecting too early after aggressive laser treatments can increase swelling, interfere with healing, and affect product placement within inflamed tissue.

Timing Treatments After Radiofrequency (RF)

Radiofrequency treatments stimulate collagen through controlled dermal heating while generally causing less surface disruption than laser resurfacing. Although downtime is often reduced, the tissue still undergoes an inflammatory response.

Typical treatment intervals following RF may include:

- Skin boosters: 5–7 days
- Polynucleotides: 5–7 days
- Biostimulants: 2–3 weeks
- Dermal filler: approximately 2 weeks
- Anti-wrinkle injections: same day or within several days

Because RF increases heat and circulation within the tissue, placing filler immediately afterwards is generally avoided.

Timing Treatments After Microneedling

Microneedling creates controlled micro-injury within the skin and is commonly combined with regenerative therapies.

One of the advantages of microneedling is that certain treatments can be applied immediately during or after the procedure to enhance penetration and tissue stimulation.

Typical treatment timing may include:

- PRP or biofiller: often performed during or immediately after treatment
- Skin boosters: depending on protocol, same day or within several days
- Polynucleotides: approximately 5–7 days
- Dermal filler: 1–2 weeks
- Biostimulants: 2–3 weeks
- Anti-wrinkle injections: approximately 3–5 days

PRP and regenerative treatments work particularly well alongside microneedling due to increased absorption and enhanced tissue stimulation during the healing phase.

When Injectables Are Performed First

Timing also matters when energy-based treatments are performed after injectables.

After Dermal Fillers

Following filler placement, it is generally advisable to allow adequate integration within the tissue before exposing the area to heat or trauma.

Typical waiting periods may include:

- Laser treatments: 2–4 weeks
- Radiofrequency: 2–3 weeks
- Microneedling: approximately 2 weeks

This allows the filler to settle appropriately and reduces the risk of displacement or altered results.

After Biostimulants

Biostimulatory products rely on a carefully controlled inflammatory response to stimulate collagen production over time.

Typical waiting periods before additional treatments may include:

- Laser: 3–4 weeks
- RF: 3–4 weeks
- Microneedling: 2–3 weeks

Allowing adequate time helps avoid disruption of the collagen stimulation process.

After Anti-Wrinkle Injections

Following anti-wrinkle injections, it is generally preferable to avoid excessive heat, pressure, or trauma immediately afterwards.
Typical waiting periods may include:

- Laser treatments: 1–2 weeks
- RF: 1–2 weeks
- Microneedling: approximately 1 week

This allows the neurotoxin to bind appropriately and reduces the risk of migration.

A Practical Treatment Sequence

In clinical practice, treatment plans are often layered progressively rather than performed all at once.
A common approach may include:

1. Improving skin quality and preparing the skin
2. Performing laser or microneedling treatments if indicated
3. Introducing regenerative therapies such as PRP, polynucleotides, or skin boosters
4. Adding structural support with biostimulants or filler where required
5. Using anti-wrinkle injections to soften excessive muscle movement
6. Maintaining results with ongoing skin and collagen-stimulating treatments

Final Clinical Considerations

There is no universal timeline that suits every patient.
Treatment intervals should always be adjusted according to:

- Skin type, Treatment intensity, Healing response, Age
- Degree of inflammation, Combination of treatments being performed

Good aesthetic medicine is not simply about selecting treatments. It is about understanding how treatments interact with tissue biology, healing, and one another over time.

Sometimes the best outcomes come not from doing more, but from knowing when to wait.

Chapter 13: Cosmetic Procedures Amongst Different Age Groups

One of the biggest changes I've seen over the past 30 years in aesthetic medicine is how differently each generation approaches cosmetic treatments.

When I first began injecting, most people waited until they looked significantly older before considering treatments. Today, younger patients are starting earlier, often focusing on prevention, skin quality, and subtle refinement rather than dramatic change.

Every age group has different concerns, different motivations, and different goals. A 25-year-old wanting lip hydration is very different from a 55-year-old experiencing facial volume loss and skin laxity. Good aesthetic medicine is never about treating everyone the same. It's about understanding the ageing process and working with the face at each stage of life.

The most natural results happen when treatments are age-appropriate, balanced, and respectful of the individual.

Ages 18–30: Prevention and Subtle Beautification

In your late teens and twenties, the skin is usually at its healthiest. Collagen production is strong, the skin is firm and elastic, and facial fat pads are still full and youthful.

Most treatments in this age group are focused on subtle enhancement rather than correction. Social media has had a huge influence on this generation, and many younger patients come in already knowing treatment names and trends. Sometimes the challenge is not doing more — it's knowing when to say less.

Preventative anti-wrinkle injections are common during this stage, especially for people who are very expressive or genetically prone to strong frown lines. The idea is not to freeze the face, but to soften repetitive muscle movement before lines become deeply etched into the skin.

Lip enhancement is also popular, but the trend has shifted away from the overfilled look. Many younger patients now want soft hydration, gentle definition, and natural balance rather than obvious volume.

Jawline contouring, chin enhancement, and cheekbone definition are often used to improve facial harmony and profile balance. Skin quality treatments such as PRP, skin boosters, microneedling, chemical peels, and laser treatments are also increasingly popular for acne scarring, pigmentation, and maintaining healthy glowing skin.

This is also the age where good skincare habits matter enormously. Daily SPF, retinol, antioxidants, hydration, and prevention will often do more long-term than excessive cosmetic procedures ever could.

The goal during this stage should always be enhancement, prevention, and maintaining natural youthful features — not trying to look like someone else.

Ages 30–45: Prevention, Correction, and Maintenance

By the thirties and forties, the ageing process starts becoming more noticeable. Collagen production slows, skin turnover decreases, and early volume loss may begin appearing around the eyes, cheeks, and mouth.

This is often the stage where patients say:

"I just look tired." "I don't look as fresh." "I still feel young, but my face is changing."

Treatments during this stage usually combine prevention with correction.

Anti-wrinkle injections continue to play an important role, not only for prevention but also for softening established expression lines. Fillers may be used more strategically in the mid-face, tear troughs, jawline, or chin to restore support and maintain facial structure. Early nasolabial folds and marionette lines may begin appearing, but it's important not to chase lines alone. Often, restoring support higher in the face creates a far more natural outcome than simply filling folds directly.

Skin tightening treatments such as radiofrequency microneedling, ultrasound treatments, and fractional lasers become more relevant as collagen and elasticity begin declining.

This is also the age where collagen-stimulating treatments like Sculptra, Radiesse, PRP, and regenerative procedures become incredibly valuable. Rather than simply filling, these treatments encourage the body to rebuild and repair its own collagen over time.

The focus during this decade is maintaining structure, supporting collagen, and ageing gracefully while still looking refreshed and natural.

Ages 45–65: Restoration and Rejuvenation

Between the mid-forties and sixties, facial ageing becomes more structural. Bone resorption increases, fat pads shrink and descend, skin laxity becomes more visible, and deeper lines begin forming.

This is often when patients notice changes in the jawline, neck, lower face, and temples. Many people say they suddenly feel like they look tired, sad, or heavier around the lower face even when they feel healthy and energetic inside.

At this stage, aesthetic treatments become more about restoration than beautification alone.

Anti-wrinkle injections are still useful, but technique becomes extremely important. Over-treating can create heaviness or an unnatural appearance in mature faces. The goal is softening, not freezing.

Full-face assessment becomes essential. Volume loss in the temples, cheeks, jawline, and chin often needs to be addressed holistically rather than treating isolated lines. This is where understanding anatomy, ligaments, fat compartments, and facial support structures becomes critical.

Biostimulators such as Sculptra and Radiesse are particularly valuable during this phase because they stimulate collagen production and improve skin quality gradually over time.

Skin resurfacing treatments including RF microneedling, CO2 laser, deeper peels, and regenerative procedures can dramatically improve texture, crepiness, and skin quality.

Some patients may also explore thread lifting or non-surgical tightening treatments for subtle lifting effects. The goal in this age group is not to look twenty again. It is to restore freshness, support the tissues, and help the face look healthier, rested, and more vibrant.

Ages 65–85: Gentle, Age-Appropriate Rejuvenation

One of the biggest misconceptions in aesthetic medicine is that mature patients should stop having treatments altogether. In reality, many people in their sixties, seventies, and beyond simply want to look fresher, healthier, and more rested — not dramatically different.

The key is respecting the ageing face.

Mature skin is thinner, more delicate, and often less forgiving. Heavy filler can look unnatural very quickly in this age group, so treatment must be conservative and strategic.

Small amounts of anti-wrinkle injections may be used to soften harsh lines while still allowing natural movement and expression. Gentle filler placement can restore facial harmony around the cheeks, lips, and mouth without creating puffiness or distortion.

Hydration treatments such as PRP, skin boosters, mesotherapy, and regenerative procedures can significantly improve skin quality, texture, and luminosity.

Collagen-stimulating treatments, RF devices, ultrasound tightening, and light laser procedures may also help improve skin laxity and support ageing tissues in a subtle, natural way.

At this stage of life, aesthetic medicine should never be about chasing youth. It should be about confidence, vitality, and helping someone look like the best version of themselves at their age.

Conclusion

There is no "perfect age" to start cosmetic treatments, and there is no single treatment plan that suits everyone. Ageing is influenced by genetics, lifestyle, stress, hormones, sun exposure, health, and emotional wellbeing. Some people age earlier, some later, and some hardly at all in certain areas.

Good aesthetic medicine is not about changing faces. It is about understanding the face at every stage of life and treating it with balance, skill, and respect. The best results are always the ones where people still look like themselves — just fresher, healthier, and more confident.

Chapter 14: Male Face

Why Male Aesthetics Require a Different Approach

Male aesthetics is very different to female aesthetics, and this is one of the biggest mistakes I see in cosmetic medicine today.

Men should not be treated using the same assessment, placement, or volumising techniques commonly used in female faces. The goal is not to soften or feminise the face, but to restore structure, maintain masculinity, and create a refreshed appearance that still looks strong and natural.

A well-treated male face should never appear overfilled, rounded, or obviously "done."

In my experience, men generally want to look:

- Less tired, Stronger, Healthier, More defined
- Refreshed without looking cosmetic

The best male aesthetic results are often the ones nobody notices.

Understanding Male Facial Anatomy

The male face differs significantly from the female face anatomically.

Men typically have:

- A broader forehead, Stronger brow projection
- Flatter cheeks, A wider lower face
- A more angular jawline
- A squarer chin, Thicker skin
- Stronger muscle activity, particularly through the masseters

Women, in contrast, tend to have softer transitions, more anterior cheek projection, and a more heart-shaped facial structure.

This distinction is critical when planning treatment.

One of the quickest ways to feminise a male face is to inject excessive anterior cheek volume or over-project the lips. Rounded cheeks and soft contouring techniques that may work beautifully in female patients can look unnatural on men.

The male face generally requires:

- Structure rather than softness
- Definition rather than roundness
- Support rather than excessive volume

How the Male Face Ages

Men age differently to women.

While women often show ageing through soft tissue volume changes and skin thinning, male ageing is frequently more structural and skeletal.

Over time, men commonly develop:

- Bone resorption through the jawline, chin, and midface
- Flattening of the cheeks, Temple hollowing
- Under-eye hollowing
- Heavier lower face changes and jowling, Skin laxity and collagen loss

The face can gradually lose strength and definition, particularly through the jawline and lower face.

This is why male rejuvenation often focuses more on structural support than simply replacing volume.

My Approach to Treating the Male Face

When treating male patients, my approach is usually more conservative, structural, and collagen-focused.

The goal is not to make the face look fuller. It is to restore support and definition while preserving masculine anatomy.

Jawline and Chin

The male jawline is one of the most important features contributing to facial masculinity.

Treatment often focuses on:

- Strengthening the mandibular angle
- Improving jawline definition
- Supporting chin projection
- Restoring lower-face structure lost through ageing

Products with stronger lifting capacity and structural support are often preferable in these areas.

Biostimulatory products such as Radiesse or collagen-stimulating treatments may create a more natural and less "puffy" outcome in male patients compared with excessive soft filler placement.

Midface Rejuvenation

Male cheeks should generally remain flatter and broader than female cheeks.

I avoid creating prominent "apple cheeks" or excessive anterior projection in men, as this can quickly feminise the face.

Instead, treatment is usually focused laterally to restore support through the zygomatic and lateral cheek region while maintaining a natural masculine contour.

Subtle support often looks far better than visible volume.

Temples and Under-Eyes

Temple hollowing and under-eye fatigue can age a man dramatically and create a tired or gaunt appearance.

Small, carefully placed amounts of filler or collagen stimulators can restore support and soften hollowness without making the face look overly polished or artificial.

In male patients, less is almost always more.

Forehead and Brows

The male brow should generally remain flatter and heavier than the female brow.

Excessive arching or over-lifting can look unnatural very quickly.

When treating the upper face in men, I aim to soften heaviness and fatigue while preserving masculine brow positioning and movement.

Fillers Versus Biostimulators in Men

In many male patients, biostimulators often produce more natural long-term outcomes than excessive filler volume.

Traditional hyaluronic acid fillers provide immediate correction and contouring, but when overused they can create heaviness and puffiness.

Biostimulatory treatments work differently by stimulating collagen production gradually over time, often producing stronger structural support without looking obviously volumised.

For this reason, treatments such as collagen stimulators are often particularly well suited to male patients who want subtle, natural rejuvenation.

The Key to Natural Male Aesthetics

The secret to treating the male face well is restraint.

A masculine face should still look masculine after treatment.

Good male aesthetics is not about making men look different. It is about helping them look healthier, stronger, and less tired while preserving their natural character and facial identity.

The best male treatments are usually invisible to everyone except the patient themselves.

That is what natural aesthetics should be.

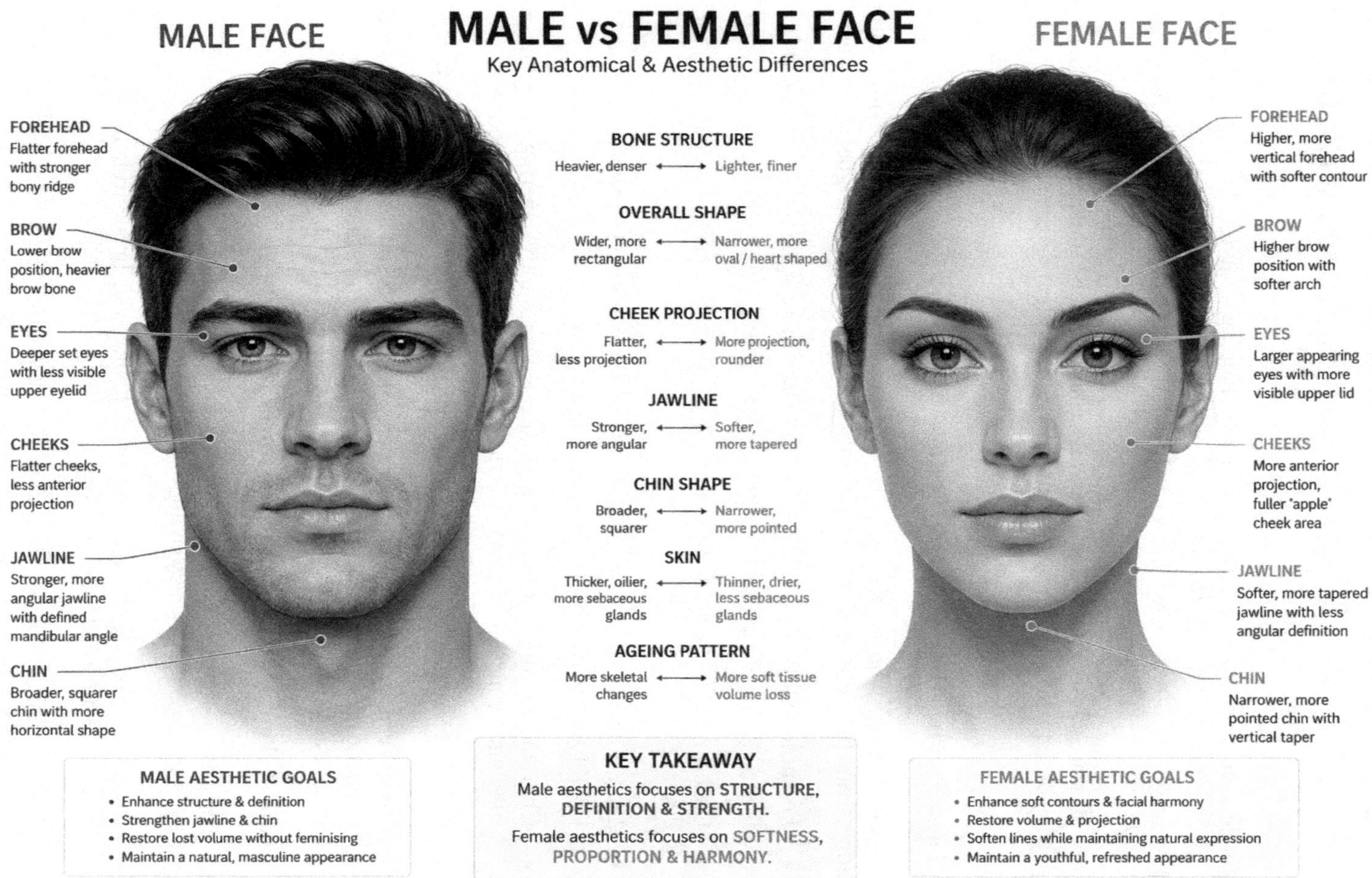
MALE FACE
MALE vs FEMALE FACE
Key Anatomical & Aesthetic Differences
FEMALE FACE
FOREHEAD
Flatter forehead with stronger bony ridge
BROW
Lower brow position, heavier brow bone
EYES
Deeper set eyes with less visible upper eyelid
CHEEKS
Flatter cheeks, less anterior projection
JAWLINE
Stronger, more angular jawline with defined mandibular angle
CHIN
Broader, squarer chin with more horizontal shape
BONE STRUCTURE
Heavier, denser ⟷ Lighter, finer
OVERALL SHAPE
Wider, more rectangular ⟷ Narrower, more oval / heart shaped
CHEEK PROJECTION
Flatter, less projection ⟷ More projection, rounder
JAWLINE
Stronger, more angular ⟷ Softer, more tapered
CHIN SHAPE
Broader, squarer ⟷ Narrower, more pointed
SKIN
Thicker, oilier, more sebaceous glands ⟷ Thinner, drier, less sebaceous glands
AGEING PATTERN
More skeletal changes ⟷ More soft tissue volume loss
FOREHEAD
Higher, more vertical forehead with softer contour
BROW
Higher brow position with softer arch
EYES
Larger appearing eyes with more visible upper lid
CHEEKS
More anterior projection, fuller 'apple' cheek area
JAWLINE
Softer, more tapered jawline with less angular definition
CHIN
Narrower, more pointed chin with vertical taper
MALE AESTHETIC GOALS
• Enhance structure & definition
• Strengthen jawline & chin
• Restore lost volume without feminising
• Maintain a natural, masculine appearance
KEY TAKEAWAY
Male aesthetics focuses on STRUCTURE, DEFINITION & STRENGTH.
Female aesthetics focuses on SOFTNESS, PROPORTION & HARMONY.
FEMALE AESTHETIC GOALS
• Enhance soft contours & facial harmony
• Restore volume & projection
• Soften lines while maintaining natural expression
• Maintain a youthful, refreshed appearance

Chapter 15: Gender Affirming Aesthetics – Aligning Features with Identity

Aesthetic medicine plays a powerful role in helping individuals express their true selves. For many, this means aligning outward features with an inner sense of identity—whether through softening, defining, or harmonising specific areas of the face and body.

Gender affirming aesthetics is not about adhering to binary standards, but rather about supporting each person's journey with precision, respect, and artistry.

For Those Seeking More Feminine Features

Many individuals who wish to present more femininely may desire softness, roundness, and harmony in their facial features. Common aesthetic goals include:

- Forehead and Brows: Creating a smoother, more open look. Botox can lift the brows to create a gentle arch and a more relaxed upper face.
- Cheeks: Adding volume to the midface with fillers creates a rounder, youthful contour.
- Lips: Enhancing volume and definition for a fuller, heart-shaped appearance using hyaluronic acid fillers.
- Chin and Jawline: Softening a square jaw or subtly tapering the chin using filler and/or masseter Botox to reduce width and create a V-shape.
- Nose: Refining nasal contours with dermal filler to create a softer profile.
- Voice-related areas: While surgical procedures address vocal resonance, aesthetic treatments like neck tightening or chin reshaping can complement vocal transition.

For Those Seeking More Masculine Features

Those desiring a more masculine appearance often seek structure, strength, and angularity in the face. Goals may include:

- Brow and Forehead: Lowering or flattening the brow arch using Botox to create a more structured, assertive look.
- Jawline: Enhancing jaw definition with structural fillers like Radiesse or high-density HA fillers to square and widen the lower face.
- Chin: Augmenting projection and width to support a strong, balanced profile.

- Cheeks: Enhancing bone structure with subtle volume to create flatter, angular contours.
- Nose: Strengthening the nasal bridge or defining the tip with non-surgical rhinoplasty.

Skin Concerns in Gender Affirming Aesthetics

Skin plays a crucial role in gender presentation. Hormonal therapy, shaving, and stress can all affect skin health. Common concerns include:

- Acne: Hormonal shifts may trigger breakouts, especially in early transition. Treatments may include salicylic acid, LED therapy, or medical-grade skincare.
- Facial Hair or Shadow: Laser hair removal, electrolysis, or pigment-correcting peels can help reduce beard shadow or excess facial hair.
- Skin Texture: Softening and smoothing the skin with PRP, microneedling, or skin boosters (like NCTF or Volite) helps enhance overall luminosity.
- Pigmentation: Hormonal changes can also trigger melasma or uneven tone; brightening agents or gentle peels can support clear, radiant skin.
- Pore Size and Oiliness: Especially relevant in testosterone therapy. Resurfacing lasers or tailored skincare can reduce excess oil and visible pores.

A Tailored Approach to Identity

Each individual has a unique vision for how they want to look and feel. Practitioners must ask thoughtful, open-ended questions such as:

“What features would you like to enhance or soften?”

“Is there a particular look or feeling you want to achieve?”

The focus should always remain on authentic expression, safety, and emotional well-being. The injector becomes not just a technician, but a partner in transformation—one who listens without assumption and acts with both skill and compassion.

Part 2- Understanding Ageing & Facial Anatomy

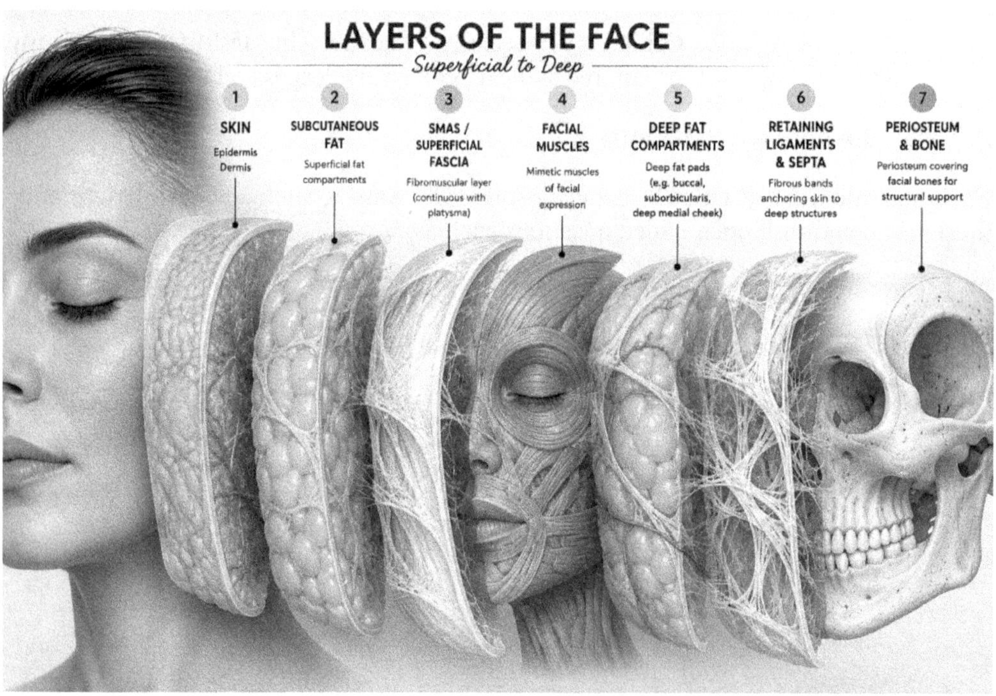

Chapter 16: Skin Structure, Ageing, and Rejuvenation Treatments

The skin is far more than just a covering. It is the body's largest organ and one of the first things people notice about us. It protects us from the environment, regulates temperature, helps prevent dehydration, and even plays a role in how we feel emotionally and socially.

In aesthetics, we spend so much time focusing on wrinkles and ageing that we sometimes forget how incredible the skin really is.

Understanding how the skin works — and what happens to it over time — is essential if we want to treat it properly and naturally.

Understanding the Skin

The skin is made up of three main layers, each with its own important role.

The epidermis is the outer layer that we see. It acts as a protective barrier against pollution, bacteria, UV damage, and environmental stress. It also helps regulate moisture and keeps hydration inside the skin.

Beneath that sits the dermis, which is where much of the magic happens. This layer contains collagen, elastin, blood vessels, nerves, and oil glands. Collagen gives the skin firmness and strength, while elastin allows it to stretch and bounce back.

The deepest layer is the hypodermis, also known as the subcutaneous layer. This contains fat and connective tissue, providing cushioning, insulation, and support for the structures above it.

When we are young, these layers work beautifully together. The skin is firm, hydrated, elastic, and luminous. But as we age, gradual changes begin to occur.

What Happens to the Skin as We Age?

Ageing happens both internally and externally.

Intrinsic ageing is the natural ageing process that occurs over time due to genetics and the slowing down of our body's repair systems.

Extrinsic ageing comes from outside influences such as sun exposure, smoking, stress, poor diet, pollution, alcohol, illness, and lifestyle factors.

One of the first changes we notice is thinning of the skin. The epidermis and dermis become thinner and more fragile, making the skin appear crepey and delicate.

Collagen production also slows dramatically with age. In fact, we begin losing collagen from our twenties onward. As collagen decreases, the skin loses firmness and fine lines begin appearing.

Elastin fibres also weaken over time, meaning the skin no longer "springs back" the way it once did. This contributes to sagging around the cheeks, jawline, neck, and eyes.

Oil production decreases as well, especially after menopause, which is why mature skin often feels drier and more sensitive.

Years of UV exposure can also create pigmentation, uneven skin tone, redness, broken capillaries, and rough texture. In many ways, the skin becomes a visual diary of our life experiences, stress, hormones, lifestyle, and environment.

Skin Rejuvenation Treatments

Modern aesthetic medicine offers many ways to support the skin and encourage regeneration rather than simply masking ageing.

The goal today is not only to look younger, but to improve skin quality, function, and health.

PRP (Platelet-Rich Plasma)

PRP uses the patient's own blood to harness natural growth factors and healing proteins. After the blood is spun in a centrifuge, the concentrated platelet-rich plasma is injected or microneedled into the skin.

PRP stimulates collagen production, improves skin texture, and helps rejuvenate dull or ageing skin naturally. It is also widely used for hair restoration.

I often describe PRP as regenerative medicine rather than cosmetic medicine because it works with the body's own healing abilities.

Microneedling

Microneedling creates tiny controlled micro-injuries in the skin using very fine needles. These microchannels stimulate the skin's natural wound-healing response, encouraging collagen and elastin production.

It can improve acne scarring, enlarged pores, fine lines, pigmentation, and overall skin texture.

When combined with PRP, exosomes, or mesotherapy solutions, results can be even more impressive.

Chemical Peels

Chemical peels help resurface the skin by removing damaged outer layers and stimulating cell turnover.

Some peels are very superficial and designed simply to brighten and freshen the skin, while others penetrate deeper to address pigmentation, acne, texture, and fine lines.

Not all peels cause visible peeling. Treatments such as PRX-T33 work differently by stimulating collagen beneath the skin without significant downtime.

Laser and Light Treatments

Laser and light therapies have transformed skin rejuvenation over the past decade.

BBL (BroadBand Light) treatments target pigmentation, redness, sun damage, and uneven skin tone using light energy.

Laser Genesis gently heats the dermis to stimulate collagen production while improving redness, texture, and fine lines with minimal downtime.

Fractional lasers and resurfacing lasers can create dramatic improvements in skin texture, wrinkles, and scarring by triggering skin renewal and collagen remodelling.

LED Light Therapy

LED light therapy is one of the gentlest yet surprisingly effective skin treatments available.

Different wavelengths of light target different concerns. Red light helps stimulate healing and collagen production, while blue light targets acne-causing bacteria.

LED is often used after treatments such as microneedling, lasers, or peels because it helps calm inflammation and accelerate recovery.

Cosmeceuticals

What patients use at home matters enormously.

Professional skincare products containing active ingredients such as retinoids, peptides, antioxidants, growth factors, and exosomes can significantly improve skin quality over time.

Daily SPF is still the single most important anti-ageing product anyone can use.

No treatment can compete with years of consistent sun protection.

Skin Boosters

Skin boosters have become increasingly popular because they improve skin quality rather than simply adding volume.

Unlike traditional filler treatments, skin boosters use microdroplets of hyaluronic acid and hydrating ingredients placed superficially into the skin to improve hydration, elasticity, and radiance.

The skin often looks fresher, glowier, and healthier rather than "filled."

Mesotherapy

Mesotherapy involves tiny injections of vitamins, amino acids, antioxidants, minerals, and hydrating ingredients directly into the skin.

One of the best-known examples is NCTF 135, which contains hyaluronic acid along with a cocktail of revitalising ingredients designed to hydrate and rejuvenate tired skin.

These treatments can improve luminosity, hydration, and overall skin vitality.

The "Glass Skin" Trend

The Korean beauty industry introduced the concept of "glass skin" — skin that appears smooth, luminous, hydrated, and almost reflective.

Rather than focusing on heavy makeup, the emphasis is on healthy, radiant skin with minimal texture and maximum hydration.

This trend has influenced aesthetic medicine worldwide and led to the popularity of treatments focused on hydration and skin quality rather than volume alone.

Skin Botox (Mesobotox)

Skin Botox, also known as mesobotox, involves injecting highly diluted botulinum toxin very superficially into the skin rather than deeply into muscles.

This technique can soften fine lines, reduce oil production, minimise pores, and create a smoother, more refined skin appearance without freezing facial expression.

The result is often described as a soft, filtered glow to the skin.

Rejuran and Polynucleotide Treatments

Rejuran, sometimes called salmon DNA therapy, contains polynucleotides derived from salmon DNA which are believed to support skin repair and regeneration.

These treatments are designed to improve hydration, elasticity, skin texture, and healing. They have become extremely popular throughout Asia and are now growing in popularity worldwide.

Patients often describe the skin as looking healthier, stronger, and more luminous after a series of treatments.

A More Natural Approach to Ageing

One of the biggest shifts happening in aesthetics today is the movement away from simply "filling faces."

Patients are becoming more educated and are increasingly seeking treatments that improve skin quality, collagen health, hydration, and regeneration rather than obvious volume or dramatic change.

The healthiest-looking skin is usually skin that has been supported over time — with good skincare, sun protection, healthy lifestyle habits, collagen stimulation, and subtle maintenance rather than overcorrection.

Beautiful skin is not about perfection.

It is about vitality, health, movement, texture, and confidence.

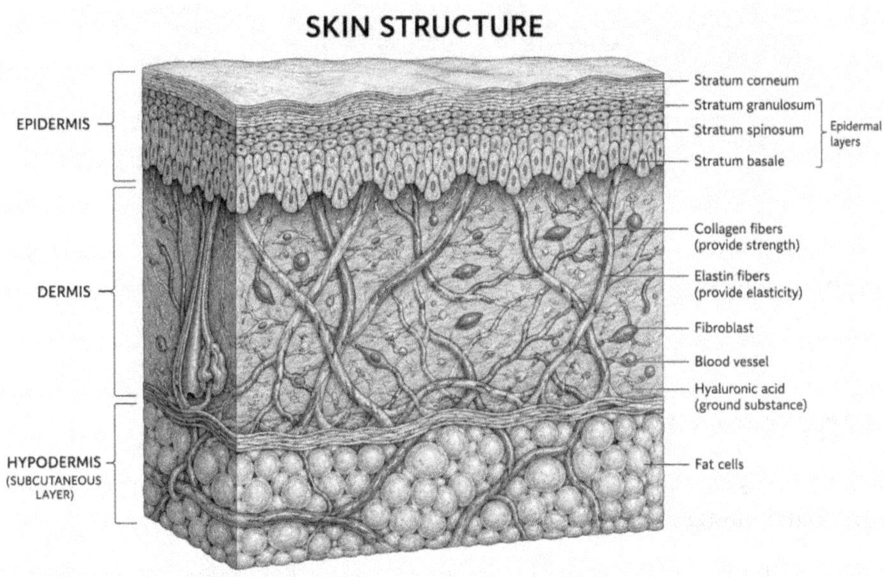

White Fat Cells: The Forgotten Foundation of Healthy Skin

For decades, the focus of skin ageing has been on two key structural proteins: **collagen** and **elastin**. Collagen provides strength and support, while elastin allows the skin to stretch and recoil. However, recent research has identified a third critical component of youthful skin—**white adipose tissue**, commonly known as white fat cells.

These specialised fat cells are not simply passive energy storage units. They are biologically active structures that play a vital role in maintaining skin health, skin quality, and facial volume.

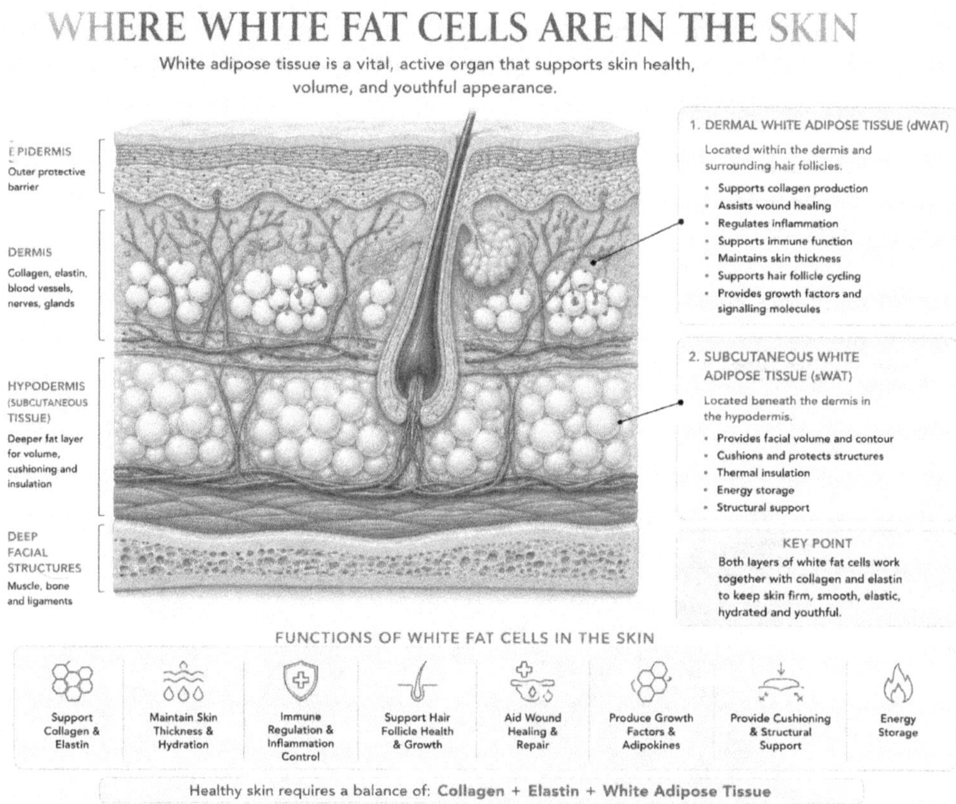

What Are White Fat Cells?

White adipose tissue (WAT) consists of specialised cells called **adipocytes**. These cells are found throughout the body and beneath the skin.

Traditionally, fat was viewed simply as a storage depot for excess calories. We now know that fat is actually an active endocrine organ that communicates with surrounding tissues through hormones, growth factors, and signalling molecules.

In the skin, white fat cells contribute to:

- Skin thickness, Hydration
- Elasticity, Wound healing, Hair follicle health

- Immune function, Collagen support, Facial volume and contour

Two Types of White Fat Found in the Skin

Dermal White Adipose Tissue (dWAT)

Dermal white adipose tissue sits directly beneath the dermis and around hair follicles.

Functions include:

- Supporting collagen production, Assisting wound healing
- Regulating inflammation, Supporting immune defence
- Maintaining skin thickness, Helping regulate hair follicle growth cycles

This layer acts as a biological support system for the skin itself.

Subcutaneous White Adipose Tissue (sWAT)

Subcutaneous white adipose tissue lies deeper beneath the skin.

Functions include:

- Facial volume support, Cushioning underlying structures, Thermal insulation
- Energy storage, Structural support of facial contours

This deeper fat layer is largely responsible for youthful facial fullness.

White Fat Cells and Hair Follicles

One of the most interesting discoveries in skin science is the close relationship between white fat cells and hair follicles.

Fat cells surrounding hair follicles release growth signals that help regulate:

- Hair growth cycles, Follicle repair
- Skin regeneration, Stem cell activity

Healthy adipose tissue contributes to healthier hair and healthier skin.

As these cells decline with ageing, hair often becomes thinner, slower growing, and less dense.

White Fat Cells as Skin Communicators

White fat cells produce chemical messengers known as: Adipokines, Cytokines, Growth factors

These substances communicate with:

- Fibroblasts, Collagen-producing cells
- Blood vessels, Immune cells, Hair follicle stem cells

This communication network helps maintain healthy skin function.

Without these signals, skin becomes thinner, less elastic, and slower to repair itself.

What Happens As We Age?

Ageing causes gradual loss and shrinkage of white adipose tissue.

As fat cells reduce:

- Skin becomes thinner, Facial support decreases
- Elasticity declines, Wrinkles deepen
- Folds become more apparent, Facial contours flatten

This process contributes significantly to the ageing face.

The cheeks lose projection.

Temples hollow. The jawline softens.

The skin begins to drape over a shrinking foundation.

White Fat Cells and Weight Loss

Rapid weight loss accelerates this process.

When body fat decreases, facial fat often decreases as well.

This may result in:

- Hollow temples, Flattened cheeks
- More visible nasolabial folds, Marionette lines
- Loose skin, Jowls, A gaunt appearance

The greater the weight loss, the greater the potential facial changes.

Ozempic Face: Why the Face Looks Like It Is Melting

One of the most common concerns associated with medications such as:

- Ozempic®, Wegovy®, Mounjaro®, Zepbound®

is the phenomenon known as **Ozempic Face**.

Contrary to popular belief, the medication itself is not damaging the face.

The issue is the rapid loss of white adipose tissue.

When weight is lost quickly, the specialised fat cells beneath the skin shrink. The skin suddenly has less structural support and begins to drape over a smaller framework.

Patients often describe the appearance as:

"My face looks like it has melted."

What they are actually seeing is:

- Loss of deep facial fat pads
- Loss of dermal white adipose tissue support, Reduced skin thickness
- Increased skin laxity, More visible wrinkles and folds

This can occur even in patients who remain healthy and are delighted with their body transformation.

Why Healthy Skin Requires Balance

Modern research suggests that healthy skin requires a balance of three essential elements:

Collagen Provides strength and structure.

Elastin Provides flexibility and recoil.

White Adipose Tissue Provides support, communication, hydration, volume, and regeneration.

Too much fat can contribute to inflammation and poor skin health.

Too little fat can lead to volume loss, skin thinning, and accelerated ageing.

The healthiest skin exists somewhere in the middle.

Restoring the Ageing Face

Understanding the role of white fat cells has changed the way aesthetic practitioners approach facial rejuvenation.

Treatment is no longer simply about filling lines.

Instead, modern approaches focus on:

- Improving skin quality, Supporting collagen production, Stimulating tissue regeneration, Restoring volume where appropriate, Maintaining facial harmony

This may involve combinations of:

- Biostimulators such as Sculptra and Radiesse
- Skin boosters, Polynucleotides, PRP and PRF, Biofiller
- Strategic filler placement, Energy-based skin tightening treatments

The goal is not to make the face larger.

The goal is to restore the healthy relationship between collagen, elastin, and the white fat cells that help keep skin youthful.

Key Point

Youthful skin depends on more than collagen and elastin. White adipose tissue is now recognised as a third essential pillar of skin health. As these specialised fat cells diminish with age or rapid weight loss, the skin loses support, elasticity, and volume—contributing to the appearance commonly known as Ozempic Face.

Subcision for Acne Scars, Tethered Scars and Facial Folds

One of the most overlooked causes of persistent facial depressions, acne scars, folds and creases is **tethering**.

As we age, or following acne, trauma, surgery, or inflammation, fibrous bands develop beneath the skin. These bands act like tiny anchor ropes, pulling the skin downward and creating a visible depression.

Simply filling these areas with dermal filler may provide temporary improvement, but if the tether remains attached, the skin continues to be pulled inward.

This is where **subcision** can be extremely effective.

What is Subcision?

Subcision is a minor procedure designed to release fibrous attachments beneath the skin.

A needle or blunt-tipped cannula is inserted beneath the skin and used to carefully break the scar bands or ligamentous tethering that are pulling the skin down.

Once these attachments are released:

- The skin can lift naturally.
- New collagen formation is stimulated.
- Blood flow to the area improves.
- The depression becomes less noticeable.
- Fillers, PRP, biofillers or biostimulants can be placed more effectively if required.

How Does Subcision Work?

Imagine a tent peg pulling a tent downward.

The skin depression is the tent fabric.

The fibrous scar band is the tent peg.

Subcision works by releasing the peg, allowing the skin to spring upward.

The small amount of controlled trauma created by the procedure also triggers the body's wound-healing response, leading to collagen production over the following weeks and months.

Conditions Treated with Subcision

Acne Scars

Particularly effective for:

- Rolling scars

- Boxcar scars with tethering
- Depressed acne scars

Less effective for:

- Ice-pick scars, Deep narrow scars

Tethered Facial Folds

Subcision may improve:

- Nasolabial folds, Marionette lines, Chin creases
- Facial depressions following surgery, Traumatic scars

Cellulite

Subcision techniques are also used to release the fibrous bands responsible for cellulite dimples.

Cannula Subcision Technique

Many practitioners now prefer a blunt cannula rather than a sharp needle because it:

- Reduces bruising
- Lowers vascular injury risk
- Is generally more comfortable
- Allows treatment of larger areas

Procedure

1. Local anaesthetic is administered.
2. A small entry point is made with a needle.
3. A cannula is inserted into the subdermal plane.
4. A fanning or windshield-wiper motion is used.
5. Fibrous attachments are gently released.
6. The area is massaged.
7. PRP, biofiller, CaHA, PLLA or HA filler may be added if indicated.

The practitioner often feels a characteristic "popping" or "snapping" sensation as the fibrous bands release.

Areas Commonly Treated

Common treatment areas include:

- Cheeks, Acne scar regions, Nasolabial folds, Marionette lines, Chin, Surgical scars, Traumatic scars

Combining Subcision with Regenerative Treatments

Subcision is often combined with:

- Platelet-Rich Plasma (PRP), Platelet-Rich Fibrin (PRF), Biofiller

- Calcium Hydroxylapatite (CaHA), Poly-L-Lactic Acid (PLLA)
- Hyaluronic Acid fillers, Microneedling

The release of the tether combined with collagen stimulation often produces better long-term results than filler alone.

Risks and Complications

Potential side effects include:

- Bruising, Swelling, Tenderness, Temporary lumpiness, Infection (rare), Haematoma, Nerve injury (very rare), Over-release resulting in contour irregularity

Most bruising settles within 7–14 days.

Clinical Pearl

One of the biggest mistakes in aesthetic medicine is repeatedly filling a depression that is actually being held down by a fibrous tether. Releasing the tether first through subcision often allows the skin to elevate naturally and can significantly reduce the amount of filler required. For many acne scars and age-related folds, subcision is the missing step that transforms a good result into an excellent one.

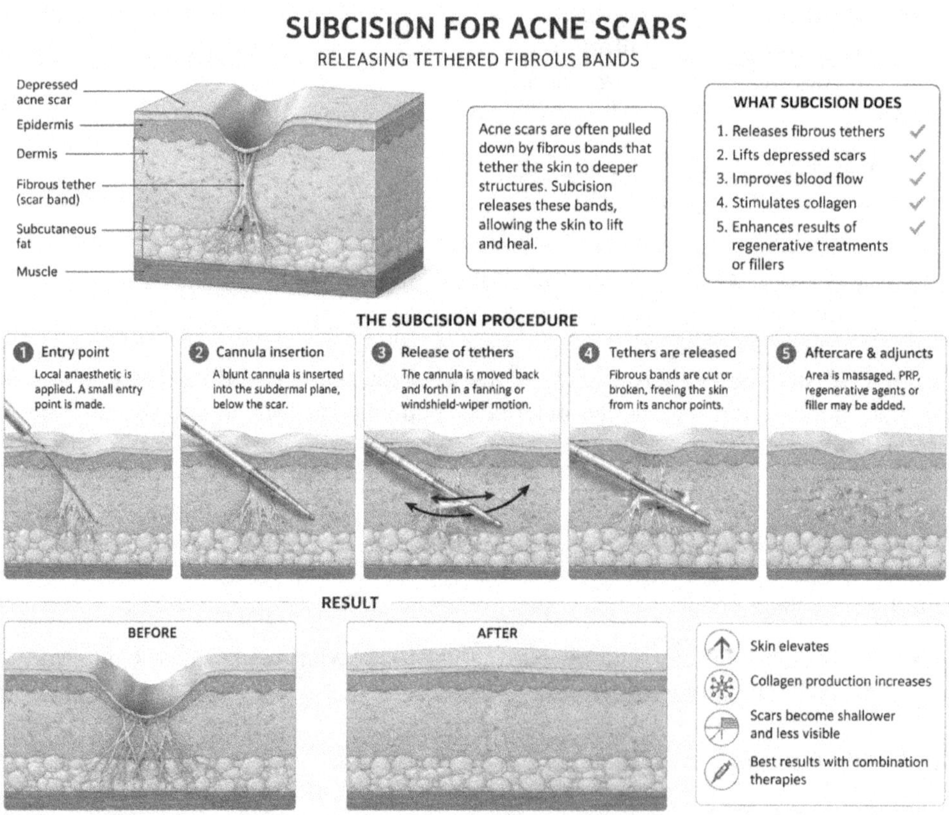

Chapter 17: Skin Renewal and the Ancient Art of Exfoliation

Skin is constantly changing.

Every single day, millions of skin cells are born, move upward through the layers of the skin, and eventually shed away. Most people never think about this process, but it is one of the reasons healthy skin can appear bright, smooth, and radiant.

When we are young, skin renewal happens quickly and efficiently. New cells rise to the surface approximately every 28 days, replacing older cells naturally. This is why youthful skin often has a glow and softness without needing much intervention.

As we age, however, this process slows down.

By our forties and fifties, skin turnover may take 40 to 60 days or longer. Dead skin cells begin to accumulate on the surface, causing skin to look dull, rough, uneven, or tired. Pores may appear more obvious, pigmentation can linger longer, and fine lines become more noticeable.

This slowing of renewal is one of the major reasons ageing skin changes in texture and brightness.

The Role of the Skin Barrier

One of the most important functions of skin is protection.

The outer layer of the skin, particularly the stratum corneum, acts like a protective wall. It keeps moisture in while defending the body against bacteria, pollution, UV radiation, chemicals, and environmental stress.

Healthy skin is not meant to be stripped raw. It needs balance.

This is why modern skincare is moving away from harsh, aggressive treatments and toward supporting the skin barrier while encouraging healthy renewal.

Why Transdermal Creams Work

Patients often ask me whether skincare creams truly penetrate the skin or whether they simply sit on the surface.

The answer lies in formulation.

Transdermal creams are designed to deliver active ingredients through the outer layers of the skin. Certain ingredients, particularly those with smaller molecular sizes, are capable of penetrating deeper into the epidermis where they can influence hydration, pigmentation, collagen production, inflammation, and barrier repair.

Ingredients such as:

- Retinol, Vitamin C

- Peptides, Niacinamide
- Growth factors, Hyaluronic acid

can all improve skin function when formulated correctly and used consistently.

Healthy skin also absorbs products more effectively than skin covered in layers of dead cells. This is one reason exfoliation can improve the effectiveness of skincare.

The Purpose of Exfoliation

Exfoliation is simply the removal of dead skin cells from the surface of the skin.

When done properly, exfoliation can:

- Brighten dull skin, Improve texture
- Help unclog pores, Enhance product penetration
- Stimulate healthier cell turnover
- Create smoother, fresher-looking skin

There are two main types of exfoliation.

Physical exfoliation uses particles, cloths, brushes, or tools to manually remove dead skin cells.

Chemical exfoliation uses acids or enzymes to dissolve the bonds between old cells so they can shed more evenly.

One of the oldest forms of chemical exfoliation dates all the way back to Cleopatra.

Legend says Cleopatra bathed in sour milk to maintain soft, radiant skin. What she likely did not realise at the time was that sour milk naturally contains lactic acid — one of the alpha hydroxy acids still widely used in skincare today.

Lactic acid gently dissolves dead skin cells while also drawing moisture into the skin, making it both exfoliating and hydrating.

Ancient cultures also used wine remnants and fermented fruits on the skin. These natural ferments contained tartaric acid and fruit acids, which acted as early forms of chemical peels.

Long before modern aesthetic clinics existed, people were already discovering ways to encourage skin renewal naturally.

More Is Not Always Better

One of the biggest mistakes I see today is over-exfoliation.

Patients often believe that if a little exfoliation is good, then more must be better. But excessive exfoliation damages the skin barrier, leading to:

- Sensitivity, Redness, Dryness, Inflammation
- Increased pigmentation, Premature ageing

Healthy skin should never feel constantly tight, burning, or irritated.

The goal is not to strip the skin. The goal is to support it.

Balanced exfoliation encourages renewal while preserving the integrity of the skin barrier.

Skin Health Before Perfection

Modern aesthetics often focuses heavily on injectables, lasers, and devices, but beautiful skin still begins with the basics:

- Protection, Hydration
- Renewal, Consistency

Good skin is not created overnight.

It is the result of daily habits, healthy cell function, barrier support, sun protection, and understanding what the skin truly needs.

When skin is healthy, everything else works better. Makeup sits better. Treatments heal better. Injectables look more natural. And the face reflects vitality rather than simply volume.

Healthy skin is not about perfection.

It is about function, balance, and respect for the remarkable organ that protects us every single day.

.

Chapter 18: Superficial Fat Pads: The Soft Contours of Youth

When we think about facial ageing, most people immediately focus on wrinkles. But beneath the skin lies another important part of facial anatomy that plays a major role in how youthful or aged the face appears — the superficial fat pads.

These soft fat compartments sit between the skin and the facial muscles and are responsible for much of the face's natural shape, softness, and contour. They give the cheeks fullness, soften transitions between facial features, and help create the balanced curves we associate with youth. When we are young, these fat pads are evenly distributed, smooth, and well supported. The face appears lifted, fresh, and naturally contoured. As we age, however, these compartments gradually lose volume, shift downward, and change shape, contributing significantly to facial ageing.

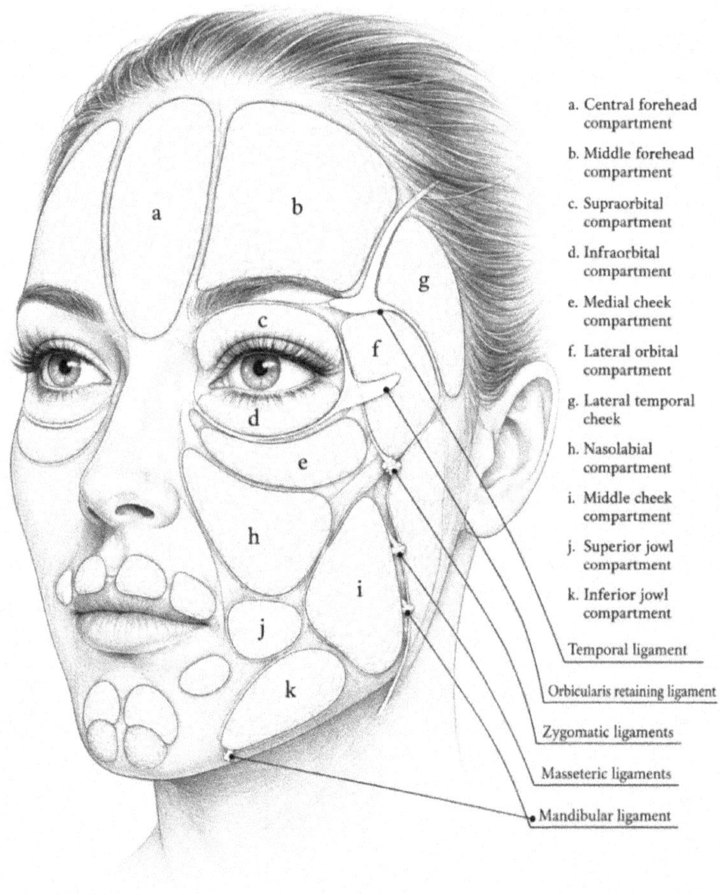

Superficial Fat Pads & Ligaments

Where Are the Superficial Fat Pads?

The face is made up of multiple superficial fat compartments, each with its own unique role in facial contouring and expression.

The infraorbital fat pad sits beneath the eyes and contributes to the smooth transition between the lower eyelid and upper cheek. When youthful and supported, this area appears soft and rested.

The malar fat pad lies over the cheekbones and is largely responsible for the fullness and projection of the midface. High, rounded cheeks are often a sign of youthful facial structure.

Beside the nose and extending toward the corners of the mouth is the nasolabial fat compartment. Changes in this area contribute to deepening smile lines and folds around the mouth.

The buccal fat pad sits within the cheek area and influences facial width and cheek hollowing. While some people naturally have fuller buccal fat pads, others have leaner cheeks with more contour.

Along the jawline lies the jowl fat compartment. As tissues descend with age, this area can become heavier and contribute to jowl formation and loss of jawline definition.

These fat compartments are separated by fibrous connective tissue structures called septa, which help maintain support and organisation within the face.

What Do Superficial Fat Pads Do?

Superficial fat pads are far more important than simply adding fullness to the face.

They create soft facial contours and help maintain balance and harmony between facial features. They also cushion underlying muscles and bones, protecting deeper structures while allowing smooth facial movement. These fat pads support the skin from underneath, helping maintain firmness and reducing the appearance of sagging. They also allow the face to move naturally during expression without looking harsh or skeletal.

In many ways, they act like the soft upholstery over the deeper framework of the face.

How Ageing Changes the Superficial Fat Pads

One of the earliest signs of facial ageing is the gradual change in the superficial fat compartments.

Over time, some fat pads shrink and lose volume, particularly in the cheeks and temples. This creates hollowness and flattening that can make the face appear tired or drawn.

At the same time, gravity and weakening ligaments allow certain fat compartments to descend. Instead of sitting high on the cheeks, tissues begin to shift downward toward the lower face.

This downward migration contributes to deeper nasolabial folds, marionette lines, and jowl formation.

Interestingly, ageing is not always about losing fat completely. In some areas, fat may actually accumulate or become heavier, while neighbouring compartments shrink. This creates imbalance and alters the natural harmony of the face.

The result is a face that gradually appears less supported, less lifted, and more bottom-heavy.

Treating Volume Loss in Superficial Fat Pads

Modern aesthetic medicine is no longer focused simply on "filling wrinkles." Instead, we now understand the importance of restoring facial structure and support by addressing changes in the fat compartments themselves.

Dermal fillers can be strategically placed to replace lost volume and restore youthful contours. Hyaluronic acid fillers are commonly used to soften folds, enhance cheeks, and improve facial balance.

Biostimulatory products such as calcium hydroxylapatite and poly-L-lactic acid work differently by stimulating collagen production and gradually improving support and skin quality over time.

Fat grafting, also known as autologous fat transfer, involves taking fat from another area of the body and injecting it into areas of facial volume loss. Because it uses the patient's own tissue, it can provide very natural and long-lasting results. Energy-based devices such as ultrasound and radiofrequency treatments can also help tighten tissues and improve skin support by stimulating collagen remodelling beneath the surface.

Emerging regenerative treatments continue to evolve, with newer approaches focusing on restoring tissue quality rather than simply replacing volume.

A More Natural Approach to Rejuvenation

One of the biggest shifts in aesthetics over the past decade has been the move away from overfilled faces.

True facial rejuvenation is not about making the face bigger. It is about restoring what has been lost in a balanced and anatomically respectful way.

When superficial fat pads are restored thoughtfully, the face looks fresher, healthier, and more supported — not swollen or artificial.

Understanding how these fat compartments age allows practitioners to create softer, more natural outcomes that respect the individual's facial anatomy rather than distort it.

Because ultimately, youthful beauty is not about perfection.

It is about balance, harmony, and healthy structure beneath the skin.

Chapter 19: Superficial Musculoaponeurotic System (SMAS) in Facial Anatomy

One of the most important structures in facial anatomy — yet one most people have never heard of — is the SMAS.

The Superficial Musculoaponeurotic System, commonly called the SMAS, is the deeper support layer of the face that connects the muscles, fat, and skin together. It sits beneath the superficial fat pads and acts almost like an internal suspension system for the face.

When we are young, the SMAS is firm, elastic, and well supported. It helps hold the cheeks higher, maintains jawline definition, and allows facial expressions to move smoothly and naturally.

But as we age, the SMAS gradually weakens and descends. This deeper structural change is one of the major reasons the face begins to sag over time.

Understanding the SMAS is essential in modern aesthetic medicine because true facial rejuvenation is not just about treating the skin. It is about understanding the deeper support structures underneath.

What Exactly Is the SMAS?

The SMAS is a thin but strong fibrous layer that lies beneath the fat pads and above the deeper facial structures.

It surrounds and connects many of the muscles responsible for facial expression while also attaching to the skin. This allows movement from the muscles to be transmitted to the surface of the face when we smile, laugh, frown, or squint.

You can think of the SMAS almost like a fabric layer beneath the skin that holds everything together.

It extends continuously from the neck into the face and forehead, blending with muscles such as the platysma in the neck and the temporalis region higher in the face.

Without the SMAS, facial movement would not appear coordinated or smooth.

The Role of the SMAS in the Face

The SMAS has several very important functions.

Its first role is structural support. It helps anchor the skin and soft tissues to the underlying facial framework, maintaining contour and facial shape.

Secondly, it allows facial expression to occur naturally. Because the facial muscles connect into the SMAS and then into the skin, muscle movement becomes visible as expression.

The SMAS also plays a role in supporting and organising the superficial fat pads of the face. This contributes to youthful fullness and smooth transitions between facial compartments.

When the SMAS is strong and lifted, the face appears firmer, fresher, and more supported.

What Happens to the SMAS With Age?

As we age, the SMAS begins to lose strength and elasticity.

Over time, gravity, repetitive facial movement, collagen loss, and weakening ligaments all contribute to stretching and descent of this support layer.

As the SMAS descends, the structures attached to it descend as well.

The cheeks begin to fall lower.

The jawline softens. Jowls develop. Nasolabial folds deepen.

The neck loses definition.

This is why simply tightening the skin alone rarely creates natural rejuvenation. The deeper support layer beneath the skin has also shifted downward.

At the same time, ageing changes in fat pads and bone structure reduce support even further. The entire facial framework slowly changes from the inside out.

The SMAS and Modern Facelifts

One of the biggest advances in facial surgery was the understanding that lifting the skin alone does not create long-lasting natural results.

Modern facelift techniques now focus heavily on the SMAS layer itself.

In a SMAS facelift, the surgeon carefully lifts and repositions the deeper support structures rather than simply pulling the skin tighter.

This allows sagging tissues to be elevated more naturally while reducing the overly stretched appearance seen in older facelift techniques.

By repositioning the SMAS, surgeons can improve:

- Midface sagging, Jowls
- Jawline definition, Neck laxity, Deep folds around the mouth

Because the deeper structures are being lifted, the results often look softer and more natural.

Micro-Botox and the SMAS

Not all SMAS treatments are surgical.

Micro-Botox is a newer technique involving very diluted botulinum toxin injected superficially into the skin and upper SMAS layer.

Rather than freezing movement, Micro-Botox aims to soften very fine muscle activity and improve overall skin quality.

Patients often notice: Smoother skin texture, Reduced pore size, Softer fine lines, Reduced oiliness, Mild tightening and lifting effects

It creates a fresher appearance without dramatically changing facial expression.

Why Understanding the SMAS Matters

The SMAS is one of the key reasons some faces age more heavily than others.

It also explains why natural rejuvenation requires more than simply filling wrinkles. If the deeper support layer has descended, treating only the surface often creates heaviness or overfilled results.

In aesthetic medicine, understanding the relationship between the skin, fat pads, ligaments, muscles, and SMAS is essential for creating balanced outcomes.

The face ages in layers. And rejuvenation must respect those layers too.

Non Surgical Smas tightening

Ultherapy® is a treatment that uses focused ultrasound energy to target the deeper structural layers of the face and neck, including the Superficial Musculoaponeurotic System (SMAS)—the same layer addressed during a surgical facelift. By delivering precise thermal energy at specific depths beneath the skin without damaging the surface, Ultherapy stimulates the body's natural production of collagen and elastin, resulting in gradual lifting and tightening of the brow, lower face, jawline, neck, and décolletage. Results typically develop over 2–6 months as new collagen forms, with improvements in skin firmness and support.

A Final Thought

One of the most important lessons I've learned over the years is this:

The skin is only the surface story.

True ageing happens deeper — in the fat pads, the ligaments, the bone, and the SMAS support system holding everything together.

That is why the most beautiful results are never about making someone look "done." They come from restoring support, balance, and harmony in a subtle and respectful way.

When the deeper structures are understood and treated properly, the face does not lose character.
It simply looks fresher, lighter, and more rested.

.

Chapter 20: Facial Muscles Movement and Formation of Wrinkles

Every expression we make — smiling, frowning, squinting, raising our eyebrows — is created by the movement of facial muscles beneath the skin. Over time, these repeated movements begin to leave their mark on the face.

In facial anatomy diagrams, red arrows often show the direction the muscle pulls, while black lines represent the wrinkles and folds that eventually form from years of repeated movement.

Understanding how facial muscles work is one of the foundations of aesthetic medicine. After all, muscles are not only responsible for expression — they also play a major role in how the face ages.

The Two Main Groups of Facial Muscles

Facial muscles can generally be divided into two categories: elevator muscles and depressor muscles.

The elevator muscles are the lifting muscles of the face. They help create an open, youthful, refreshed appearance.

The frontalis muscle lifts the eyebrows and creates a more awake and alert expression. The zygomaticus major and minor muscles elevate the cheeks and corners of the mouth when we smile. The levator labii superioris lifts the upper lip and influences smile shape and lip movement. The levator anguli oris helps elevate the corners of the mouth, while the upper fibres of the orbicularis oculi assist in lifting the cheeks during smiling. These are the muscles associated with youthfulness, expression, and lift.

The depressor muscles, on the other hand, pull the face downward. As these muscles become stronger and more dominant with age, they contribute to heaviness, sagging, and a tired appearance.

The depressor anguli oris (DAO) pulls down the corners of the mouth, often creating a sad or unhappy expression. The depressor labii inferioris lowers the bottom lip, particularly during speaking or frowning. The platysma, a thin sheet-like muscle in the neck, pulls the jawline downward and contributes to jowls and neck banding over time.

The lower fibres of the orbicularis oris contribute to vertical lip lines, while the mentalis muscle in the chin can become overactive and create dimpling or puckering of the chin.

How Muscles Change With Age

One of the most important things to understand about facial ageing is that it is not simply the skin getting older. The muscles themselves also change over time.

As we age, the elevator muscles gradually weaken. The brows begin to descend, the cheeks lose support, and the corners of the mouth may start to turn downward.

At the same time, the depressor muscles often remain strong and active. This creates an imbalance where the downward pull on the face becomes greater than the lifting support.

The face quite literally begins to get pulled downward.

Certain muscles also become overworked as the body tries to compensate for ageing changes.

For example, as the brows begin to droop, many people unconsciously overuse the frontalis muscle in an attempt to keep the eyes looking open. Over time, this repeated movement creates horizontal forehead lines.

The orbicularis oculi muscle around the eyes contracts thousands of times through squinting and smiling, eventually forming crow's feet.

The platysma becomes increasingly active with age, contributing to neck bands and loss of jawline definition.

At the same time, bone resorption and shrinking fat pads reduce the structural support beneath the muscles. Without proper support, tissues descend even further.

This is why ageing is never caused by just one thing. It is the combined effect of changes in muscle, fat, ligaments, bone, and skin.

How Botulinum Toxin Works

Botulinum toxin works by temporarily interrupting communication between nerves and muscles.

Normally, when a nerve wants a muscle to contract, it releases a neurotransmitter called acetylcholine. This chemical messenger tells the muscle to move.

Botulinum toxin blocks the release of acetylcholine at the neuromuscular junction. Without this signal, the muscle cannot contract as strongly.

As the muscle relaxes, the overlying skin smooths out and repetitive folding decreases. This softens dynamic wrinkles and reduces excessive downward pull on the face.

The result is not paralysis when done correctly. The goal should always be softening, balancing, and natural movement.

Common Treatment Areas

Botulinum toxin is commonly used in areas where muscle movement creates repetitive wrinkles or downward pull.

In the forehead, relaxing the frontalis softens horizontal lines.

In the glabella, treatment of the corrugator and procerus muscles reduces frown lines between the brows.

Around the eyes, relaxing portions of the orbicularis oculi softens crow's feet.

Treating the DAO muscles can reduce the downward pull at the corners of the mouth, helping the face appear less sad or heavy.

Strategic placement around the brows can create a subtle brow lift by weakening depressor muscles while allowing the elevator muscles to function more effectively.

In the neck, treating the platysma can soften neck bands and improve jawline definition.

The Art of Balance

One of the biggest misconceptions about botulinum toxin is that it is simply about freezing wrinkles.

In reality, good aesthetic treatment is about balance.

A youthful face is not wrinkle-free. It is balanced. The lifting muscles and depressing muscles work in harmony, creating natural movement and support.

As we age, that balance shifts.

By carefully relaxing overactive depressor muscles, we can reduce heaviness and allow the natural elevator muscles to function more effectively again.

When performed well, the face should not look frozen or artificial. It should simply look softer, fresher, and more rested — like a better version of yourself.

FACIAL MUSCLES
(SUPERFICIAL MUSCLES OF FACIAL EXPRESSION)

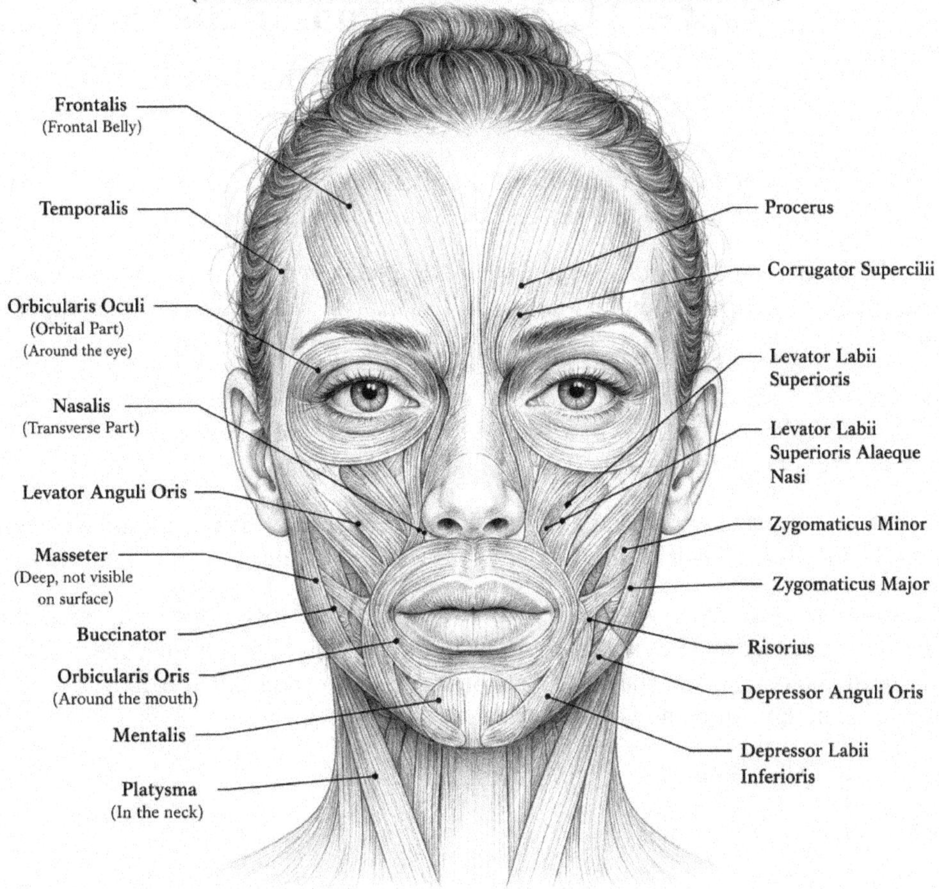

ELEVATOR (LIFTING) MUSCLES

1. **Frontalis** – lifts the eyebrows
2. **Zygomaticus Major** – elevates the corners of the mouth (smiling)
3. **Zygomaticus Minor** – elevates the upper lip
4. **Levator Labii Superioris** – lifts the upper lip
5. **Levator Labii Superioris Alaeque Nasi** – lifts the upper lip and widens the nostril
6. **Levator Anguli Oris** – elevates the corners of the mouth
7. **Orbicularis Oculi (Upper Fibers)** – helps raise the cheeks when smiling

DEPRESSOR (PULLING DOWN) MUSCLES

1. **Depressor Anguli Oris (DAO)** – pulls down the corners of the mouth
2. **Depressor Labii Inferioris** – lowers the lower lip
3. **Platysma** – pulls the jawline and mouth downward, causing neck bands
4. **Orbicularis Oris (Lower Fibers)** – pulls the lips downward, causing vertical lip lines
5. **Mentalis** – pulls the chin upward, causing chin dimpling

COMMON DYNAMIC LINES AND WRINKLES CAUSED BY MUSCLE MOVEMENT

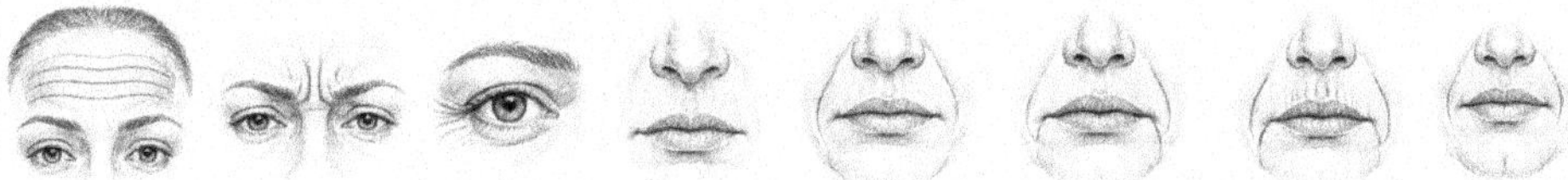

Forehead Lines (Frontalis) | **Frown Lines** (11 Lines) (Corrugator, Procerus) | **Crows Feet** (Orbicularis Oculi) | **Bunny Lines** (Nasalis) | **Nasolabial Folds** (Levator Labii Superioris, Zygomaticus Minor) | **Marionette Lines** (Depressor Anguli Oris) | **Vertical Lip Lines** (Orbicularis Oris) | **Chin Dimpling** (Mentalis)

Chapter 21: Deep Fat Pads in the Face: The Foundation of Volume

One of the biggest misconceptions about facial ageing is that wrinkles are the main problem. In reality, ageing often begins much deeper beneath the surface.

Under the muscles of the face lie structures called deep fat pads. These hidden compartments are the true foundation of youthful facial shape. They create support, softness, and contour long before lines and wrinkles appear on the skin.

When we are young, these fat pads are full, hydrated, and positioned high on the face. They give the cheeks gentle projection, soften the transition between the eyes and cheeks, and help maintain smooth, balanced facial proportions.

Over time, however, these fat pads shrink, shift, and descend. This is one of the major reasons the face begins to look tired, hollow, or heavy with age.

Understanding deep fat pads completely changed the way aesthetic medicine approaches rejuvenation. Years ago, treatments focused mainly on filling lines. Today, experienced injectors understand that restoring structure beneath the muscles often creates a far more natural and youthful result.

What Are Deep Fat Pads?

Facial fat exists in two main layers.

The superficial fat pads sit just beneath the skin and move with facial expression. These are the compartments that contribute to surface fullness and softness.

The deep fat pads lie underneath the muscles of facial expression, closer to the bone. They act almost like the scaffolding of the face, supporting the overlying tissues and helping maintain youthful shape and contour.

Because these fat pads sit deeper, they are not usually the first thing people notice when ageing begins. Yet when they shrink, the effects ripple throughout the face.

The cheeks flatten. The under-eyes hollow. The mouth area starts to fold. The jawline loses definition.

Much of what people think is "skin ageing" is actually deep structural volume loss.

The Most Important Deep Fat Pads

The midface contains some of the most significant deep fat compartments.

The deep medial cheek fat pad is one of the key structures responsible for youthful cheek projection. When it is full, the face appears lifted, rested, and supported. As it shrinks with age, the cheeks flatten and the nasolabial folds become more noticeable.

Beside it sits the deep lateral cheek fat pad, which supports the outer cheek and cheekbone region. Loss of volume here contributes to a tired or drawn appearance.

Under the eyes is the Sub-Orbicularis Oculi Fat pad, commonly called the SOOF. This fat pad lies beneath the orbicularis oculi muscle and plays a major role in maintaining smooth under-eye contours. As it descends with age, the under-eye area can begin to look hollow, shadowed, or puffy.

In the lower face, the deep premaxillary fat pad supports the upper lip and the area beside the nose. Volume loss here contributes to flattening around the mouth and deeper smile lines.

Under the chin lies the deep submental fat compartment, which influences jawline definition and neck contour.

Why Deep Fat Pads Matter

Deep fat pads are not simply "fat." They are essential support structures.

They provide foundational volume beneath the muscles and skin, helping the face maintain shape and balance. They also cushion movement, soften facial transitions, and contribute to the smooth contours associated with youth.

Healthy fat compartments also contain important lipids that support skin quality and elasticity.

When these structures begin to shrink, the face loses more than volume. It loses support.

What Happens With Ageing?

Ageing affects the deep fat pads in several ways.

The first is atrophy, meaning the fat pads slowly shrink over time. This loss of volume is one of the earliest signs of facial ageing, even before significant wrinkles develop.

The second change is descent. Gravity, repeated facial movement, ligament weakening, and bone resorption all contribute to the downward migration of facial tissues. The fat that once sat high over the cheekbones slowly shifts lower.

This creates heaviness around the mouth and jawline while simultaneously leaving hollowness higher in the face.

The under-eye area is particularly vulnerable. As the SOOF descends, the transition between the lower eyelid and cheek becomes more pronounced. This can create shadows, hollows, and the appearance of eye bags even in people who are well rested.

Bone loss also plays a major role. As the facial skeleton gradually resorbs with age, there is less structural support holding the fat pads in place. Ligaments weaken, tissues slide downward, and folds deepen further.

This is why ageing is never just about the skin. It involves changes in bone, ligaments, fat, muscle, and skin all occurring together.

Deep Fat Pads and Facial Anatomy

Deep fat pads sit beneath important facial muscles and close to major nerves and blood vessels. This is why anatomy knowledge is critical in aesthetic medicine.

The infraorbital nerve lies beneath the deep medial cheek fat pad and supplies sensation to the midface.

Branches of the facial nerve travel through deeper cheek tissues and control facial movement.

In the lower face, the marginal mandibular nerve runs near the jawline and chin region.

For injectors, understanding these anatomical relationships is essential. Placing filler too deeply or incorrectly can increase the risk of complications, nerve irritation, or unnatural outcomes.

This is why facial assessment should never simply focus on "where the wrinkle is." A skilled injector must understand the deeper architecture of the face.

Restoring Deep Volume

One of the most effective ways to create natural rejuvenation is to restore support within the deep fat compartments rather than overfilling superficial lines.

Strategic placement of dermal fillers can recreate structural support and restore youthful proportions. Small amounts placed deeply in the cheeks, temples, or chin can often create a more refreshed appearance than large amounts placed superficially.

Biostimulatory injectables such as calcium hydroxylapatite or poly-L-lactic acid may also help improve structural support by stimulating collagen production over time.

Fat grafting is another option, where a patient's own fat is transferred from another part of the body into areas of facial volume loss. While more invasive, it can provide longer-lasting restoration.

Regenerative treatments such as PRP may also help improve tissue quality and support collagen health.

A Final Thought

When I look at a face now, I don't just see wrinkles. I see structure.

I see where support has been lost.

I see where volume has shifted.

I see how the face has changed from the inside out.

This is why natural rejuvenation is never about chasing lines with syringes. It is about understanding the deeper foundations of the face and restoring balance carefully and respectfully.

The deep fat pads are the hidden architecture of youth. When they are supported properly, the face looks fresher, softer, and healthier — not overfilled or artificial.

In aesthetic medicine, less is often more.

The art lies in knowing where to place it.

.

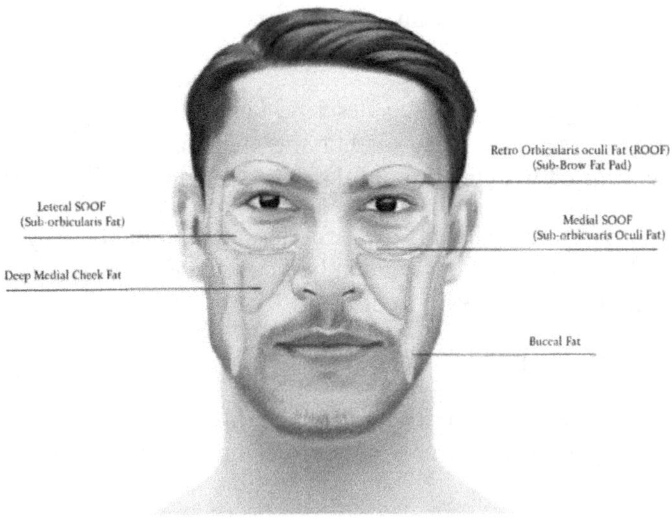

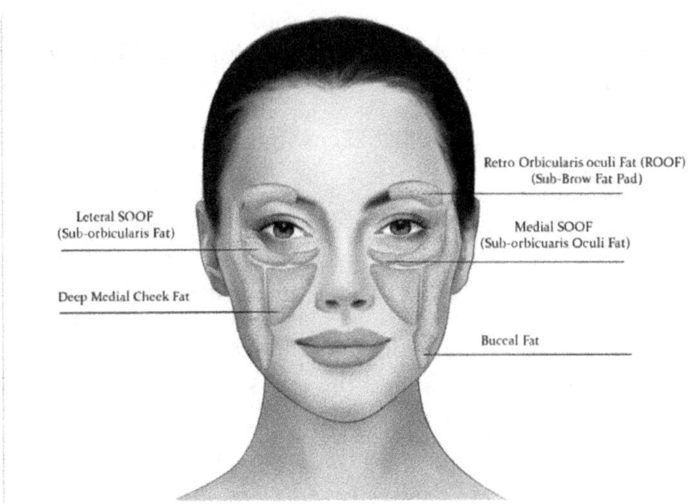

Chapter 22: Facial Ligaments: The Framework of Youth

When people think about ageing, they often focus on wrinkles, sagging skin, or volume loss. But beneath the surface lies an entire support system quietly holding the face together.

These are the facial ligaments. I often describe facial ligaments as the scaffolding or suspension cables of the face. They anchor the skin, fat pads, and soft tissue to the underlying bone, helping maintain youthful shape, structure, and support.

When we are young, these ligaments are firm, strong, and tight. They hold everything neatly in place. But as we age, they gradually weaken and stretch. The support system loosens, and the tissues above begin to descend.

This is one of the major reasons the face starts to sag.

Understanding the facial ligament system is incredibly important in modern aesthetic medicine because ageing is not simply about lines on the surface. It is about structural support changing underneath.

What Are Facial Ligaments?

Facial ligaments are bands of connective tissue that stabilise and support the face.

Some attach firmly from bone to skin, acting like strong anchors. Others form softer partitions within the face, helping suspend fat pads and separate facial compartments.

Together, they create the architecture that keeps the face lifted and balanced.

True Retaining Ligaments

The true retaining ligaments are the strongest support structures in the face. These ligaments attach directly from the bone to the skin and act like anchor points.

One of the most important is the orbital retaining ligament around the eyes. This ligament helps support the tissues around the eye socket and maintains the transition between the lower eyelid and cheek.

As it weakens over time, patients begin noticing hollowness, crepey skin, under-eye bags, and drooping around the eyes and brows.

The zygomatic ligaments are located around the cheekbone area. These ligaments support the midface and help maintain youthful cheek position.

When they weaken, the cheeks descend and the nasolabial folds become more prominent.

The mandibular and masseteric ligaments support the lower face and jawline. These structures play a major role in maintaining jawline definition.

As these ligaments lose strength, jowls begin forming and the lower face appears heavier and less defined.

False Retaining Ligaments and Septa

The face also contains softer ligamentous structures known as septal or false retaining ligaments.

These structures do not attach directly to bone but instead act like fibrous partitions that separate and support the facial fat compartments.

The SMAS system — the superficial musculoaponeurotic system — is part of this network. It connects muscles, fat, and connective tissue together and plays a major role in facial movement and ageing.

As these support structures weaken, fat pads shift downward, facial contours change, and folds deepen.

How Ligaments Age

Like collagen and elastin in the skin, ligaments also age.

Over time, the collagen within the ligaments breaks down and the tissues become thinner, weaker, and more stretched.

This laxity allows the fat pads and skin above them to descend downward under gravity.

At the same time, facial fat compartments shrink and shift position, further exaggerating hollows and sagging.

Bone resorption also contributes to the problem. As the facial skeleton shrinks with age, ligaments lose some of their original support and attachment points.

Everything becomes less supported.

The result is the ageing changes we commonly see: deeper nasolabial folds, hollow eyes, jowls, heavier lower face, marionette lines, and loss of jawline definition.

Why This Matters in Aesthetic Medicine

This is why simply filling lines often does not create natural results.

If you only chase wrinkles without understanding ligament support and facial structure, the face can quickly become puffy, overfilled, or distorted.

Modern aesthetic medicine focuses more on restoring support than simply adding volume.

In many cases, strategic placement of filler near ligament attachment points can create subtle lifting and repositioning effects.

PRP and Ligament Rejuvenation

PRP, or Platelet-Rich Plasma, is becoming increasingly valuable in regenerative aesthetics because it works with the body's own healing response.

PRP contains growth factors that stimulate collagen production, tissue repair, and improved skin quality.

When used around weakened ligament structures, PRP may help improve tissue quality, hydration, and support over time.

Rather than simply masking ageing, regenerative treatments aim to strengthen and improve the quality of the tissues themselves.

Fillers as Structural Support

Dermal fillers can also be used strategically to support ageing ligaments and recreate lost structural support.

For example, placing filler around the cheekbone area can support the zygomatic ligaments and create a subtle lifting effect through the midface.

Jawline and chin filler can restore definition lost through weakening mandibular support and bone resorption.

Under-eye and midface treatments can help compensate for changes around the orbital retaining ligament and surrounding fat compartments.

Good filler placement should never look obvious. The goal is support, balance, and restoration — not overfilled cheeks or exaggerated contours.

The Tree Analogy

I often explain facial ageing using the analogy of a tree.

Imagine the ligaments are the roots of the tree, anchoring it firmly into the ground. The skin, fat, and soft tissue are like the branches and leaves above.

When the roots are strong, the tree stands upright and supported.

But over time, if the roots weaken and the soil erodes, the branches begin drooping downward.

Strategic filler placement is like restoring the support around the roots, helping lift and stabilise the structure again.

A More Natural Approach to Ageing

The future of aesthetics is moving away from simply "chasing lines" and toward understanding the anatomy of ageing properly.

The most natural results come from respecting the architecture of the face — the bone, ligaments, fat pads, skin, and muscles all working together.

When treatments are done thoughtfully and conservatively, patients do not look “done.”

They simply look fresher, healthier, and more supported.

HOW LIGAMENT TETHERING CREATES FOLDS

THE HIDDEN ANCHORS THAT SHAPE AND AGE THE FACE

Retaining ligaments are strong bands of fibrous tissue that anchor the skin to the underlying bone and deep fascia. With age, fat pads descend and volume is lost, but these ligaments remain fixed, creating tethering points that pull the skin inward and downward — forming visible lines, folds and hollows.

1. YOUTHFUL FACE | 2. EARLY AGING | 3. PROGRESSIVE AGING | 4. VISIBLE FOLDS

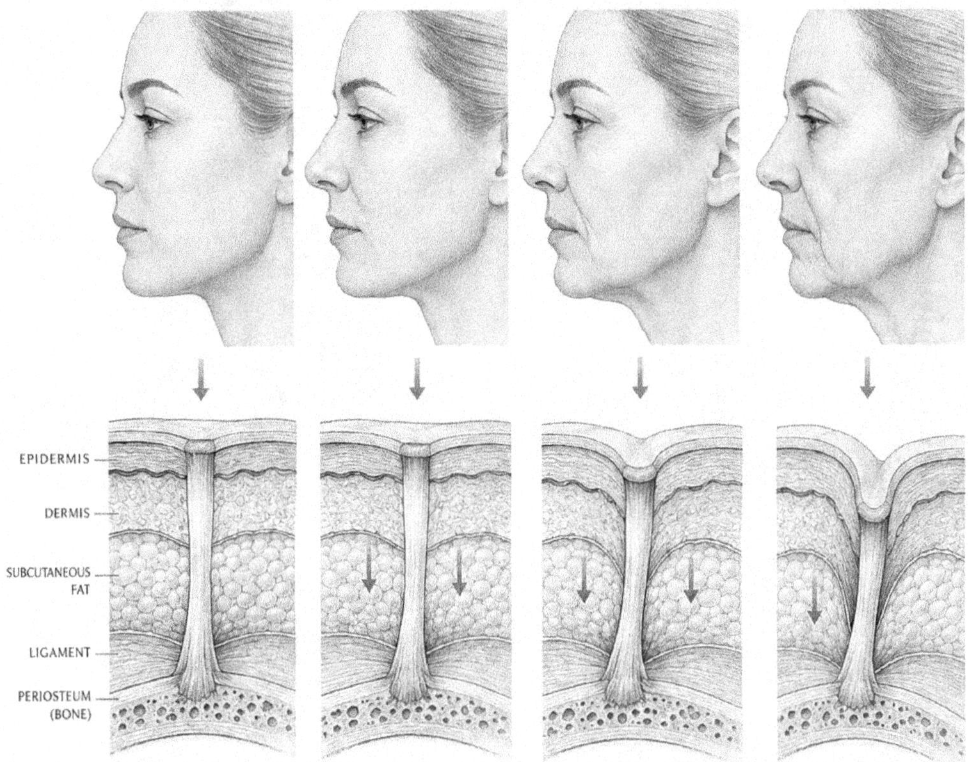

1. Fat pads are full and ligaments support the skin without creating depressions. The skin surface is smooth and transitions are seamless.

2. Fat pads begin to descend with volume loss. Ligaments remain fixed to bone, creating tethering points.

3. Descending tissue is caught at ligament attachments. The skin is pulled inward at these points, creating lines and shadows.

4. Skin folds inward at the ligaments, forming visible lines, creases and hollows. The depth increases with age.

FACIAL LIGAMENTS

True (Bone–Anchored) and False (Septal) Retaining Ligaments

TRUE (BONE–ANCHORED) RETAINING LIGAMENTS

1. **ORBITAL RETAINING LIGAMENT (ORL)**
   Anchors the skin and muscle of the eyelid and brow to the orbital rim.
2. **ZYGOMATIC LIGAMENT (ZL)**
   Extends from the zygomatic bone to the skin, supporting the midface and nasolabial region.
3. **MASSSETERIC LIGAMENT (MaL)**
   Connects the masseter muscle to the skin and parotid fascia, defining the jawline and preventing jowls.
4. **MANDIBULAR RETAINING LIGAMENT (MRL)**
   Anchors the skin and soft tissue of the lower face to the mandible, maintaining lower face firmness.

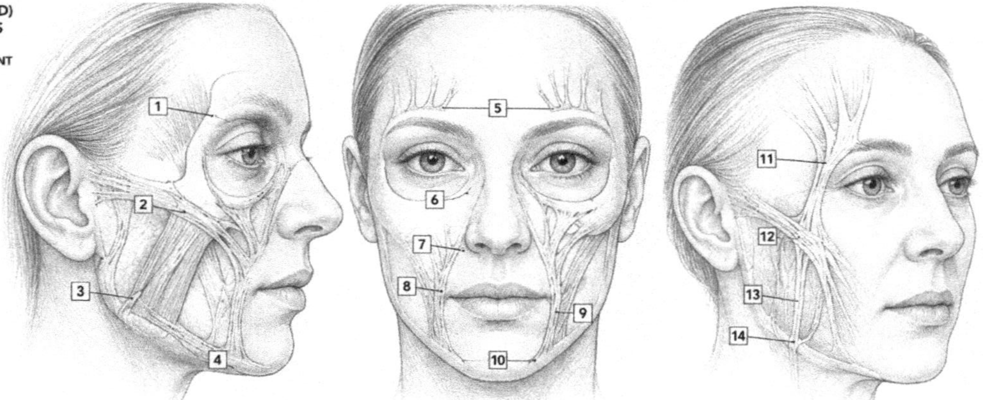

SUPERFICIAL MUSCULOAPONEUROTIC SYSTEM (SMAS) LIGAMENTS (SEPTA)

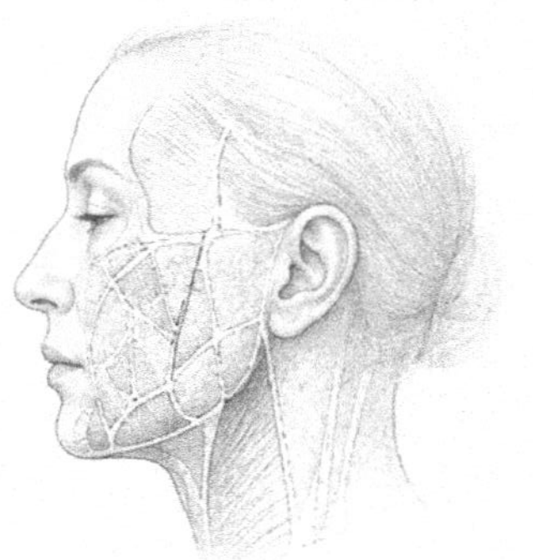

- The SMAS septa are fibrous connections between the SMAS and the overlying skin.
- They form vertical retaining structures that suspend soft tissue and fat compartments.
- Key SMAS septa correspond to many of the ligaments listed above.

DEEP VIEW – LIGAMENTS AND SEPTA

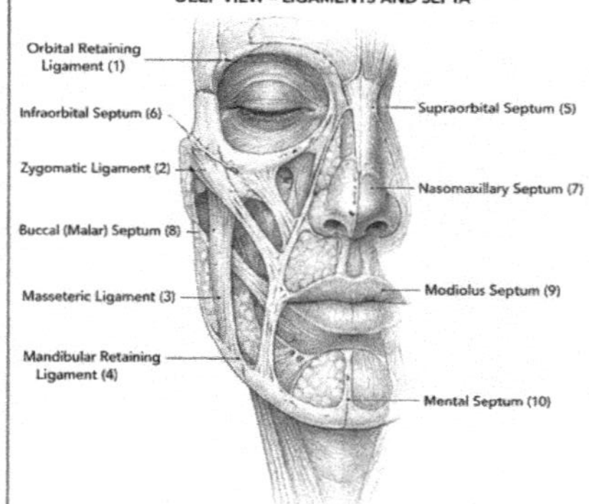

LIGAMENTS IN RELATION TO FACIAL FAT COMPARTMENTS

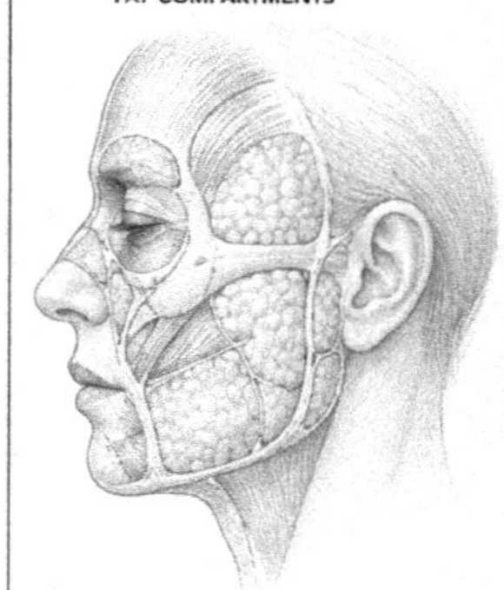

FALSE (SEPTAL) RETAINING LIGAMENTS (SEPTA)

5. **SUPRAORBITAL SEPTUM**
   Blends with the brow soft tissues, contributing to brow position.
6. **INFRAORBITAL SEPTUM**
   Attaches to the orbital rim and blends with cheek soft tissue, supports the lower eyelid.
7. **NASOMAXILLARY SEPTUM**
   Extends from the side of the nose to the maxilla and skin, supporting the nasal sidewall.
8. **BUCCAL (MALAR) SEPTUM**
   Extends over the cheek fat pad, maintaining cheek contour.
9. **MODIOLUS SEPTUM**
   Attaches around the corner of the mouth, supporting the upper lip and preventing downturn.
10. **MENTAL SEPTUM**
    Extends from the chin region to the skin, helping define the chin and lower lip.
11. **TEMPORAL SEPTUM**
    Extends from the temporal fascia to the skin, blending with the SMAS.
12. **PAROTIDOMASSETERIC SEPTUM**
    Separates the parotid and masseteric fat compartments.
13. **ANTERIOR JUXTAMANDIBULAR SEPTUM**
    Runs along the anterior border of the jaw, separating cheek and jowl fat.
14. **POSTERIOR JUXTAMANDIBULAR SEPTUM**
    Runs along the posterior border of the jaw, supporting the jowl area.

Chapter 23: Septa and the Architecture of Facial Ageing

One of the most misunderstood aspects of facial ageing is the difference between ligaments and septa. Although both are connective tissue structures beneath the skin, they have very different roles in facial anatomy.

Understanding how they work — and how they change with age — is essential in aesthetic medicine because many folds, hollows, and shadows are not simply caused by "loose skin." They are created by deeper structural changes occurring beneath the surface.

Facial ligaments are strong fibrous bands that anchor the skin and soft tissues to deeper structures such as bone or deep fascia.
You can think of ligaments as the major support cables of the face.

Their role is to hold facial tissues in position and maintain structural stability. They help suspend the cheeks, support the jawline, and keep facial compartments organised.

Important retaining ligaments include:

- Orbital retaining ligament, Zygomatic ligaments
- Masseteric ligaments, Mandibular ligament

When we are young, these ligaments are firm and supportive. They hold the fat pads higher on the face and maintain youthful contour.

As we age, however, ligaments weaken and stretch. The tissues attached to them begin to descend, contributing to sagging cheeks, jowls, and deeper facial folds.

Septa are very different from ligaments.

Rather than acting like major anchor cables, septa are thin fibrous walls that separate and organise the facial fat compartments.

They run between the fat pads like internal partitions or dividers, helping maintain structure and compartmentalisation within the face.

Septa attach from deeper tissues upward toward the skin and help guide the movement and positioning of facial fat.

If ligaments are the tent poles holding everything up, septa are the internal walls separating the rooms.

They help:

- Organise facial fat compartments
- Maintain smooth transitions between areas
- Support skin tension
- Allow natural facial movement
- Stabilise the relationship between fat, muscle, and skin

The Difference Between Ligaments and Septa

Although they work together, ligaments and septa serve different purposes.

Ligaments are stronger, more fixed anchoring structures. Their main job is support and suspension.

Septa are softer connective tissue partitions that separate fat compartments and influence how tissues move and age.

Ligaments hold.
Septa organise.

Both play enormous roles in facial ageing.

What Happens to Septa With Age?

As collagen decreases with age, septa begin to change.

Some septa stretch and weaken, allowing fat pads to descend. Other septa tighten and tether tissues inward.

At the same time:

- Fat compartments shrink, Bone resorbs
- Ligaments weaken, Skin thins
- Muscle movement changes

This creates the complex patterns we associate with ageing:

- Hollows, Shadows, Grooves
- Puffiness beside hollow areas, Uneven facial contours

This is why ageing is never just about sagging skin. It is the changing relationship between fat pads, septa, ligaments, muscle, bone, and skin.

How Septa Create Grooves and Shadows

One of the fascinating things about septa is how they influence the visible lines and folds we see on the surface of the face.

As surrounding fat shrinks or descends, the septal boundaries become more visible. These tethering points can create grooves, depressions, and shadows.

Tear Troughs

The tear trough, also called the nasojugal groove, forms partly because of septal tethering between the under-eye fat compartments. As deep support decreases and the skin thins, the groove between the lower eyelid and cheek becomes more obvious.

This is why simply filling the hollow directly is often not the best solution. Without restoring cheek support first, the area can become heavy or prone to filler migration.

Nasolabial Folds

Nasolabial folds are rarely caused by "too much skin."

They develop because:

- Midface fat descends, Deep structural support shrinks
- Septal attachments tether the skin inward

The fold forms at the boundary between facial compartments.

This is why overfilling the fold itself often looks unnatural. The real issue usually lies higher in the cheek structure.

Mid-Cheek Grooves

As superficial fat compartments lose volume, septal divisions within the cheek become more visible.

This can create hollow grooves across the midface and contribute to a tired or flattened appearance.

Marionette Lines

Around the mouth and chin, septal tethering combines with:

- Bone resorption, Chin shortening
- Jawline changes, Tissue descent

The result is the downward grooves known as marionette lines.

The septa remain relatively fixed while surrounding tissues shift downward.

Temple Hollowing

The temple is anatomically complex, containing multiple fascial layers, ligaments, septa, and vascular structures.

As deep fat and bone volume decrease, hollowing develops and the septal architecture becomes more apparent.

This area requires advanced anatomical knowledge because filler can spread unpredictably through these planes if injected incorrectly.

Septa and Filler Migration

One of the reasons filler sometimes migrates is because of the anatomical pathways created by septa and fascial planes.

Filler movement is influenced by:

- Facial movement, Gravity
- Injection depth, Product selection
- Muscle action, Septal pathways
- Ligaments and tissue planes

Certain areas such as:

- Lips, Tear troughs, Temples, Nasolabial folds

are more prone to filler spreading because of their anatomical structure.

This is why understanding anatomy is far more important than simply placing product into lines.

Treating Facial Folds Holistically

Natural rejuvenation is not about chasing every crease with filler.

Sometimes the visible fold is not the true problem.

The real issue may be:

- Loss of deep cheek support
- Fat pad descent, Tight septal tethering
- Bone resorption, Collagen depletion, Ligament weakening

Treating the face holistically creates softer, more natural outcomes.

Subcision and Facial Fold Release

In some cases, tethering septa can be released using a technique called subcision.

Subcision involves inserting a blunt cannula beneath the skin to carefully release fibrous attachments pulling the skin inward.

This technique can:

- Improve depressed grooves, Soften folds
- Stimulate collagen production
- Improve skin texture over time

Using a blunt cannula is generally safer than sharp needles because it reduces trauma, bruising, and vascular risk.

Combining Subcision With Fillers

After releasing tethered septa, dermal fillers may be used to restore support and volume.

Hyaluronic acid fillers can provide immediate softening and hydration.

Biostimulatory fillers such as calcium hydroxylapatite may stimulate collagen production while restoring structure.
The combination of releasing tethered tissue and restoring lost support often creates far more natural results than simply overfilling folds alone.

A Final Thought

The more I studied facial anatomy, the more I realised that wrinkles are only the surface story.
Beneath every fold is an architectural change occurring within the face.
Ligaments weaken., Septa tighten or stretch.
Fat shifts. Bone shrinks. Skin thins.

Everything is connected.

This is why the best aesthetic results come from understanding the face as a living structure rather than simply treating isolated lines.

True rejuvenation is about restoring harmony beneath the skin — not just filling what we see on the surface.

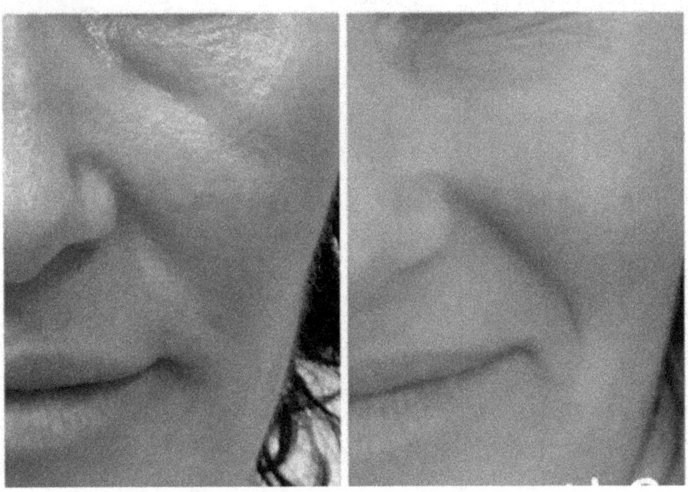

Before and after filler and subsicion of naso jugal groove caused by septa tethering.

Chapter 24: The Bone Beneath the Beauty

When we think about ageing, we often focus on the skin—wrinkles, sagging, volume loss. But what if I told you that the true culprit behind an ageing face is something you don't see? The bones of your skull.

Yes, just like the rest of your body, your skull changes over time. It shrinks, shifts, and resorbs (meaning the body breaks it down and reabsorbs it). This isn't just a random process—it's nature's way of recycling materials. But when it happens in the face, it dramatically affects how we look.

Let's break it down by age.

The Youthful Skull (Teens to Early 30s)

In our younger years, the skull is strong, structured, and proportionate. The eye sockets are relatively smaller, the cheekbones are well-defined, and the jawline is sharp and prominent.

The bone structure acts as a sturdy frame that keeps the soft tissues, like skin and fat, lifted and taut—like a queen-sized quilt perfectly placed on a queen-sized bed. Everything is in balance.

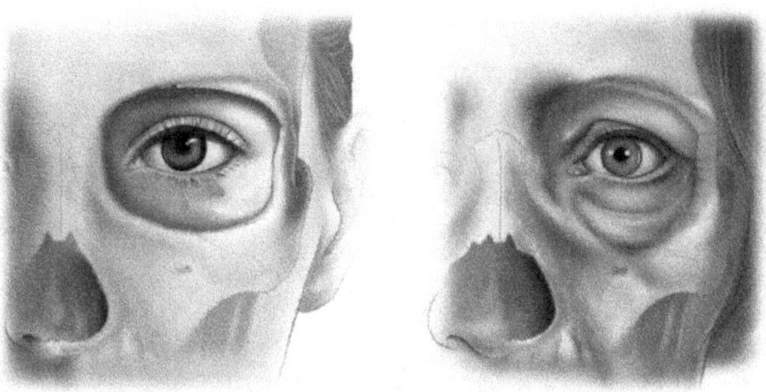

Orbital ageing. The superomedial and inferolateral aspects of the orbit have the greatest tendency to resorb. This contributes to the stigmata of periorbital ageing such as increased prominence of the medial fat pad, elevation of the medial brow, and langthening of the lid cheek junction.

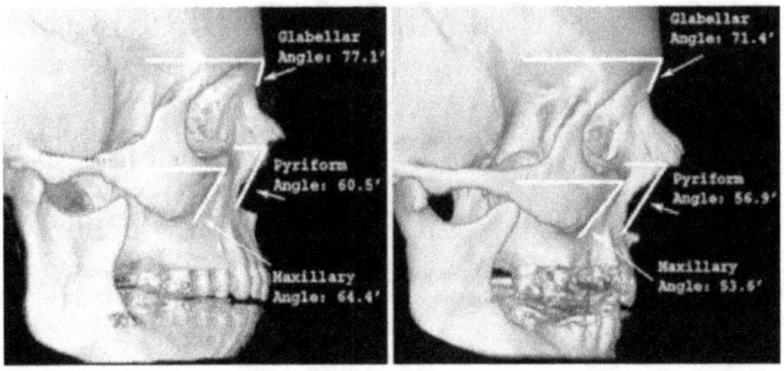

The piriform (piriform angle) and the maxilla (maxillary angle) significantly recede with ageing, from youth (left) to old age (right)

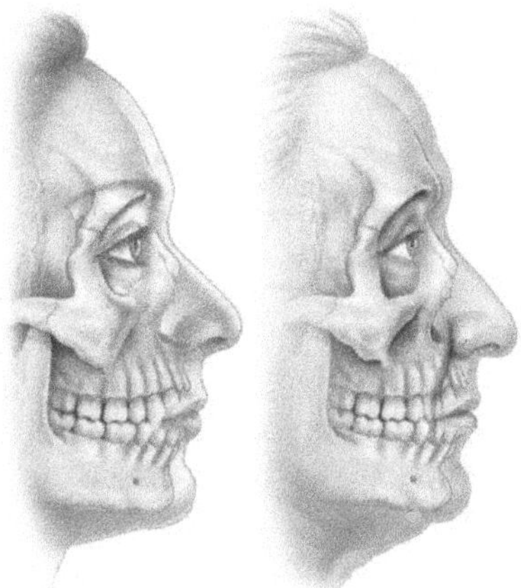

The Loss of bone in the pyriform area weakens the support of the lateral crura. Deepening of the maxilla results in posterior positioning of the nasolabial crease and adjacent upper lip.

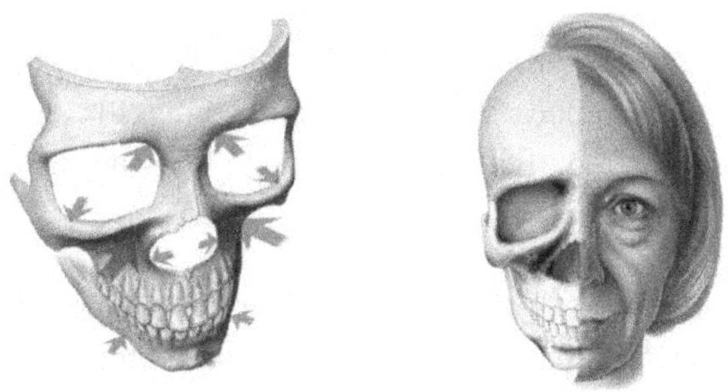

(image left) Arrows indicate the areas of the facial skeleton susceptible to resorption with ageing. The size of the arrow correlates with the amount of resorption.

(Image right) The Darker areas are those of the greatest bone loss. The stigmata of ageing , manifested by the facial soft tissues, corresponds with the areas of weakened skeletal support.

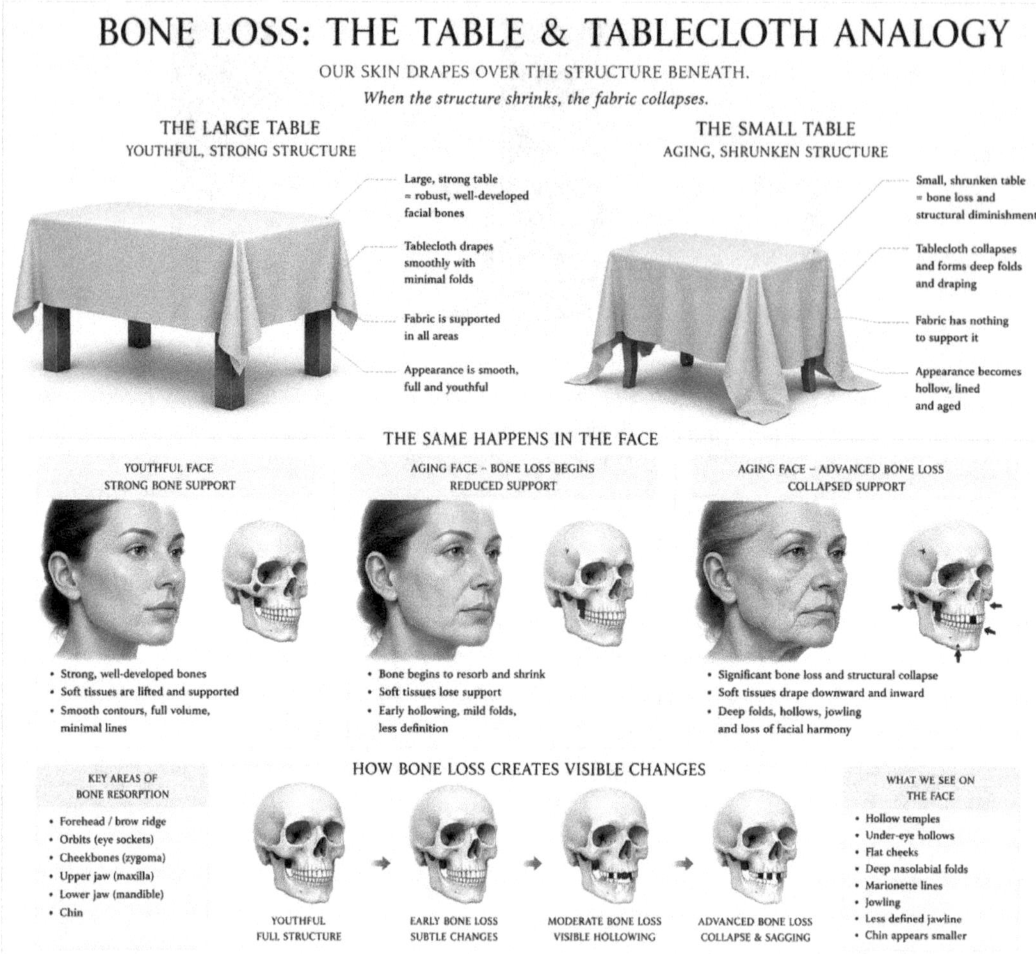

The 30s and 40s: The Beginning of Bone Loss

As we enter our 30s, bone resorption subtly begins. The orbits (eye sockets) start to enlarge, causing the eyes to appear more sunken. The maxilla (midface bone) recedes slightly, making the cheeks look flatter. The jawbone loses density, softening the once-defined jawline.

The chin and mouth area also start to change. The bone supporting the lips recedes, which can make the mouth appear smaller and less structured. This contributes to the development of marionette lines (the lines running from the corners of the mouth downward) and a less defined chin.

Think of it like slightly deflating a balloon—it's not drastic yet, but the structure is starting to weaken. This is when early signs of ageing start to appear, like under-eye hollows, nasolabial folds (smile lines), and a less-defined jawline.

The 50s and Beyond: The Skull Shrinks, The Face Falls

Now the changes become more obvious. The skull has further resorbed, especially in key areas:

Eye sockets: Widen and deepen, making eyes look hollow and tired.

Cheekbones: Flatten further, contributing to sagging skin.

Jawbone: Becomes smaller and less structured, leading to jowls and a receding chin.

Nasal bone: Shrinks slightly, altering the nose shape and making it appear more prominent.

Chin and mouth: The bone surrounding the mouth recedes further, leading to a loss of lip support, increased wrinkling around the mouth, and a downturn of the lips, giving a more aged or sad appearance.

Remember that queen-sized quilt? Imagine putting it on a double bed. Suddenly, it looks oversized and droopy. This is what happens to our face—the skin, muscles, and fat pads no longer fit snugly over the shrinking bone, leading to sagging, folds, and wrinkles.

Why This Matters in Aesthetics

Understanding the role of bone in ageing is crucial when considering cosmetic treatments. Many people think fillers and injectables only address the skin, but the goal is actually to restore the underlying structure.

For example:

Temple and cheek fillers help replace lost volume where bone has resorbed, lifting the face naturally.
Jawline contouring restores definition lost due to bone shrinkage.
Under-eye fillers compensate for the widening of the eye sockets, reducing hollows and shadows.
Chin and lip fillers help restore structure and support lost due to bone resorption, improving lip definition and mouth contour.
Modern aesthetics isn't about just chasing lines and wrinkles—it's about rebuilding the foundation.

Conclusion: The Secret to a Youthful Face?

A youthful appearance isn't just about good skin; it's about a strong, structured base. Bone loss is a natural part of ageing, but understanding it allows us to make more informed decisions about aesthetic treatments. So next time you look in the mirror, remember—it's not just about what's on the surface. The real secret to beauty lies beneath.

Chapter 25: Arteries and Veins of the Face

Understanding the Highways Beneath the Skin

One of the most important responsibilities of any cosmetic injector is understanding the vascular anatomy of the face. Beneath the skin lies an intricate network of arteries and veins carrying oxygen, nutrients, and blood to every structure of the face. These vessels are not just anatomy textbook material. They are the difference between a safe treatment and a potentially devastating complication. When we inject fillers, biostimulants, or even perform certain skin procedures, we are working around these vascular pathways constantly. Knowing where they travel, how deep they sit, and where danger zones exist is essential for safe aesthetic practice.

The face is highly vascular because it requires an enormous blood supply to support facial expression, skin health, healing, temperature regulation, and the delicate structures of the eyes, nose, lips, and brain connections.

Arteries carry oxygenated blood away from the heart into the face. Veins return deoxygenated blood back toward the heart. While both are important, arteries are the vessels injectors fear most because accidental injection into an artery can obstruct blood flow and cause tissue death or blindness.

The Major Arteries of the Face

Facial Artery: The facial artery is one of the most important arteries in aesthetic medicine.

It branches from the external carotid artery and travels upward along the side of the mouth toward the nose and inner eye.

It typically: Crosses the jawline just in front of the masseter muscle, Travels beside the nasolabial fold, Gives branches to the lips and nose, Continues upward as the angular artery

This artery can be tortuous and variable, meaning it twists and changes position from person to person. This is why the nasolabial fold and lower face require careful injecting.

Angular Artery: The angular artery is the terminal branch of the facial artery. It runs beside the nose toward the inner corner of the eye.

Location: Side of the nose, Medial cheek, Inner canthus area

This is one of the highest-risk areas for vascular occlusion because of connections to the ophthalmic artery and retinal circulation.

Superior and Inferior Labial Arteries: These arteries supply the lips.

Location: Run within the upper and lower lips, Usually sit deep within the wet-dry border region, Course horizontally from the corners toward the centre

Lip injections require extreme care because these vessels can vary greatly between individuals.

Dorsal Nasal Artery: This artery supplies the bridge and tip of the nose.

Location: Along the nasal dorsum, Connected to ophthalmic circulation

The nose is considered one of the most dangerous areas for filler because of limited collateral circulation and direct links to vessels supplying the eye.

Supratrochlear Artery: This artery emerges from the orbit and travels upward through the forehead.

Location: Medial forehead, Between the brows moving upward

This vessel is relevant in glabella and forehead injections.

Supraorbital Artery: This artery exits through the supraorbital notch and supplies the forehead and scalp.

Location: Upper orbital rim, Central forehead

Often found approximately in line with the pupil.

Temporal Artery (Superficial Temporal Artery): This artery supplies the temple and scalp.

Location: Side of the forehead, Temple region above the zygomatic arch

Temple filler requires anatomical precision because vessels here can sit superficially.

Transverse Facial Artery: This artery runs horizontally across the cheek.

Location: Below the zygomatic arch, Across the lateral cheek

It supplies the cheek tissues and parotid region.

Infraorbital Artery: This artery exits through the infraorbital foramen.

Location: Under-eye region, Mid-cheek

Important in tear trough and midface treatments.

Mental Artery: The mental artery exits from the mental foramen.

Location: Chin region, Lower lip and chin area

Relevant in chin augmentation procedures.

DANGER ZONES: FACIAL ARTERIES

KNOW THE ARTERIES. RESPECT THE FLOW. PROTECT THE PATIENT.

Accidental arterial injection can lead to vascular occlusion, tissue ischemia, necrosis, or even blindness. Always use aspiration, inject slowly, know your anatomy, and avoid high-risk zones.

KEY

- **HIGH RISK** (Avoid Injection)
- **MODERATE RISK** (Use Caution)
- **LOWER RISK BRANCHES** (Small Caliber)

1 SUPRAORBITAL ARTERY
Terminal branch of the ophthalmic artery.
Emerges from the orbit through the supraorbital foramen/notch.
Supplies the forehead and scalp.
Risk: Blindness, skin necrosis.

2 SUPRATROCHLEAR ARTERY
Terminal branch of the ophthalmic artery.
Emerges from the orbit medial to the supraorbital artery.
Supplies the medial forehead and glabella.
Risk: Skin necrosis, visual loss.

3 DORSAL NASAL ARTERY
Branch of the ophthalmic artery.
Runs down the dorsum of the nose.
Anastomoses with the angular artery.
Risk: Skin necrosis.

4 ANGULAR ARTERY
Terminal branch of the facial artery.
Ascends along the side of the nose.
Anastomoses with the dorsal nasal and infraorbital arteries.
Risk: Skin necrosis.

5 INFRAORBITAL ARTERY
Branch of the maxillary artery.
Exits the infraorbital foramen to supply the lower eyelid, nose, upper lip.
Risk: Skin necrosis, visual complications.

6 FACIAL ARTERY
Main arterial supply to the face.
Courses along the mandible, crossing the inferior border.
Gives multiple branches to the face.
Risk: Skin necrosis.

7 SUPERFICIAL TEMPORAL ARTERY
Branch of the external carotid artery.
Runs within the superficial temporal fascia, anterior to the ear.
Risk: Scalp necrosis.

8 MENTAL ARTERY
Branch of the inferior alveolar artery.
Exits the mental foramen to supply the chin and lower lip.
Risk: Lip/chin ischemia.

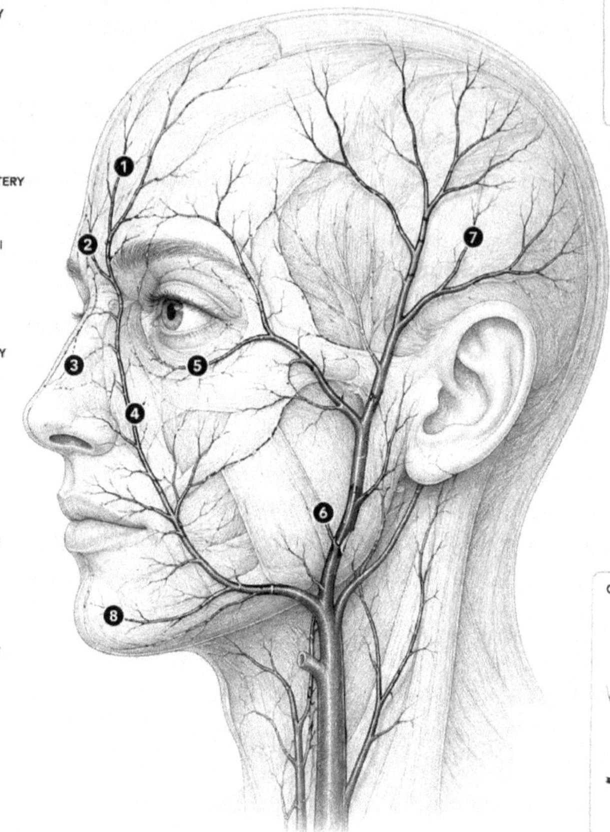

ARTERIAL SOURCES

EXTERNAL CAROTID ARTERY

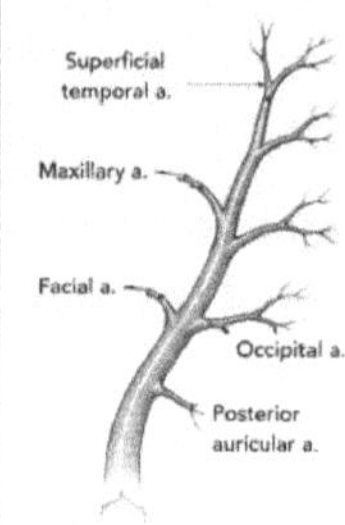

COMMON CAROTID ARTERY

OPHTHALMIC ARTERY BRANCHES

(Internal Carotid System)

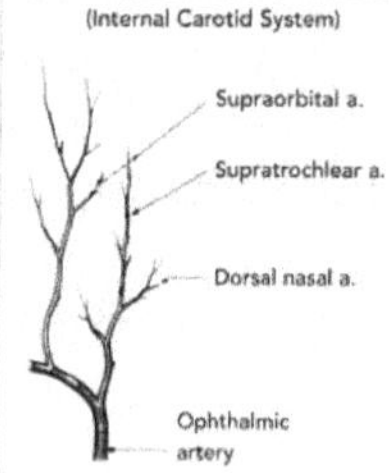

MAJOR ANASTOMOSES (COMMUNICATIONS)

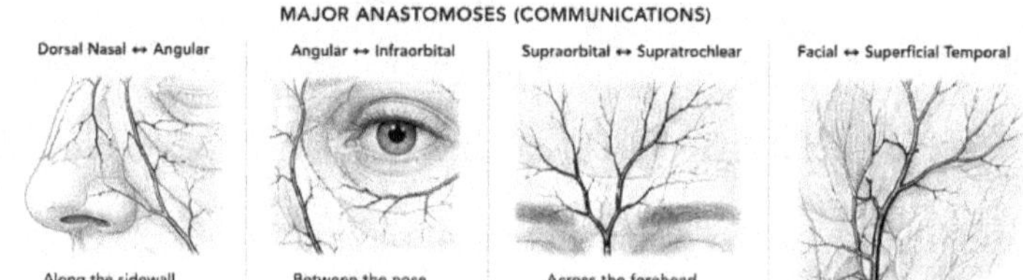

Dorsal Nasal ↔ Angular: Along the sidewall and tip of the nose.

Angular ↔ Infraorbital: Between the nose and lower eyelid.

Supraorbital ↔ Supratrochlear: Across the forehead and glabella.

Facial ↔ Superficial Temporal

POTENTIAL COMPLICATIONS

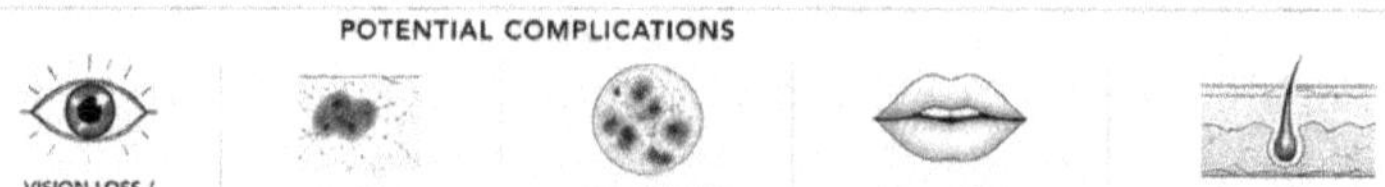

- **VISION LOSS / BLINDNESS** From retrograde flow into the ophthalmic artery.
- **SKIN ISCHEMIA** Reduced blood flow to skin and soft tissue.
- **TISSUE NECROSIS** Progression to ulceration and scarring.
- **LIP / CHIN ISCHEMIA** Pain, blanching, ulceration, necrosis.
- **SCALP NECROSIS** From compromise of the superficial temporal artery.

The Major Veins of the Face

Facial veins are thinner-walled and more variable than arteries. Although venous injection is usually less catastrophic than arterial injection, veins can still contribute to bruising, swelling, and vascular complications.

Facial Vein

The facial vein travels alongside parts of the facial artery but is generally straighter and deeper.

Location: Side of nose, Cheek, Jawline

It drains blood from much of the face.

Angular Vein

Located beside the nose and connected to veins around the eye.

Importance:
This vein communicates with deeper orbital veins and indirectly with the cavernous sinus inside the skull.

This anatomical connection explains why infections in the "danger triangle" of the face historically carried serious risks.

Retromandibular Vein

Located near the parotid gland and jaw.

Superficial Temporal Vein

Runs through the temple and scalp region alongside the superficial temporal artery.

Supraorbital and Supratrochlear Veins

Drain the forehead and upper facial region.

External Jugular Vein

Drains portions of the face and neck into larger cervical circulation.

High-Risk Injection Zones

Some areas of the face carry greater vascular risk because arteries are superficial, tightly confined, or connected to the eye circulation.

These include: Glabella, Nose, Nasolabial folds, Tear troughs, Temple, Lips

Understanding vascular depth is just as important as knowing the vessel name. In some areas vessels lie deep on bone, while in others they become superficial within fat compartments.

Why Anatomy Knowledge Matters

Good aesthetic medicine is not simply about placing product. It is about understanding living anatomy beneath the skin.

Every injector should know:

- Where vessels emerge from foramina
- Which areas have limited collateral circulation
- Which arteries communicate with the ophthalmic system
- How ageing changes vascular position
- How previous surgery or filler alters anatomy

A beautiful result means nothing if safety is compromised.

The more experienced I become, the more respect I have for anatomy. The face is not just skin and wrinkles. It is a sophisticated map of vessels, nerves, muscles, ligaments, fat pads, and emotion all layered together.

As injectors, we are not merely treating lines. We are navigating living anatomy millimetre by millimetre..

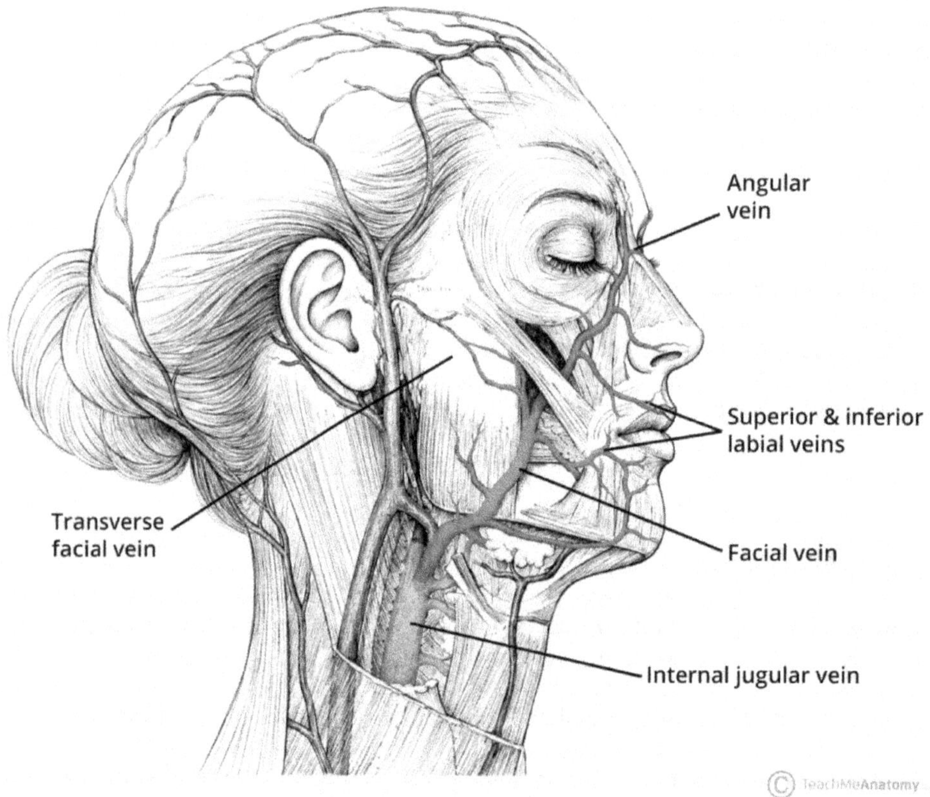

Chapter 26: Facial Nerves: The Body's Electrical Wiring

One of the most important subjects for any injector to understand is the nerve anatomy of the face.

While much attention is given to blood vessels and avoiding vascular complications, nerves are equally important. They control facial expression, provide sensation, allow us to smile, frown, blink, chew, and feel touch, temperature, and pain.

I often describe nerves as the body's electrical wiring system. They carry messages between the brain and the face. Some nerves make muscles move, while others allow us to feel.

For cosmetic injectors, understanding where these nerves travel is essential. It improves assessment, helps avoid complications, and allows us to provide effective pain relief during treatments.

The Two Types of Facial Nerves

Facial nerves can be divided into two major groups:

Motor Nerves

Motor nerves control movement.

These nerves tell muscles when to contract and relax. Every smile, frown, blink, kiss, and raised eyebrow is controlled by motor nerves.

When we inject botulinum toxin, we are not targeting the nerve itself. We are targeting the muscle that receives messages from the nerve. The toxin temporarily blocks the communication between the nerve ending and the muscle, reducing movement.

Sensory Nerves

Sensory nerves allow us to feel. They carry information from the skin, lips, nose, cheeks, and forehead back to the brain.

Without sensory nerves we would not feel: Touch, Pressure, Temperature, Pain, Vibration

These are the nerves we target when performing local anaesthetic blocks before procedures.

The Facial Nerve

(Cranial Nerve VII)

The facial nerve is the primary motor nerve of the face.

After leaving the skull near the ear, it travels through the parotid gland and divides into five major branches.

A useful memory aid is:

"To Zanzibar By Motor Car"

- Temporal, Zygomatic, Buccal, Marginal Mandibular, Cervical

These branches control the muscles of facial expression.

1. Temporal Branch

Travels upward toward the forehead.

Controls: Frontalis muscle, Upper orbicularis oculi, Corrugator muscles

Functions: Raising the eyebrows, Wrinkling the forehead, Frowning

Damage may result in: Brow droop , Forehead asymmetry, Difficulty raising the eyebrow

2. Zygomatic Branch

Travels across the cheekbone.

Controls: Orbicularis oculi

Functions: Blinking, Closing the eyes, Squinting

Damage may result in: Inability to close the eye completely, Dry eye symptoms

3. Buccal Branch

Crosses the mid-cheek.

Controls: Buccinator, Upper lip elevators, Nasal muscles

Functions: Smiling, Showing teeth, Puffing out the cheeks

Damage may result in: Uneven smile, Difficulty eating or drinking

4. Marginal Mandibular Branch

Travels along the jawline.

Controls: Depressor anguli oris (DAO), Depressor labii inferioris, Mentalis

Functions: Lower lip movement, Expression of sadness, Mouth symmetry

Damage may result in: Crooked smile, Lower lip weakness

This is one of the branches injectors must be particularly aware of when treating the jawline.

5. Cervical Branch

Travels into the neck.

Controls: Platysma muscle

Functions: Neck bands, Lower facial pull

This nerve becomes relevant when treating platysmal bands and lower face rejuvenation.

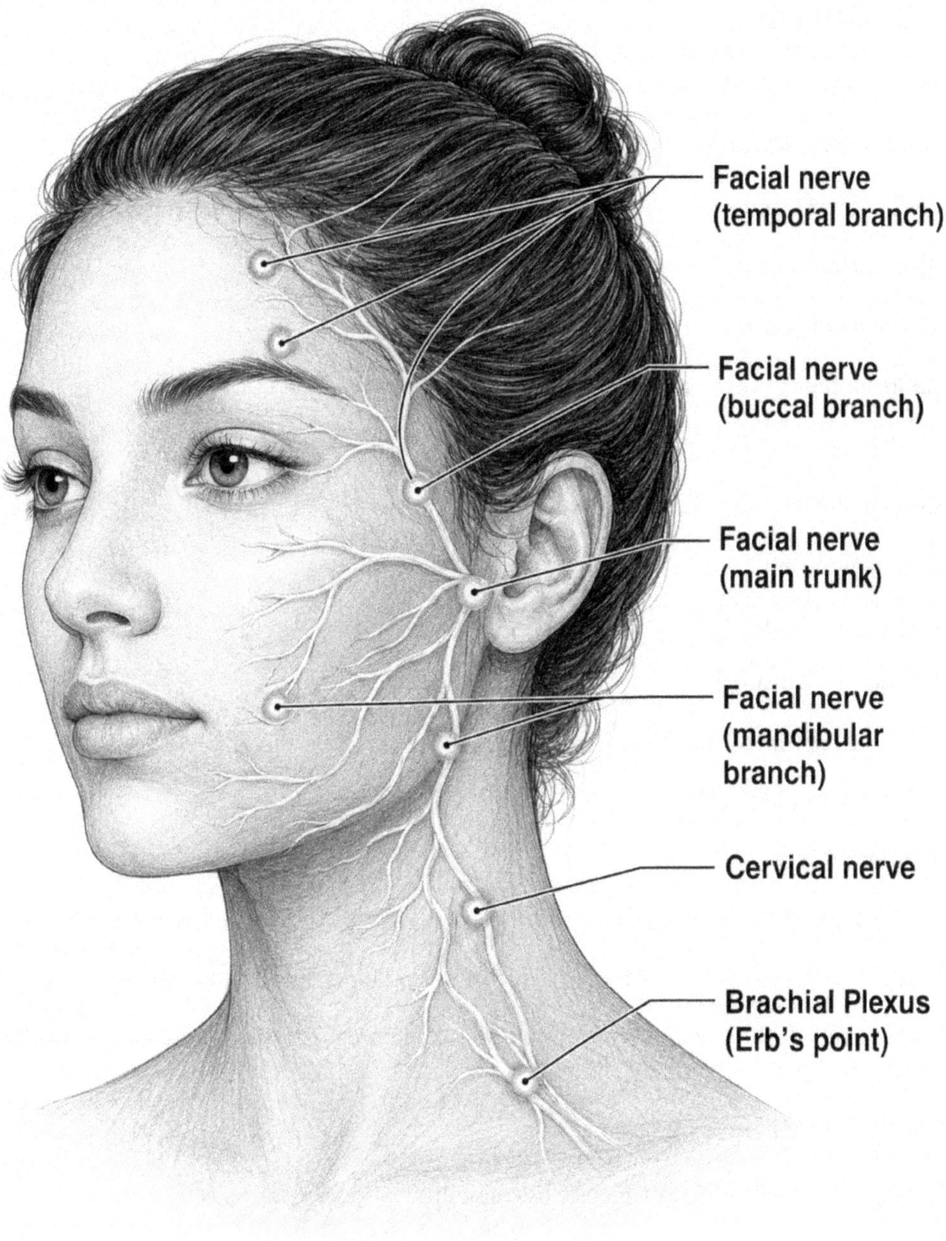

The Trigeminal Nerve

(Cranial Nerve V)

The trigeminal nerve is the major sensory nerve of the face.

Almost all facial sensation comes from this nerve.

It divides into three branches:

1. Ophthalmic (V1)
2. Maxillary (V2)
3. Mandibular (V3)

Think of these as three major sensory highways supplying the face.

Ophthalmic Branch (V1)

Supplies sensation to: Forehead, Scalp, Upper eyelids, Bridge of the nose

Major branches include:

Supraorbital Nerve

Exits from the supraorbital notch above the eyebrow.

Provides sensation to: Forehead, Frontal scalp

Supratrochlear Nerve

Provides sensation to: Central forehead, Glabella region

These nerves are often involved in forehead procedures.

Maxillary Branch (V2)

Supplies sensation to: Midface, Lower eyelid, Nose, Upper lip, Cheeks

Major branches include:

Infraorbital Nerve

Exits through the infraorbital foramen approximately 7–10 mm below the orbital rim.

Provides sensation to: Lower eyelid, Side of nose, Upper lip, Central cheek

This is one of the most commonly blocked nerves for pain control in aesthetic procedures.

Mandibular Branch (V3)

Supplies sensation to: Lower face, Chin, Jawline

Major branches include:

Mental Nerve

Exits through the mental foramen in the lower jaw.

Provides sensation to: Chin, Lower lip

This nerve is frequently targeted when treating lips and chin areas.

Nerve Blocks in Aesthetic Medicine

One of the best ways to improve patient comfort is through nerve blocks.

Rather than injecting anaesthetic repeatedly throughout the treatment area, we can numb an entire region by depositing local anaesthetic near a sensory nerve.

When performed correctly, patients often experience minimal discomfort.

Supraorbital Nerve Block

Used for: Forehead procedures, PRP, Skin treatments Forehead filler dissolving

Area numbed: Forehead, Anterior scalp

Infraorbital Nerve Block

Used for: Upper lip treatments, Midface procedures, Nasolabial folds

Area numbed: Upper lip, Side of nose, Central cheek

Mental Nerve Block

Used for: Lower lip treatments, Chin treatments, Marionette lines

Area numbed: Chin, Lower lip

Greater Palatine Block

Used for: Lip augmentation

Anaesthetic is placed inside the mouth near the palate.

Provides profound numbness of: Upper lip

Many experienced lip injectors favour this technique because it produces excellent anaesthesia without distorting the lips.

Why Nerve Anatomy Matters

A thorough understanding of facial nerve anatomy improves both safety and outcomes.

Motor nerves allow us to assess muscle function, understand facial movement patterns, and perform botulinum toxin treatments more accurately.

Sensory nerves help us manage patient comfort through targeted anaesthesia and assist in recognising nerve-related complications should they occur.

The more you understand facial nerves, the more confidently you can assess, treat, and care for your patients.

After all, behind every expression, every smile, every blink, and every sensation lies an intricate network of nerves silently carrying messages between the face and the brain. Understanding that network is one of the foundations of safe and effective aesthetic practice.

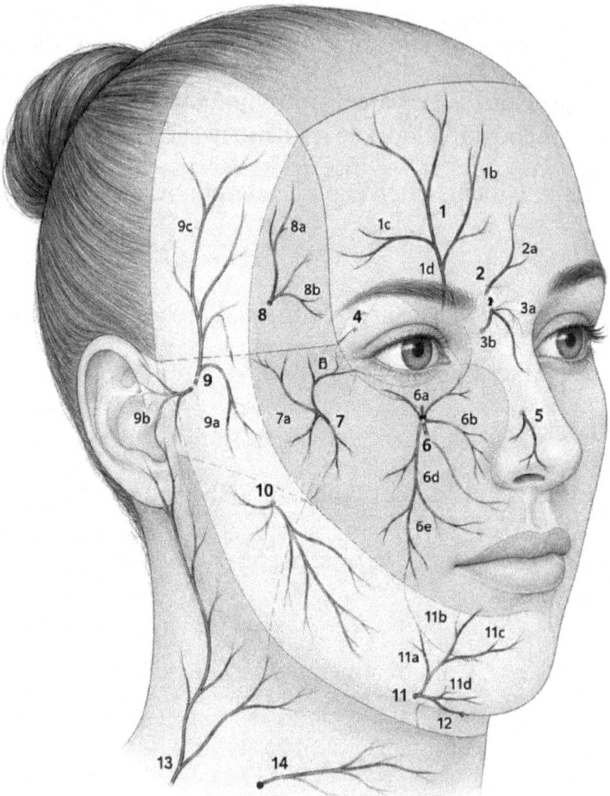

Illustration of the cutaneous, sensory nerves of the face. 1 = supraorbital nerve (1 a = medial branch, 1 b = lateral branch, 1 c = horizontal branch, 1 d = palpebral branches); 2 = supratrochlear nerve (2 a = forehead branches, 2 b = palpebral branch); 3 = infratrochlear nerve (3 a = nasal branches, 3 b = palpebral branch); 4 = palpebral branches of lacrimal nerve; 5 = external nasal branch of anterior ethmoidal nerve; 6 = infraorbital nerve (6 a = inferior palpebral branches, 6 b = external nasal branch, 6 c = internal nasal branch, 6 d = medial branch of superior labial branch, 6 e = lateral branch of superior labial branch); 7 = zygomaticofacial nerve (7 a = zygomatic branch, 7 b = palpebral branch); 8 = zygomaticotemporal nerve (8 a = temporal branches, 8 b = palpebral branch); 9 = auriculotemporal nerve (9 a = zygomatic branches, 9 b = auricular branches, 9 c = temporal branches); 10 = long buccal nerve; 11 = mental nerve (11 a = angular branch, 11 b = lateral labial branch, 11 c = medial labial branch, 11 d = mental branch); 12 = mental branch of mylohyoid nerve; 13 = great auricular nerve; 14 = transverse cervical nerve

Chapter 27: Lymphatic Anatomy & Facial Puffiness

The Lymphatic System

Why the Face Becomes Puffy and What You Can Do About It

One of the most overlooked systems in facial ageing and facial appearance is the lymphatic system.

Many people assume facial fullness is always fat or ageing, when often it is fluid retention, inflammation or sluggish lymphatic drainage. Understanding the lymphatic system is important not only for consumers, but also for aesthetic practitioners assessing facial puffiness, heaviness and inflammation.

What Is the Lymphatic System?

The lymphatic system is the body's drainage and waste removal network.

It consists of: Lymph fluid, Lymph vessels, Lymph nodes

Its role is to:

- Remove waste products, Remove excess fluid
- Help immune function, Reduce inflammation, Support circulation.

Unlike the blood circulation system, the lymphatic system does not have a pump like the heart.

It relies on:

- Muscle movement, Breathing, Massage, Body movement , Manual stimulation

When lymphatic flow becomes sluggish, fluid can accumulate in the tissues — particularly in the face and under-eye area.

Why Does the Face Become Puffy?

Puffiness can occur for many reasons.

Common Causes of Facial Puffiness

Fluid Retention Excess salt, alcohol, poor sleep and hormonal fluctuations can all increase water retention.
Inflammation: Inflammation from stress, allergies, poor diet or illness may cause swelling in the face.
Poor Lymphatic Drainage When lymphatic flow slows down, fluid stagnates within the tissues.
Lack of Sleep Tiredness often shows first around the eyes.

Allergies and Sinus Congestion These can create swelling and heaviness around the eyes and cheeks.
Crying Emotional tears often leave fluid trapped around the delicate eye area.
Heat and Hormones Hormonal fluctuations and hot weather can worsen swelling.
Cosmetic Treatments After injectables, surgery or some energy-based treatments, temporary swelling is common.

Areas Most Affected

The face commonly retains fluid in: Under-eye area, Jawline, Jowls, Cheeks Around the nose, Neck

Some people wake with a noticeably swollen face in the morning that improves throughout the day as movement stimulates drainage.

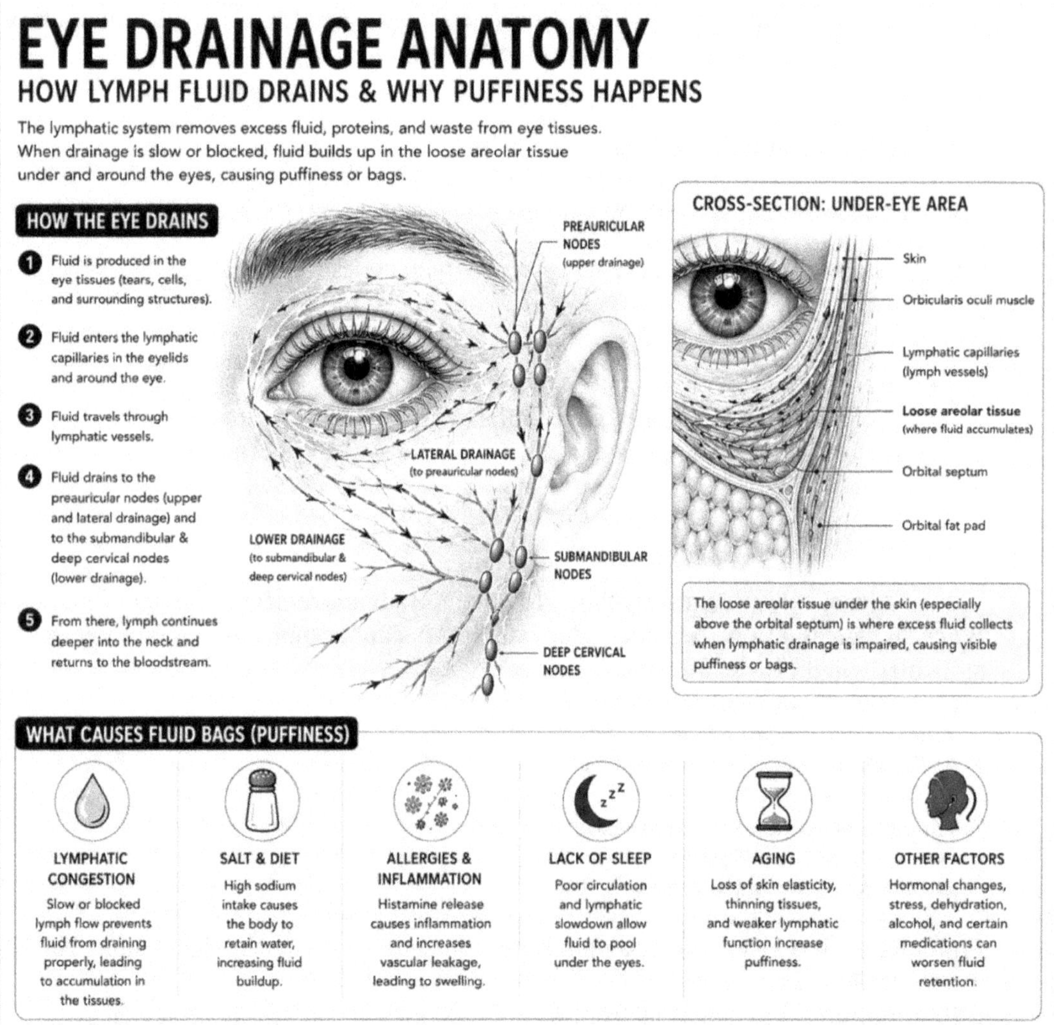

Signs of Sluggish Lymphatic Drainage

- Puffy eyes, Heavy-looking face
- Morning facial swelling, Soft jawline definition
- Fluid pockets under eyes
- Feeling "inflamed"
- Skin looking dull or congested

How to Improve Lymphatic Drainage

Small daily rituals can make a visible difference.

Consistency is more important than intensity.

Facial Massage

Gentle facial massage encourages movement of lymphatic fluid.

Always massage:

- Upward, Outward
- Then down the sides of the neck toward the collarbone

The neck is important because this is where lymphatic drainage pathways empty.

Use gentle pressure only. The lymphatic vessels sit very close to the surface of the skin.

Daily Gua Sha Stone Massage

A gua sha stone is one of my favourite tools for lymphatic drainage.

The curved edges fit beautifully around: Jawline, Cheekbones, Neck, Under-eye area

Used regularly, it may help:

- Reduce puffiness, Encourage drainage
- Improve circulation, Relax facial tension
- Create a more sculpted appearance

Apply facial oil first.

I personally like: Argan Oil, Castor Oil

Never drag a gua sha stone over dry skin.

Morning and night use can become a calming self-care ritual.

Ice Rollers

Ice rollers have become extremely popular and can feel wonderful first thing in the morning.

Cooling the skin may temporarily:

- Reduce swelling, Tighten superficial blood vessels
- Refresh tired eyes, Wake up the skin

Roll gently over:

- Under eyes, Jawline, Cheeks, Forehead

Always move outward and downward toward drainage points.

Many people keep their ice rollers in the fridge.

The Ice Water Bowl Trick

One old beauty trick that still works beautifully is the ice water bowl ritual.

Fill a bowl with: Cold water, Ice cubes

Then briefly immerse the face for a few seconds.

This may:

- Wake up the skin, Reduce morning puffiness
- Tighten the appearance of pores, Refresh tired eyes

It is simple, inexpensive and surprisingly effective.

Ice Cubes in a Soft Towel

Another easy home remedy is wrapping ice cubes in a soft towel or cloth and gently pressing around: Eyes, Cheeks, Jawline

Never place ice directly onto the skin for prolonged periods.

Cold therapy can temporarily reduce swelling and help the face feel firmer and fresher.

Lifestyle Tips for Puffiness

Sometimes the simplest changes make the biggest difference.

Helpful habits include:

- Drinking enough water, Reducing excess salt
- Limiting alcohol, Improving sleep
- Manageing stress, Regular movement and exercise
- Treating allergies if present

Aesthetic Perspective

As injectors, it is important to recognise the difference between:

- Fluid retention, Fat pads
- Structural ageing, Skin laxity

Not every "heavy face" requires filler.

Sometimes improving lymphatic flow, reducing inflammation and addressing lifestyle factors creates a fresher and more natural result than adding more volume.

Natural beauty is not always about adding — sometimes it is about reducing stagnation and restoring flow.

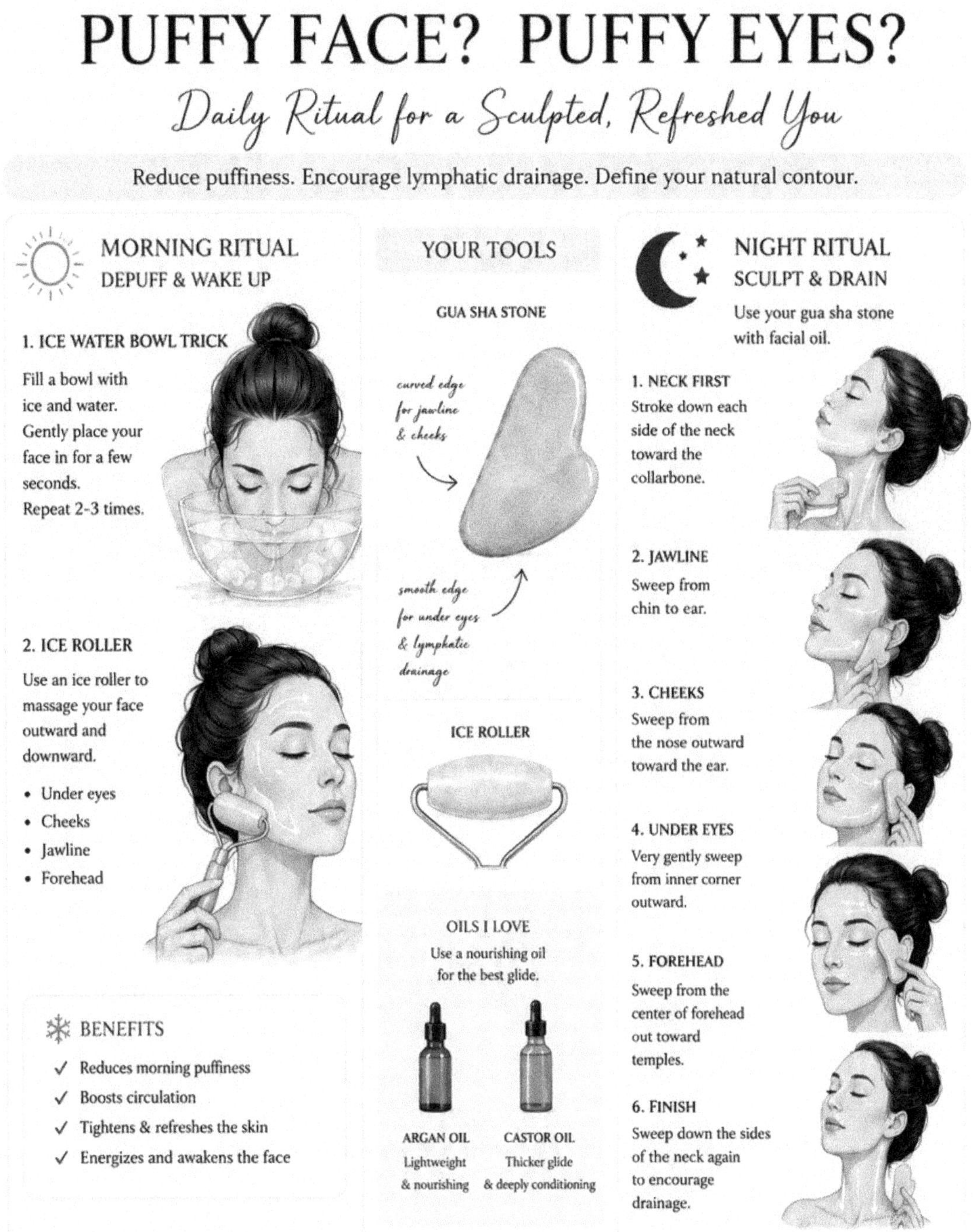

PUFFY FACE? PUFFY EYES?
Daily Ritual for a Sculpted, Refreshed You
Reduce puffiness. Encourage lymphatic drainage. Define your natural contour.
MORNING RITUAL
DEPUFF & WAKE UP
1. ICE WATER BOWL TRICK
Fill a bowl with ice and water. Gently place your face in for a few seconds. Repeat 2-3 times.
2. ICE ROLLER
Use an ice roller to massage your face outward and downward.
• Under eyes
• Cheeks
• Jawline
• Forehead
BENEFITS
✓ Reduces morning puffiness
✓ Boosts circulation
✓ Tightens & refreshes the skin
✓ Energizes and awakens the face
YOUR TOOLS
GUA SHA STONE
curved edge for jawline & cheeks
smooth edge for under eyes & lymphatic drainage
ICE ROLLER
OILS I LOVE
Use a nourishing oil for the best glide.
ARGAN OIL
Lightweight & nourishing
CASTOR OIL
Thicker glide & deeply conditioning
NIGHT RITUAL
SCULPT & DRAIN
Use your gua sha stone with facial oil.
1. NECK FIRST
Stroke down each side of the neck toward the collarbone.
2. JAWLINE
Sweep from chin to ear.
3. CHEEKS
Sweep from the nose outward toward the ear.
4. UNDER EYES
Very gently sweep from inner corner outward.
5. FOREHEAD
Sweep from the center of forehead out toward temples.
6. FINISH
Sweep down the sides of the neck again to encourage drainage.

Part 3- Facial Ageing by Region

Chapter 28: Wrinkles, Lines And Folds

Let's face it-lines happen. We smile, we squint, we sleep (hopefully), and our faces keep score. But not all lines are created equal. In this chapter, we'll decode the different types of wrinkles, what causes them, and what can be done-clinically and cleverly-to soften or even erase their presence.

Dynamic Lines: The Lines of Expression These are the first ones to show up, often while you're still young and animated. They're called dynamic because they appear with movement-when you frown, laugh, or raise your brows.

Forehead lines: Those horizontal "surprise!" lines from raising your eyebrows.- Glabellar lines (the '11s'): Between the brows-thanks, frowning.- Crow's feet: The fan of fine lines at the outer corners of the eyes from smiling or squinting.

Treatment: These respond beautifully to wrinkle relaxers like Botox, Dysport, or Xeomin. By calming the muscles, you soften the lines-and yes, you can still express yourself (just minus the furrows).

Static Lines: When They Stick Around Over time, dynamic lines become static-meaning they're visible even when your face is resting. But wait, there's more: We also develop sleep lines, those vertical creases that have nothing to do with emotion and everything to do with how you face-plant your pillow.

Sleep Lines: The Quiet Saboteurs- Common spots: Between the brows, across the top lip, along the cheeks, and the dreaded marionette lines.- They often appear worse on one side-yes, the side you sleep on.- Tip: If you're married, it's usually the side facing away from your husband (insert dramatic sigh here).

These lines don't respond well to wrinkle relaxers, because they're not caused by movement-they're etched into your skin like creases in satin from years of being smooshed into a pillow.

Line Work: Filling in the Story When relaxers can't help, dermal fillers step in. But not just any filler-you need one that's soft, flexible, and designed for fine superficial lines.

Top Products for Line Work:

Teosyal RHA 1: A standout for treating fine lines thanks to its high stretch and low viscosity. Great around the lips and eyes.

Belotero Balance: Excellent for feathering into superficial lines without Tyndall effect.

Restylane Fynesse or Vital Light: Especially helpful for crepey areas with fine etched lines.

Juvéderm Volbella (used lightly): Can work under the eyes or lips with caution.

NCTF 135 HA (for skin quality): Not a filler per se, but supports hydration and fine line softening.

The Fern Technique:

One of the most refined approaches to line work is the fern technique, developed to mimic the natural direction of collagen and elastin fibers in the dermis. The injector creates tiny, branching lines of filler-like fern leaves-along the wrinkle's path.

This technique disperses the filler in a way that supports the skin without creating bulk. It works especially well for smokers' lines, accordion lines, and sleep creases, particularly around the top lip, chin, and cheeks. It's delicate work-think calligraphy for the face-and best done with soft fillers like RHA 1 or Belotero Soft. It requires finesse, and not all injectors are trained in this technique, so always seek out someone experienced.

Takeaway Tips:

Relaxers work best for movement lines-get in early before they etch in.

Fillers are for lines that don't move but refuse to leave.

Soft, stretchy fillers and techniques like the fern method offer natural results when done right.

And yes-how you sleep matters. A silk pillowcase helps, but maybe don't roll away from your spouse every single night.

Sleep Smart, Not Scrunched

Want to reduce those pesky sleep lines? Try this:

Place a pillow under your knees and a travel pillow under your neck—you'll feel like you're in a side-sleeping, fetal position, but you're actually on your back. This position is surprisingly comfortable and reduces pressure on your face.

If you must sleep on your side, use a C-shaped travel pillow and rest your face in the open space. Your cheek stays free-floating—not squished—helping prevent those deep creases from forming overnight.

Facial Folds

One of the biggest mistakes in aesthetics is treating folds as if they are simply lines in the skin.

Most folds are actually signs of deeper structural ageing.

As we age, the face undergoes gradual changes involving:

- Bone resorption, Fat pad shrinkage, Ligament tightening
- Collagen loss, Skin thinning, Muscle imbalance, Tissue descent

The fold is usually the visible symptom — not the true cause.

Beautiful rejuvenation comes from understanding what has been lost underneath the skin.

The Nasojugal Fold (Tear Trough)

What Is It?

The nasojugal fold is the hollow running from the inner corner of the eye diagonally into the upper cheek.

It is commonly called the tear trough.

When this area deepens it can create:

- Tired-looking eyes, Hollowing, Dark shadows
- Puffiness beside hollowness, An aged or exhausted appearance

What Causes It?

The under-eye area is one of the thinnest and most delicate areas of the face.

The fold develops due to:

- Orbital bone resorption, Shrinkage of deep medial cheek fat
- Tightening of retaining ligaments, Skin thinning, Collagen loss, Tissue descent
- Lymphatic congestion and fluid retention

The supporting structures underneath the eye gradually weaken and shrink.

How to Treat It

One of the biggest mistakes is placing large amounts of filler directly into the tear trough.

This may create:

- Puffiness, Swelling, Water retention
- Migration, A heavy under-eye appearance

The key is to support the surrounding structures first.

Treatment may include:

- Deep medial cheek support, Zygomatic support
- Conservative tear trough filler, Biostimulators such as CaHA or Sculptra
- PRP and skin boosters, Skin tightening procedures
- Improving lymphatic drainage

Sometimes less filler under the eye creates the most natural and youthful result.

The Nasolabial Fold (NLF)

What Is It?

The nasolabial fold is the crease running from the side of the nose toward the corner of the mouth.

Everyone has nasolabial folds, but ageing causes them to deepen and become heavier.

What Causes It?

The fold itself is usually not the real problem.

The deeper issue is loss of structural support in the midface.

Contributors include:

- Maxillary bone resorption, Pyriform aperture shrinkage
- Deep cheek fat loss, Midface descent
- Ligament contraction, Skin laxity
- Repetitive facial movement

As the cheek loses support and volume, the tissues descend downward and inward, creating a heavier fold.

How to Treat It

Overfilling the fold directly can create:

- Puffiness around the mouth
- Heaviness, A bulky lower face
- Filler build-up over time, Distortion when smiling

The better approach is restoring the structures that have shrunk first.

Treatment may include:

- Structural cheek support, Pyriform support
- Midface restoration, Collagen stimulation
- Biostimulators, Skin tightening treatments
- Conservative filler in the fold only if required

Marionette Folds

What Are They?

Marionette folds run downward from the corners of the mouth toward the chin and jawline.

These folds can create:

- A sad appearance, Downturned mouth corners, Jowling
- Heaviness in the lower face, Shadowing beside the chin

What Causes Them?

Marionette folds are usually caused by lower-face structural collapse.

Contributors include:

- Jawbone shrinkage, Chin retrusion
- Prejowl hollowing, Fat pad loss
- Collagen depletion, Skin laxity
- Downward pull from depressor muscles

As the jaw and chin lose support, the tissues begin collapsing inward and downward.

How to Treat Them

One of the biggest mistakes is placing excessive filler directly into the marionette lines.

This may create:

- Bulging beside the mouth, Puffiness
- A widened lower face, Heavy unnatural results

Treatment should focus on rebuilding the framework underneath the lower face.

Treatment approaches may include:

- Jawline support, Chin projection, Prejowl correction

- High G-prime structural fillers, Sculptra or CaHA
- DAO muscle relaxation, Skin tightening procedures
- RF microneedling, PRP and collagen stimulation

Often, improving jawline support softens the marionette folds naturally.

My Side Sleeping Tip

One thing many people do not realise is that chronic side sleeping may gradually worsen facial folds over time.

Constant compression of the face against a pillow can deepen:

- Nasolabial folds, Marionette folds
- Under-eye creasing, Facial asymmetry

After filler treatments especially, I encourage patients to try sleeping on their back where possible.

My little trick

I place a pillow under my knees to relieve pressure on my lower back.

Then I use a small travel pillow around my neck.

It gives the sensation of slight side support while helping keep the face off the pillow.

Many patients find this far more comfortable than forcing themselves flat on their back.

Little habits over time can make a surprisingly big difference to facial ageing.

The Golden Rule of Rejuvenation

Do not chase the fold.

Ask instead: "What support has been lost underneath?"

When the underlying framework is restored properly:

- The face appears lighter, The tissues sit higher
- The folds soften naturally, Results look fresher and more natural

Beautiful aesthetics should restore harmony — not create heaviness or puffiness.

Chapter 29: Forehead Structure, Ageing, and Rejuvenation Strategies

The forehead plays a pivotal role in facial aesthetics and expressions. As we age, structural changes in the forehead can lead to concerns such as eyebrow drooping (brow ptosis) and the formation of wrinkles. Understanding the anatomy of the forehead, the ageing process, and available rejuvenation treatments can aid in maintaining a youthful and refreshed appearance.

Anatomy of the Forehead

The forehead comprises several key components:

Skin: The outermost layer, providing protection and housing sensory receptors.

Subcutaneous Fat: A thin layer of fat beneath the skin that offers minimal cushioning.

Frontalis Muscle: A broad, flat muscle responsible for elevating the eyebrows and creating horizontal forehead lines during contraction.

Galea Aponeurotica: A tough, fibrous tissue layer connecting the frontalis muscle to the occipitalis muscle at the back of the head.

Periosteum: A dense layer of connective tissue covering the frontal bone, providing attachment points for muscles and ligaments.

Ageing of the Forehead

With advancing age, the forehead undergoes several notable changes:

Skin Laxity: Decreased collagen and elastin production lead to reduced skin elasticity, resulting in sagging.

Volume Loss: Diminished subcutaneous fat and bone resorption contribute to a hollowed or sunken appearance.

Muscle Weakness: Over time, the frontalis muscle may weaken, exacerbating sagging and the descent of the eyebrows.

Wrinkle Formation: Repetitive muscle contractions and skin laxity cause the development of horizontal forehead lines and vertical glabellar lines (frown lines).

Eyebrow Droop (Brow Ptosis)

Brow ptosis refers to the downward displacement of the eyebrows, often resulting in a tired or stern appearance. This condition is primarily due to:

Soft Tissue Descent: Age-related weakening and stretching of the soft tissues lead to the downward movement of the brow.

Frontalis Muscle Weakness: Reduced muscle tone diminishes the ability to elevate the eyebrows effectively.

Bone Resorption: Loss of bone mass in the frontal bone can contribute to the descent of the forehead and brow structures.

The lateral (outer) portion of the eyebrow often exhibits ptosis earlier than the medial (inner) portion, contributing to a fatigued appearance.

Rejuvenation Treatments

To address the signs of ageing in the forehead and brow region, several treatment options are available:

1. Sculptra® (Poly-L-Lactic Acid) Injections

Sculptra is a biostimulatory injectable that stimulates the body's natural collagen production, restoring volume and improving skin texture.

Application: While Sculptra is commonly used in areas such as the temples, cheeks, and chin, its use in the forehead is less typical due to anatomical considerations.

Benefits: When appropriately applied, Sculptra can address volume loss and enhance skin elasticity, contributing to a more youthful forehead contour.

Considerations: Treatment effects develop gradually over several months, with results lasting up to two years.

2. Hyaluronic Acid Fillers

Dermal fillers with specific rheological properties can be used to smooth forehead wrinkles and restore volume.

Application: Fillers are injected into targeted areas to fill in deep lines and compensate for volume loss.

Benefits: Immediate improvement in the appearance of wrinkles and enhanced skin hydration.

Considerations: Choosing fillers with appropriate viscosity ensures even distribution and minimizes the risk of lumpiness.

3. Neuromodulators (e.g., Botulinum Toxin)

Injectables like botulinum toxin temporarily relax the frontalis muscle, reducing the appearance of dynamic wrinkles.

Application: Administered into specific points of the forehead to diminish muscle activity.

Benefits: Effective in smoothing horizontal forehead lines and preventing the formation of deeper wrinkles.

Considerations: Overuse can lead to brow ptosis; thus, treatments should be performed by experienced practitioners.

4. Brow Lift Surgery

For more pronounced brow ptosis, surgical intervention may be considered.

Procedure: Involves repositioning the brow to a more elevated position, addressing both functional and aesthetic concerns.

Benefits: Provides long-lasting results and can significantly rejuvenate the upper face.

Considerations: Surgical risks and recovery time should be discussed with a qualified surgeon.

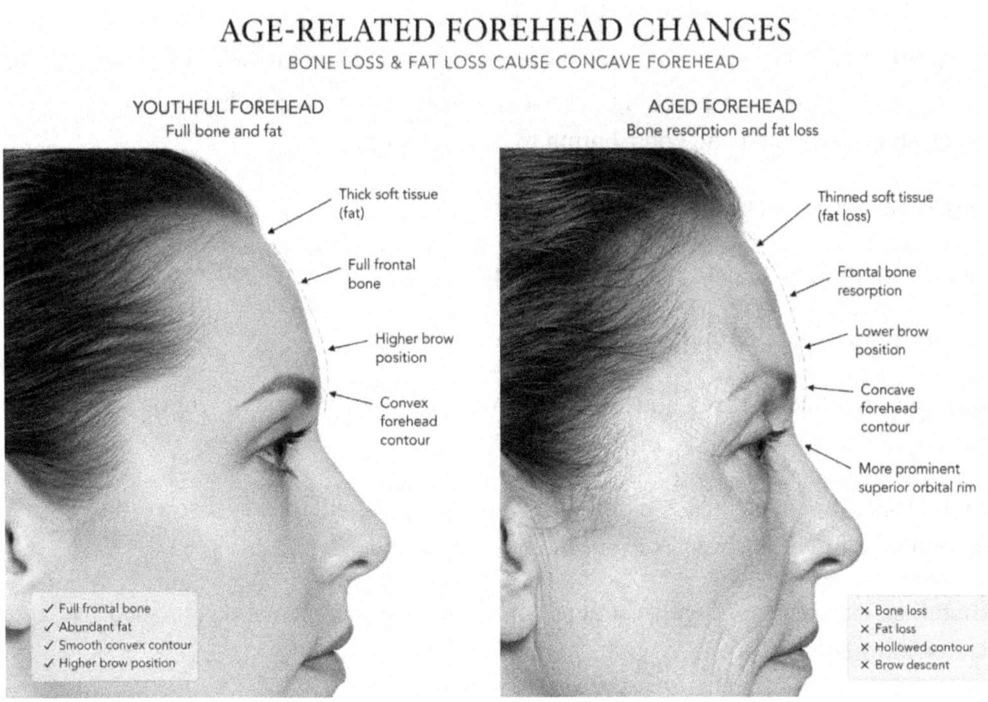

Chapter 30: Eyebrows: Ageing Changes and Rejuvenation Strategies

Eyebrows play a crucial role in facial expression, symmetry, and aesthetics. As we age, various changes occur in the eyebrows that can affect overall facial appearance. Understanding these changes and exploring effective rejuvenation strategies can help maintain a youthful and balanced look.

Ageing and the Eyebrows

Several factors contribute to the ageing of eyebrows:

Thinning and Hair Loss: Over time, eyebrows may become sparser due to hormonal changes and the natural ageing process. This can result in a less defined brow, impacting facial expression.

Greying: Just like scalp hair, eyebrow hairs can lose pigment, leading to greying. This change can make the brows appear less prominent.

Drooping: The lateral (outer) portion of the eyebrow tends to sag with age due to the lack of muscle support in that area, contributing to a tired or stern appearance.

Over-Plucking: Trends from past decades, such as the thin brows popular in the 1970s, have led to over-plucking. This can result in permanent thinning, making the brows appear outdated and contributing to an aged look.

Rejuvenation Strategies

To counteract these ageing effects, several approaches can be considered:

1. Botulinum Toxin (Botox) for Brow Lift

Injecting botulinum toxin into specific muscles can provide a subtle lift to the eyebrows.

Procedure: Botox is injected into the muscles that pull the eyebrows downward, allowing the forehead muscles to lift the brows naturally.

Benefits: This non-invasive treatment can create a more open and refreshed eye area without surgery.

Considerations: Results are temporary, typically lasting 3 to 4 months, and maintenance treatments are necessary to sustain the effect.

2. Cosmetic Tattooing (Microblading)

For those with sparse or over-plucked eyebrows, cosmetic tattooing offers a semi-permanent solution.

Procedure: Microblading involves using fine needles to deposit pigment into the skin, creating the appearance of fuller, well-shaped eyebrows.
Benefits: This technique can restore the look of natural brows, enhancing facial symmetry and framing the eyes effectively.
Considerations: It's essential to choose a skilled and experienced technician to achieve natural-looking results. Regular touch-ups are required to maintain the desired appearance.

3. Eyebrow Growth Serums

Topical serums can promote eyebrow hair growth and improve density.

Application: Applied daily, these serums contain ingredients that stimulate hair follicles.
Benefits: Over time, users may notice thicker and fuller eyebrows.
Considerations: Results vary among individuals, and consistent use is necessary to see improvements.

4. Makeup Techniques

Utilizing makeup can provide an immediate enhancement to eyebrow appearance.

Application: Brow pencils, powders, and gels can fill in sparse areas, define shape, and add color to greying hairs.
Benefits: Makeup offers a non-permanent way to achieve the desired brow look, allowing for flexibility and daily adjustments.
Considerations: Proper application techniques are essential to achieve a natural appearance.

Nita in 1970s over plucked eyebrows	*2025 Eyebrows tattooed to restore more balanced shape for face*
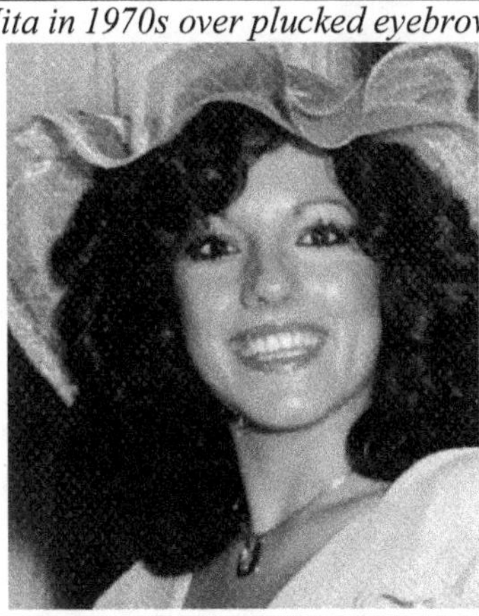	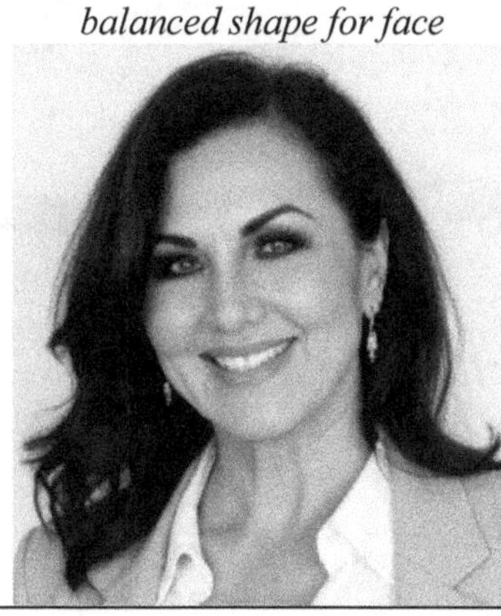

PERFECT EYEBROW MAPPING

The 3 Point Rule

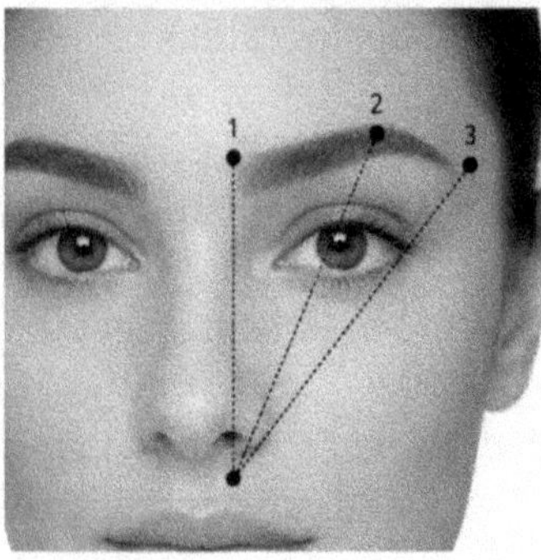

1. **START**
   Align with the side of your nose
2. **ARCH**
   Align with the outer edge of your iris
3. **END**
   Align with the outer corner of your eye

KEY POINTS

- Start of the brow should be in line with the side of the nose.
- Arch should be in line with the outer edge of the iris.
- End of the brow should be in line with the outer corner of the eye.
- Eyebrows should be sisters, not twins – they don't have to be identical but should be balanced.

ANATOMY OF A PERFECT EYEBROW

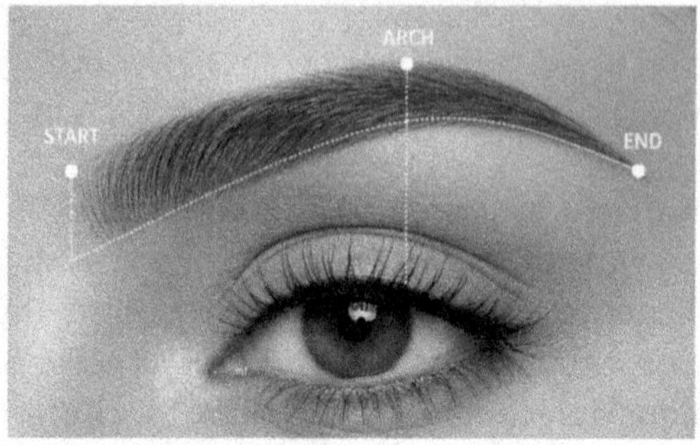

START (HEAD): The beginning of the brow, aligned with the side of the nose.

ARCH: The highest point of the brow, aligned with the outer edge of the iris.

END (TAIL): The end of the brow, aligned with the outer corner of the eye.

BOTTOM LINE: The brow should follow the natural shape of the eye and slightly lift at the arch.

TOP LINE: The top of the brow should have a soft natural curve.

EXAMPLE OF WELL MADE EYEBROWS

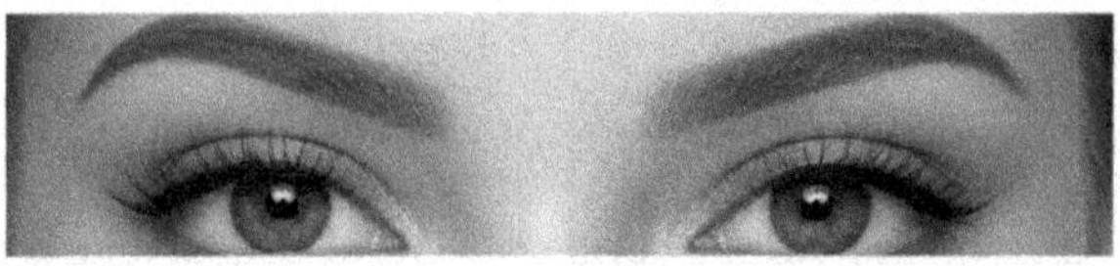

- ✓ Symmetrical
- ✓ Natural shape and proportion
- ✓ Clean, well-defined arch
- ✓ Complements the eye shape
- ✓ Frames the face beautifully

FEMALE vs MALE EYEBROWS: KEY DIFFERENCES

SHAPE, ANGLE & STRUCTURE COMPARISON

FEMALE EYEBROWS

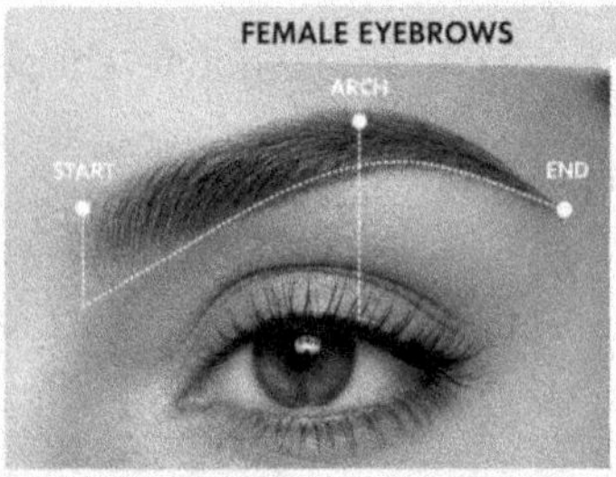

1. START
   Align with the side of your nose
2. ARCH
   Align with the outer edge of your iris
3. END
   Align with the outer corner of your eye

- Higher arch
- More defined peak
- Tapered, slimmer tail
- Softer overall shape with a gentle curve

MALE EYEBROWS

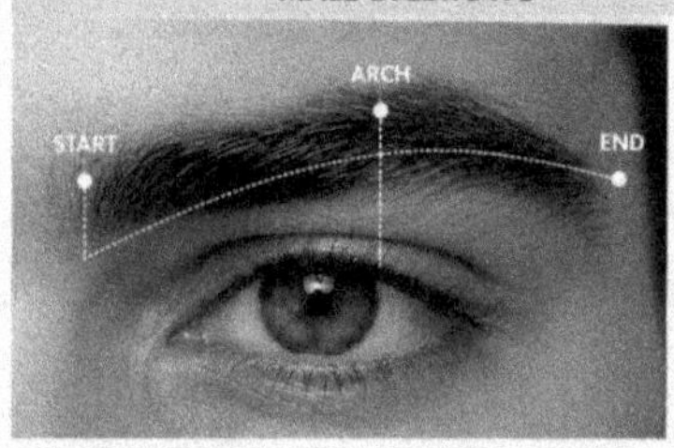

1. START
   Align with the side of your nose
2. ARCH
   Align with the outer edge of your iris
3. END
   Align with the outer corner of your eye

- Lower, flatter arch
- Less pronounced peak
- Thicker, straighter tail
- Stronger, more rectangular shape

SHAPE PROFILE COMPARISON

FEMALE (MORE ARCHED)

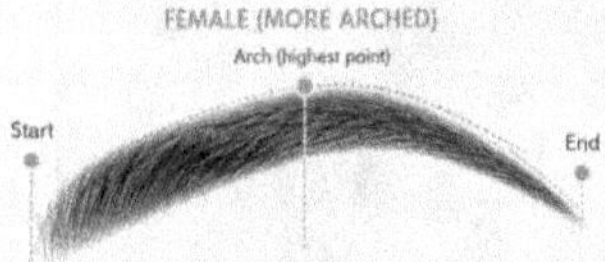

MALE (FLATTER)

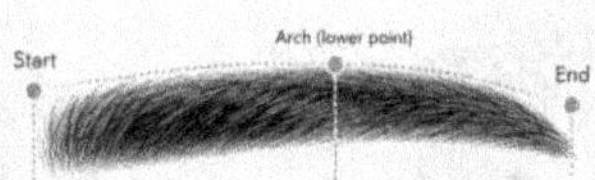

AT A GLANCE

	FEMALE	MALE
Arch	Higher	Lower / Flatter
Shape	Curved	Straighter
Tail	Tapered	Thicker
Overall Look	Soft, defined	Strong, natural
Thickness	Medium	Thick
Grooming	More refined	Natural, clean

- Keep brows balanced and symmetrical
- Follow your natural growth pattern
- Groom regularly but don't over-pluck
- Choose a shape that suits your face

Chapter 31: Ears, Eyes, and Nose: Ageing Changes and Rejuvenation Treatments

As we age, our ears, eyes, and nose undergo various structural and functional changes. Understanding these alterations and the available treatments can help maintain a youthful appearance and optimal function.

Ageing of the Ears

Changes Observed:

Elongation and Sagging: Over time, the skin and cartilage of the ears lose elasticity, leading to elongation and sagging, particularly in the earlobes.

Wrinkling: The reduction in collagen and elastin contributes to the formation of wrinkles on the earlobes.

Treatment Options:

Dermal Fillers: Injecting hyaluronic acid-based fillers can restore volume and reduce the appearance of wrinkles in the earlobes.

Platelet-Rich Plasma (PRP) Therapy: PRP injections stimulate collagen production, enhancing skin texture and firmness in the earlobes.

Earlobe Lift Surgery: For more pronounced sagging, surgical procedures can reshape and reduce the size of the earlobes.

Ageing of the Eyes

Changes Observed:

Periorbital Wrinkles: Commonly known as crow's feet, these fine lines develop around the eyes due to repetitive facial expressions and thinning skin.

Dark Circles and Hollows: Volume loss and decreased skin thickness can lead to a sunken appearance and darkening under the eyes.

Puffiness: Fluid retention and weakening of the tissues around the eyes can cause puffiness.

Eye Bags from Fluid Retention: Can Hyalase Help?

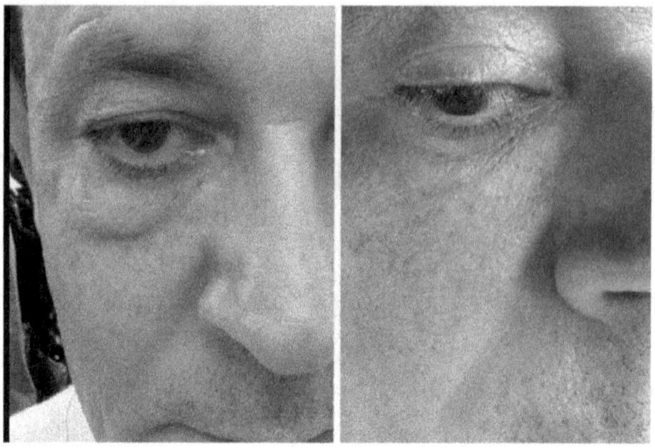

25 iu of hyalase drained the fluid build up (no filler present).

Some under-eye puffiness is caused not by fat pads but by fluid retention due to poor lymphatic drainage. This can worsen with hay fever and allergies, as inflammation can affect drainage channels around the eyes—possibly linked to valve-like structures in the lymphatic vessels.

While true fat pads or permanent eye bags typically require lower blepharoplasty surgery for correction, fluid-based puffiness may respond to Hyalase (hyaluronidase). This enzyme can help dissolve any lingering HA filler or excess glycosaminoglycans that may be obstructing lymphatic flow, improving drainage.

Worth a trial: If there is a history of prior filler or persistent puffiness that fluctuates, a conservative dose of Hyalase may reduce swelling by improving drainage—even if no obvious filler is present.

Treatment Options:

Platelet-Rich Plasma (PRP) Therapy: PRP injections under the eyes can improve skin texture, reduce dark circles, and promote a more youthful appearance.

Laser Resurfacing: Fractional CO 2 and erbium lasers can reduce fine lines and wrinkles by promoting collagen production and resurfacing the skin.

Dermal Fillers: Hyaluronic acid-based fillers can restore volume to under-eye hollows, reducing the appearance of dark circles and providing a rejuvenated look.

Upper blepharoplasty , surgically removing excess sagging skin, and lower blepharoplasty surgically addressing fat pads that cause bags and removing excess skin .

Lifestyle Modifications: Wearing sunglasses to protect against UV rays, reducing consumption of ultra-processed foods, manageing allergies, and applying retinol eye cream can help maintain youthful-looking eyes.

Ageing of the Nose

Changes Observed:

Drooping Tip: The nasal tip may droop due to weakening of the supporting cartilage, leading to a lengthened appearance.

Prominent Nasolabial Folds: Volume loss around the nose can deepen the folds between the nose and mouth.

Treatment Options:

Dermal Fillers: Injecting fillers into areas like the pyriform fossa can provide support, lift the nasal tip, and soften nasolabial folds.

Rhinoplasty: Surgical intervention can correct structural changes in the nose, addressing both aesthetic and functional concerns.

Consulting with qualified medical professionals is essential to determine the most appropriate treatment plan based on individual needs and anatomical considerations.

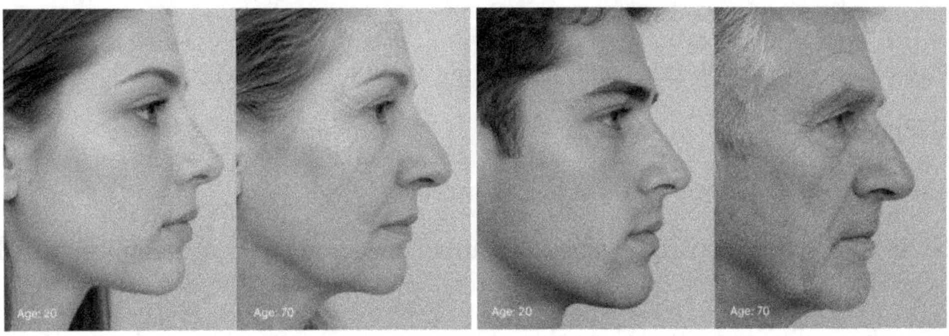

Age 20- Elevated nasal tip, strong cartilage support, shorter nose appearance, firm skin and soft tissue. Age 70- Nasal tip droop, Weakened cartilage support, apparent nose lengthening, Reduced skin elasticity, increased columella show, longer upper lip.

Chapter 32: The Ageing Temples- Why Some Faces develop a "Peanut Shape"

One of the most overlooked signs of facial ageing occurs in the temples.

Patients often focus on their cheeks, jawline, neck, or nasolabial folds, yet the temples can quietly lose volume for decades before anyone notices. Once significant temple hollowing develops, the face can begin to take on what many aesthetic practitioners refer to as a **"peanut shape."**

Instead of the youthful oval or heart-shaped face, the forehead and temples narrow while the midface remains wider, creating an inward hollow on either side of the forehead.

The result can make a person appear older, tired, gaunt, or even unwell.

Why Do Temples Hollow?

Temple hollowing is not caused by a single factor.

It is the result of age-related changes occurring at multiple anatomical levels.

Skeletal Changes

As we age, the skull undergoes gradual remodelling.

The temporal fossa enlarges and the surrounding bony support diminishes. The forehead and lateral orbital rim lose projection, creating a larger hollow space.

Just as the jawline and eye sockets change with age, the temporal bone also contributes to facial volume loss.

Fat Loss

The temple contains superficial and deep fat compartments.

Over time these fat pads shrink and redistribute, reducing the soft contours that once connected the forehead, brow, cheek and hairline.

Muscle Changes

The temporalis muscle can undergo age-related atrophy.

In some patients who clench their teeth heavily, the muscle may remain bulky. In others it gradually loses volume, contributing to temple hollowing.

Skin Changes

Collagen, elastin and hydration decline with age.

The overlying skin becomes thinner and less resilient, making underlying skeletal changes more visible.

The Peanut Shape

When temple volume is lost, the upper face narrows.

Viewed from the front, the cheeks may remain relatively full while the temples collapse inward.

This creates a shape resembling a peanut shell: Hollow temples, Wider midface, Narrow upper face, Loss of youthful facial balance

Temple rejuvenation often restores harmony to the face far more dramatically than patients expect.

Many patients cannot identify exactly what has changed after treatment, but they frequently describe looking healthier, fresher and less tired.

Temple Anatomy

Understanding temple anatomy is essential because the temple contains important blood vessels.

Although temple filler can be highly rewarding, it must be approached with respect.

From Bone to Skin

The layers of the temple can be simplified as:

1. **Temporal Bone**: The deepest layer providing skeletal support.

2. **Deep Temporal Fascia**: A dense fibrous layer covering the temporalis muscle.

3. **Temporalis Muscle**: The chewing muscle occupying much of the temporal fossa.

4. **Loose Areolar Plane**: A potential space between fascial layers.

5. **Superficial Temporal Fascia:** (continuous with the SMAS)

6. **Subcutaneous Fat**: Contains superficial fat compartments and vessels.

7. **Skin**: The visible outer layer.

Important Temple Arteries

The temple contains several significant blood vessels.

Superficial Temporal Artery

The major artery of the temple.

It emerges just in front of the ear and divides into: Frontal branch, Parietal branch

The frontal branch is particularly important because it travels across the temple and communicates with vessels around the eye.

Middle Temporal Artery

A branch supplying deeper temporal tissues.

Zygomatico-Orbital Artery

A variable vessel that may cross the temple toward the lateral orbital region.

Sentinel Vein

While not an artery, it is an important landmark indicating nearby vascular structures.

Because of the extensive vascular connections between the temple and orbital circulation, inadvertent intravascular injection can potentially cause serious complications.

Temple Filling Techniques

Temple rejuvenation can be performed at different anatomical depths.

The chosen technique depends on the patient's anatomy, severity of hollowing and injector preference.

Deep Temple Filling

Many practitioners prefer a deep supraperiosteal approach.

A high G-prime filler is placed directly onto bone using a needle.

Often referred to as a "swift spot" technique, the filler acts almost like an implant, restoring skeletal support.

Benefits include Excellent lift, Predictable projection, Minimal product required, Long-lasting support

Typical products include firmer structural fillers designed for deep placement.

Subdermal Cannula Technique

For broader hollowing, filler may be placed more superficially using a cannula.

The cannula is advanced through the subdermal plane and filler is distributed gradually throughout the hollow.

Benefits include:

- Smoother contour correction, Wider coverage, Reduced bruising
- Less risk of vessel penetration compared with a needle

Many injectors combine deep structural support with superficial contouring for optimal results.

Safety Considerations

The temple is often considered an advanced treatment area.

Safe treatment requires:

- Thorough anatomical knowledge, Careful patient assessment
- Awareness of vascular pathways, Slow injection technique
- Minimal injection pressure, Constant needle or cannula awareness
- Aspiration where appropriate according to injector preference

Patients should always be informed that the temple contains important blood vessels and that treatment should only be performed by experienced medical practitioners trained in facial anatomy.

Clinical Pearl

Temple rejuvenation is one of the most powerful yet underappreciated treatments in facial aesthetics.

A small amount of strategically placed filler can transform a hollow, ageing upper face into a softer, more youthful contour. When combined with forehead, brow and cheek assessment, temple restoration often becomes the missing piece that restores facial balance and eliminates the characteristic "peanut shape" associated with ageing.

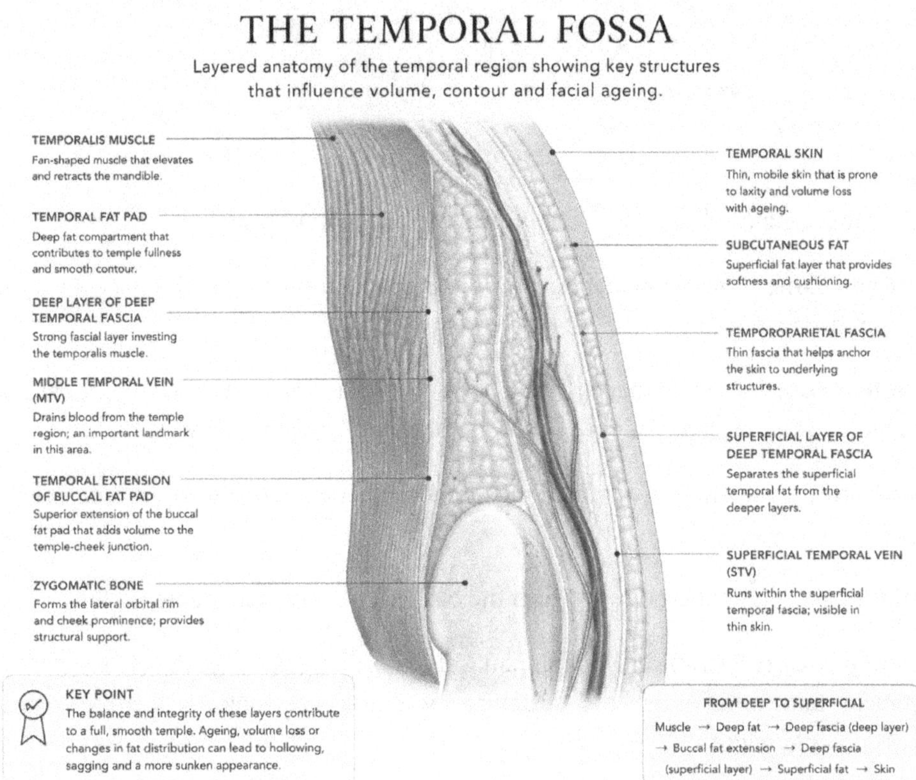

Chapter 33: Lips: Ageing Changes, and Rejuvenation Treatments

The lips are a central feature of facial aesthetics, playing a significant role in expressions and overall appearance. Understanding their anatomy, the ageing process, and available treatments can aid in maintaining or restoring their youthful allure.

Anatomy of the Lips

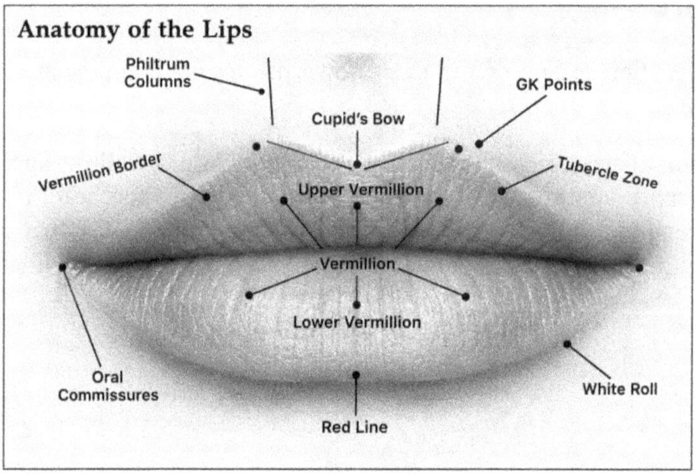

The lips are composed of several distinct anatomical components:

Vermilion Zone: The pigmented area of the lips, lacking sweat and sebaceous glands, making it prone to dryness.

Vermilion Border: The demarcation line between the vermilion zone and the surrounding skin, often highlighted by a subtle ridge known as the white roll.

Cupids Bow: The double-curve of the upper lip, contributing to its characteristic shape.

Philtrum: The vertical groove between the base of the nose and the upper lip.

Orbicularis Oris Muscle: A circular muscle encircling the mouth, essential for lip movement and function. These structures work in harmony to facilitate speech, expression, and ingestion.

Ageing of the Lips

As individual's age, the lips undergo several changes:

Volume Loss: A decrease in collagen and elastin leads to thinner lips and diminished fullness.

Lengthening of the Upper Lip: The upper lip tends to elongate over time, contributing to a flatter appearance.

Development of Fine Lines: Vertical lines, often referred to as lipstick lines • or smoker's lines • emerge due to repetitive movements and skin thinning.

Loss of Definition: The vermilion border and Cupid's bow become less distinct, reducing lip contour clarity

These alterations can result in a less youthful and vibrant appearance.

Rejuvenation Treatments

To counteract the effects of ageing on the lips, several treatments are available:

1. Platelet-Rich Plasma (PRP) Therapy

PRP involves injecting concentrated platelets from the patient blood into the lips to stimulate collagen production and tissue regeneration.

Benefits: Enhances lip texture, reduces fine lines, and promotes natural fullness.

Procedure: Blood is drawn, processed to isolate platelets, and then injected into the lips.

Considerations: Results develop gradually over several weeks, with minimal risk of allergic reactions since the patient's own blood is used.

2. Dermal Fillers

Hyaluronic acid-based fillers are commonly used to restore volume and define lip contours.

Benefits: Immediate enhancement of lip fullness and shape, with the ability to target specific areas for balanced results.

Procedure: Fillers are injected into designated lip regions to achieve the desired augmentation.

Considerations: Results are temporary, typically lasting 6 to 12 months, and treatments can be adjusted to achieve subtle or more pronounced enhancements.

Consultation with a qualified medical professional is essential to determine the most appropriate treatment plan based on individual goals and anatomical considerations.

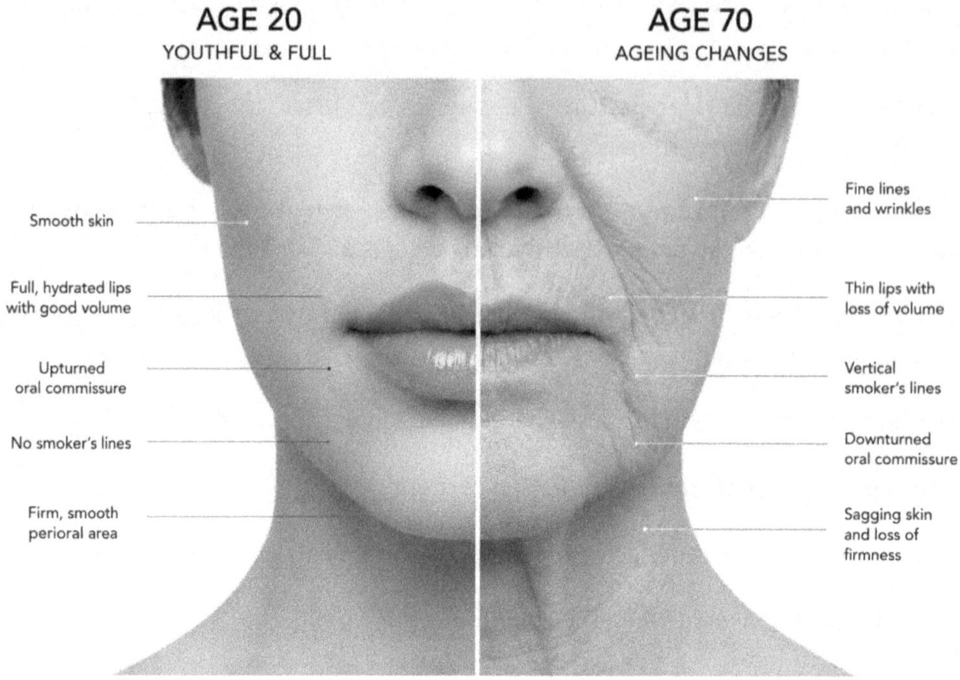

Oral Commissures – The Corners of the Mouth

The oral commissures are the corners where the upper and lower lips meet. Although they are small anatomical structures, they play a significant role in facial expression, attractiveness, and the perception of age. In youth, the commissures naturally sit in a neutral or slightly upward position, contributing to a rested, approachable, and happy appearance. As we age, a combination of bone resorption, loss of soft tissue support, weakening of retaining ligaments, repetitive muscle movement, and skin laxity can cause the corners of the mouth to gradually turn downward.

This downward pull creates what is often referred to as a "sad mouth" appearance, even when the person feels perfectly happy. The depressor anguli oris (DAO) muscle contributes to this process by pulling the corners of the mouth downward, while loss of support from the cheeks, marionette area, jawline, and chin further exaggerates the effect. Over time, fine lines, smoker's lines, volume loss within the lips, and the formation of marionette folds can make the oral commissures appear heavier and more downturned.

When assessing a patient, it is important not to focus solely on the lips themselves. Treating the corners of the mouth often requires a full-face approach. Support may be needed in the cheeks, prejowl area, marionette region, chin, or jawline before directly addressing the commissures. Small amounts of filler can be strategically placed around the oral commissure to provide support, while neuromodulators can sometimes be used to soften the downward pull of the DAO muscle.

A successful treatment does not necessarily create an exaggerated smile. Rather, it restores a neutral or slightly elevated corner of the mouth, helping patients look more refreshed, approachable, and less tired without appearing overtreated. The goal is always balance and support, not simply adding volume. As with all aesthetic treatments, understanding the underlying cause of the downturn is more important than treating the visible symptom alone.

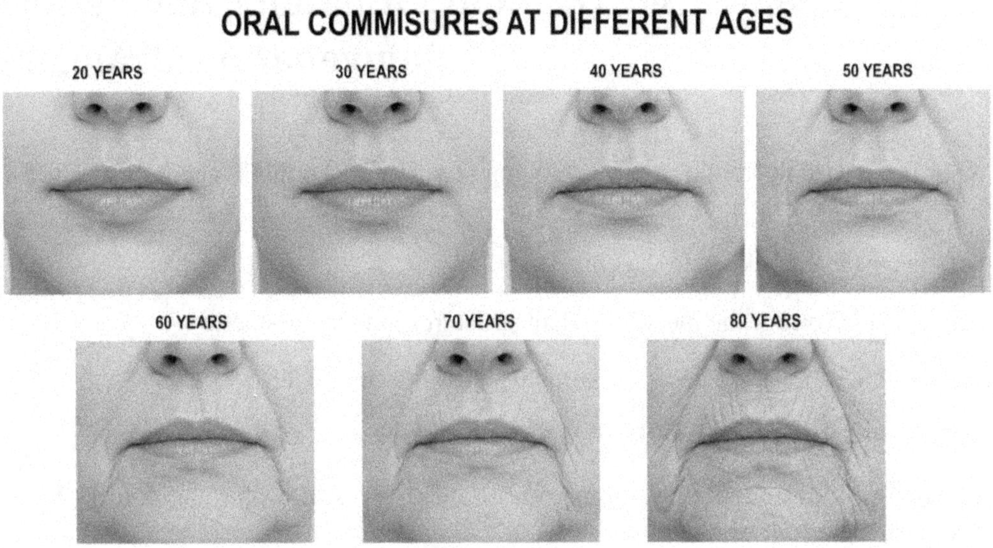

Chapter 34: The Chin's Anatomy, Ageing, and Rejuvenation Strategies

When most people think about facial rejuvenation, they think about lips, cheeks, jawlines, or perhaps the eyes.

Very few people think about the chin.

Yet the chin is one of the most important structures in facial aesthetics.

A weak chin can make a perfectly attractive nose appear too large.

A small chin can make the neck appear fuller.

An ageing chin can contribute to marionette lines, jowls, downturning corners of the mouth, and loss of jawline definition.

The chin is the anchor of the lower face.

Without adequate support, the entire lower face can lose harmony.

As injectors, we often say:

"The chin is small, but its influence is enormous."

Understanding the Chin

The chin is not simply a piece of bone projecting from the front of the face.

It is a complex structure made up of:

- Bone, Ligaments, Muscles, Fat pads, Skin, Arteries, Veins, Nerves

All of these structures change as we age.

The result is often a chin that becomes shorter, weaker, wider, less defined, and less supportive.

The Five Dimensions of the Chin

Professor Mauricio de Maio describes the chin in five dimensions:

1. Projection

How far the chin projects forward.

Insufficient projection can:

- Create a retruded profile

- Make the nose appear larger, Reduce jawline definition, Increase the appearance of a double chin

2. Height

The vertical length of the chin.

A chin may be: Too short, Too long, Well proportioned

The ideal height contributes to balanced facial thirds.

3. Width

The horizontal width of the chin.

Generally:

- Female chins tend to be softer and narrower
- Male chins are often wider and squarer

However, ethnicity and personal preference play significant roles.

4. Animation

The chin is constantly moving.

The mentalis muscle contracts during: Speech, Eating, Smiling, Lip closure

This movement influences treatment planning and product selection.

5. Time

The chin changes dramatically with age.

Bone resorption, ligament laxity, muscle changes, and skin ageing all contribute to the ageing lower face.

How the Chin Ages

Ageing is a multidimensional process.

Bone Changes

The mandible undergoes gradual resorption.

Common changes include:

- Loss of anterior mandibular projection, Widening of the mandibular angle
- Enlargement and migration of the mental foramen, Reduced support for soft tissues

As the bony foundation shrinks, the overlying tissues begin to descend.

Muscle Changes

The mentalis muscle becomes increasingly active over time.

This often produces: Cobblestone chin, Orange-peel texture (peau d'orange), Horizontal chin creases

In some patients the muscle may weaken, resulting in chin pad descent.

Fat Pad Changes

The chin fat pad also changes.

With age: Fat compartments descend, Support diminishes, Volume becomes uneven

This contributes to: Marionette lines, Pre-jowl hollowing, Chin ptosis

Skin Changes

The skin becomes: Thinner, Less elastic, More wrinkled

This further accentuates the ageing process.

The Muscles of the Chin

Mentalis

The mentalis is the primary chin muscle.

Functions: Elevates the lower lip, Everts the lower lip, Compresses the chin pad

Overactivity produces: Dimpling, Cobblestone texture, Chin wrinkles

This muscle is commonly treated with botulinum toxin.

Depressor Anguli Oris (DAO)

The DAO pulls the corners of the mouth downward.

Overactivity creates: Sad appearance, Downturned oral commissures, Marionette line exaggeration

Depressor Labii Inferioris (DLI)

The DLI lowers the lower lip.

Because it overlaps with the DAO, treatment requires caution.

Over-treatment may result in: Lip asymmetry, Difficulty smiling, Speech changes

Vascular Anatomy of the Chin

The chin possesses a rich and highly variable vascular network.

No two patients are identical.

This is why injectors should never assume vessels are exactly where textbooks place them.

Mental Artery

The mental artery emerges from the mental foramen.

It supplies: Chin skin, Soft tissues, Lower lip

The mental foramen represents an important danger zone.

Inferior Labial Artery

Supplies: Lower lip, Labiomental region

It often anastomoses with adjacent vessels.

Submental Artery

A branch of the facial artery.

It supplies: Chin, Floor of mouth, Submental region

The submental artery is particularly important because of its communication with vessels supplying the tongue.

Ascending Mental Artery

An important branch that contributes to the rich arterial network around the lower face.

Why the Chin Can Be Dangerous

One of the most serious complications of chin filler is vascular occlusion.

The chin has extensive connections to:

- The facial artery, The submental artery
- The lingual circulation, The floor of mouth vasculature

A retrograde embolisation event can theoretically travel through the submental arterial system into the lingual circulation.

This may compromise blood flow to the tongue.

Although rare, cases of: Tongue ischaemia, Tongue necrosis, Floor of mouth necrosis have been reported in the medical literature following filler-related vascular compromise.

Safety Principles for Chin Injections

To minimise risk:

Always Know Your Anatomy

Understand:

- Mental foramen location, Facial artery course, Submental artery position, Labiomental groove anatomy

Inject Slowly

High-pressure injections increase risk. Small aliquots are safer.

Aspirate When Appropriate

While aspiration is not foolproof, it remains one component of safe practice.

Respect Depth

For projection: Deep supraperiosteal placement is often preferred.

Avoid unintentionally injecting within muscle layers.

Use Conservative Volumes

The chin responds beautifully to subtle correction. More product is not always better.

Chin Assessment

When assessing the chin, ask: **Is it projected enough?**, **Is the vertical height appropriate?**, **Is the width balanced?**, **How does it move?**, **How has ageing changed it?**

Only after answering these questions should treatment planning begin.

A beautifully balanced chin can:

- Improve the profile, Support the lips, Improve jawline definition, Reduce marionette lines, Improve facial proportions

Ageing of the Chin

With ageing, the chin experiences several notable changes:

Bone Resorption: The mandible undergoes resorption, leading to a reduction in chin projection and a less defined jawline.

Muscle Activity: Overactivity of the mentalis muscle can cause chin dimpling, often referred to as an "orange peel" appearance.

Soft Tissue Changes: Loss of subcutaneous fat and skin elasticity contributes to sagging and the formation of marionette lines (melomental folds) extending from the mouth corners to the chin.

Rejuvenation Treatments

To address these ageing-related changes, several treatment options are available:

1. Botulinum Toxin Injections

Injecting botulinum toxin into the mentalis muscle can relax overactivity, reducing chin dimpling and creating a smoother appearance.

Procedure: A small amount of botulinum toxin is injected directly into the mentalis muscle.

Benefits: Improves the Orange peel texture and softens the mental crease.

Considerations: Effects are temporary, typically lasting 3 to 4 months, requiring repeat treatments for maintenance.

2. Dermal Fillers

Dermal fillers can restore lost volume, enhance chin projection, and smooth marionette lines.

Procedure: Fillers are injected into specific areas of the chin and surrounding regions to add volume and structure.

Benefits: Immediate improvement in chin contour and reduction of wrinkles.

Considerations: Choosing fillers with appropriate rheological properties ensures a natural look and minimizes lumpiness.

3. Calcium Hydroxylapatite (Radiesse)

Radiesse is a filler that provides immediate volume and stimulates collagen production, making it suitable for enhancing chin structure and addressing bone loss.

Procedure: Injected into deeper layers of the chin to provide structural support.

Benefits: Restores volume, improves skin texture, and offers longer-lasting results compared to some other fillers.

Considerations: Results can last up to a year or more; some patients may experience temporary swelling or bruising.

4. Subcision with Cannula ("Happy Lift")

Marionette lines can be treated using a subcision technique with a cannula, sometimes referred to as the "Happy Lift"

Procedure: A blunt-tipped cannula is inserted under the skin to release fibrous bands causing the marionette lines, followed by filler injection to maintain the lifted appearance.

Benefits: Reduces the depth of marionette lines and restores a smoother transition between the mouth corners and chin.

Considerations: The term "happy lift" is associated with thread lifting techniques; however, in this context, it refers to the subcision method using a cannula.

5. Lip Support and Projection

As the chin bone recedes with age, the lower lip may turn inward, leading to a thinner appearance.

Procedure: Injecting fillers into the upper part of the chin can provide support and outward projection to the lower lip.

Benefits: Enhances lip fullness and restores a balanced profile.

Considerations: Careful assessment is required to achieve natural-looking results without overcorrection.

Consultation with a qualified medical professional is essential to determine the most appropriate treatment plan based on individual anatomy and aesthetic goals. Combining multiple treatments may yield optimal results in restoring a youthful chin appearance..

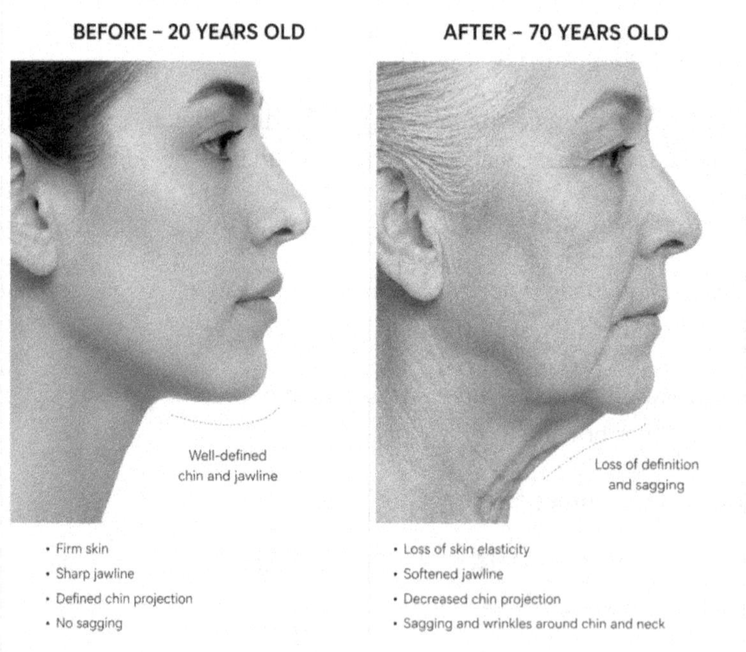

Chapter 35: The Neck: Anatomy, Ageing, and Rejuvenation Treatments

The neck, a vital yet often overlooked region, exhibits unique anatomical features and ageing patterns distinct from the face. Understanding its layered structure and the available treatments can aid in maintaining its youthful appearance.

Anatomy of the Neck

The neck's anatomy comprises several layers, each contributing to its function and aesthetics:

1. Skin: The outermost layer, providing a protective barrier.

2. Superficial Cervical Fascia: Located just beneath the skin, this layer contains:

Neurovascular structures supplying the skin

Superficial veins, such as the external jugular vein

Superficial lymph nodes, Fat, The platysma muscle

3. Platysma Muscle: A broad, superficial muscle extending from the chest and shoulder region upward to the lower face, playing a role in facial expressions and contributing to the neck's contour.

4. Deep Cervical Fascia: Situated beneath the superficial fascia and platysma, this fascia is organized into several layers:

Investing Layer: Encircles the entire neck, enclosing the trapezius and sternocleidomastoid muscles.

Pretracheal Layer: Surrounds the trachea, esophagus, and thyroid gland.

Prevertebral Layer: Envelops the vertebral column and associated deep muscles.

These fascial layers compartmentalize neck structures, providing support and facilitating movement. In comparison, the face features the superficial musculoaponeurotic system (SMAS), a continuous fibromuscular layer that differs from the neck's fascial composition.

Ageing of the Neck

The neck undergoes specific changes as part of the ageing process:

Skin Laxity: Decreased collagen and elastin production lead to looser, sagging skin.

Muscle Banding: The platysma muscle may become more prominent, forming vertical bands.

Fat Accumulation or Loss: Uneven fat distribution can result in a double chin or a gaunt appearance.

Sun Damage: Chronic exposure contributes to wrinkles, pigmentation changes, and a leathery texture.

These changes can cause the neck to age differently from the face, often becoming a noticeable indicator of ageing.

Rejuvenation Treatments for the Neck

Various treatments aim to address the signs of neck ageing, focusing on skin tightening, volume restoration, and texture improvement:

1. Platelet-Rich Plasma (PRP) Therapy

PRP involves injecting concentrated platelets from the patient's blood into the neck skin to stimulate collagen production and enhance skin quality.

Benefits: Improved skin texture, increased elasticity, and a more youthful appearance.

Procedure: Blood is drawn, processed to concentrate platelets, and then injected into targeted areas.

Considerations: Multiple sessions may be required for optimal results.

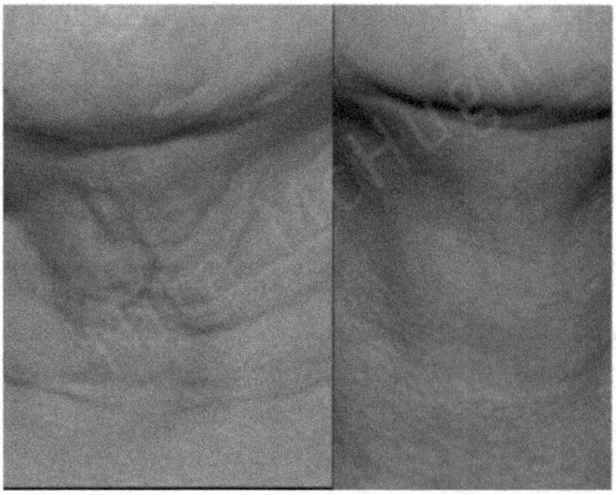

Neck after 3 sessions of PRP

2. Hyperdiluted Sculptra (Poly-L-Lactic Acid)

Sculptra is a biostimulatory filler that, when hyperdiluted, can be used to treat larger surface areas like the neck.

Benefits: Stimulates collagen production, leading to gradual skin tightening and improved texture.

Procedure: The diluted solution is injected into the dermis, promoting collagen synthesis over time.

Considerations: Results develop gradually over several months, with effects lasting up to two years.

3. Hyperdiluted Radiesse (Calcium Hydroxylapatite)

Radiesse, another biostimulatory filler, can be diluted for use in the neck area.

Benefits: Provides immediate volume and stimulates collagen production for long-term improvement.

Procedure: The hyperdiluted filler is injected to cover larger areas, enhancing skin texture and firmness.

Considerations: Typically requires multiple treatments spaced weeks apart.

4. Skin Boosters

Injectable treatments that deliver hyaluronic acid and other nutrients to the skin.

Benefits: Deep hydration, improved skin elasticity, and a radiant appearance.

Procedure: Microinjections are administered into the superficial dermis.

Considerations: Maintenance treatments are often needed to sustain results.

5. Profhilo

A unique injectable hyaluronic acid treatment designed to improve skin laxity.

Benefits: Enhances skin hydration and stimulates collagen and elastin production, resulting in firmer skin.

Procedure: Injected into specific points, allowing the product to diffuse and rejuvenate the skin.

Considerations: Typically involves two sessions spaced a month apart, with effects lasting up to six months.

6. Fine Line Fillers

Utilizing very fine fillers designed to integrate smoothly into the tissue.

Benefits: Targets horizontal lines and creases without creating lumps, resulting in a natural look.

Procedure: Injected superficially to smooth out lines and creases.

Submental Fat (Double Chin)

Submental fat, commonly known as a "double chin," can be caused by various factors, including:

Causes of Submental Fat

1. **Genetics** – Some people are predisposed to storing fat under the chin.

2. **Ageing** – Loss of skin elasticity and fat redistribution can contribute.

3. **Weight Gain** – Excess fat deposits accumulate in various areas, including the submental region.

4. **Posture** – Poor posture can weaken neck muscles, making fat more noticeable.

5. **Hormonal Changes** – Hormones and metabolism shifts can impact fat storage.

Treatment Options for Reducing Submental Fat

1. Belkyra (Kybella in the USA)

• Active ingredient: Deoxycholic Acid (DCA)

• Works by breaking down fat cells, which are then absorbed by the body.

• Sessions Required: Usually 3 to 4 sessions (4-6 weeks apart)

• Downtime: Swelling is common for 1-2 weeks, with tenderness and firmness in the treated area.

• Best For: Small-to-moderate fat pockets.

2. Compounded PPC + Deoxycholic Acid (Mesotherapy)

• Similar to Belkyra/Kybella but may have a different formulation.

• Main ingredients: Phosphatidylcholine (PPC) + Deoxycholic Acid (DCA).

• Swelling/Downtime: Similar to Belkyra, with noticeable swelling lasting 5-14 days.

• Sessions Required: Typically 3+ sessions.

3. CoolSculpting (Cryolipolysis)

• Freezes fat cells, which are naturally eliminated over time.

• Non-invasive, minimal downtime but may take 8-12 weeks for full results.

• Sessions Required: Usually 2+ sessions.

• Best For: Mild-to-moderate fat deposits.

4. Liposculpture (Liposuction for Chin)

• Surgical option to suction out excess fat.

• Downtime: Bruising and swelling for 1-2 weeks.

• Best For: Significant fat deposits or those seeking immediate, permanent results.

5. FaceTite (Radiofrequency-Assisted Liposuction)

• Uses RF energy to melt fat and tighten skin simultaneously.

• Minimally invasive with 1-2 weeks of downtime.

• Best For: Fat reduction with skin laxity improvement.

6. PRP for Small Fat Deposits & Skin Tightening

• Platelet-Rich Plasma (PRP) can tighten skin and improve collagen around the jawline.

• Works best for mild cases or in combination with other treatments.

• Sessions Required: Usually 3+ sessions.

Choosing the Right Treatment

• For minimal fat + skin laxity: PRP or FaceTite.

• For moderate fat: Belkyra/Kybella, PPC/Deoxycholic, or CoolSculpting.

• For large fat deposits: Liposuction or FaceTite.

• For immediate results: Liposculpture or FaceTite.

• For gradual, non-invasive reduction: CoolSculpting or Belkyra.

Tech Neck

Tech neck lines are horizontal wrinkles on the neck caused by constantly looking down at screens, leading to collagen breakdown and premature ageing. Factors such as poor posture, skin dehydration, and repetitive movement contribute to their formation.

Since the neck has thinner skin and fewer oil glands, it is more prone to wrinkles and laxity.

While ageing plays a role, lifestyle habits accelerate the process. Addressing these lines requires a combination of treatments that hydrate, tighten, and stimulate collagen production to restore skin smoothness and elasticity.

A powerful approach to treating tech neck lines is combining PRP (Platelet-Rich Plasma) and Skin Boosters. PRP stimulates collagen production and strengthens skin over time, while skin boosters provide deep hydration, smoothing static wrinkles.

Together, they enhance skin elasticity, hydration, and overall texture.

A recommended treatment plan involves three sessions spaced over a few months, with visible improvements in hydration within weeks and long-term collagen repair over several months.

Alongside treatment, good posture, sun protection, retinol, and hydration play key roles in prevention.

With the right combination of treatments and lifestyle changes, tech neck lines can be significantly reduced, leaving the neck looking youthful and rejuvenated.

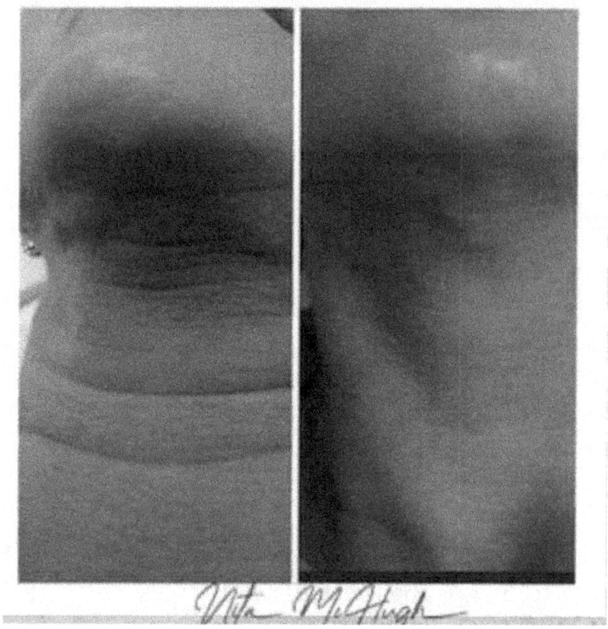

Chapter 36: The Décolletage

The décolletage , encompassing the upper chest area between the neck and the breasts, is often exposed yet frequently neglected in skincare routines. Understanding its anatomy, the effects of ageing, and preventive measures can help maintain its youthful appearance.

Anatomy of the Décolletage

The skin of the décolletage is notably thin and delicate, with fewer oil glands and less subcutaneous fat compared to other body areas. This makes it more susceptible to environmental damage and the early onset of wrinkles. The underlying structures include the pectoral muscles and connective tissues that provide support to the skin and breast tissue.

Ageing of the Décolletage

As we age, the décolletage undergoes several changes:

Loss of Elasticity: Decreased collagen and elastin production lead to skin laxity and the formation of wrinkles.

Hyperpigmentation: Prolonged sun exposure can cause age spots and uneven skin tone.

Volume Loss: Reduction in subcutaneous fat can result in a less plump appearance.

Wrinkling from Sleep Positions: Sleeping on one's side can cause the breasts to press together, leading to vertical creases in the décolletage area.

Preventive Measures for Side Sleepers

For individuals who prefer side sleeping, the following strategies can help prevent sleep-induced chest wrinkles:

Breast Support Pillows: Specialized pillows, such as the Intimia Breast Pillow, are designed to be worn between the breasts during sleep. They help maintain breast separation, reducing skin creasing and discomfort.

Supportive Sleepwear: Wearing a supportive bra or specially designed sleepwear can minimize breast movement and skin folding during sleep.

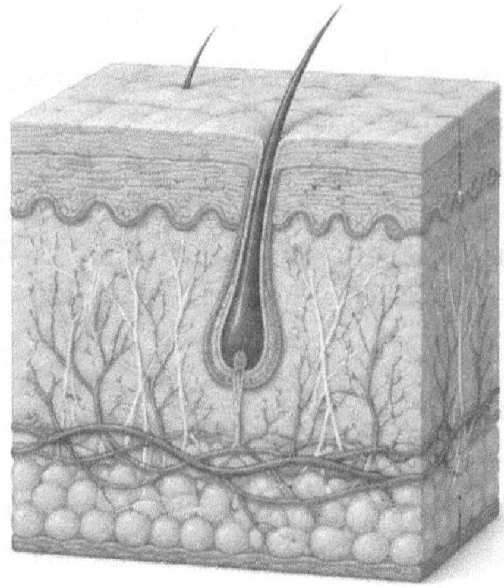

Various treatments can address signs of ageing in the décolletage:

Topical Retinoids: Applying retinoid creams can stimulate collagen production, improving skin texture and reducing fine lines.

Chemical Peels: Controlled application of chemical solutions exfoliates the skin, promoting the growth of new, smoother skin and reducing pigmentation issues.

Laser Resurfacing: Laser treatments can resurface the skin, remove discoloration, smooth lines, and tighten loose skin.

Micro needling : This procedure creates micro-injuries in the skin, stimulating collagen production and improving skin texture.

Injectable Fillers: Hyaluronic acid-based fillers, can effectively reduce the appearance of lines and wrinkles on the chest.

Sculptra (Poly-L-Lactic Acid): Sculptra injections stimulate collagen production, improving wrinkles and crepey skin in the décolletage area with natural, long-lasting results.

Silicone Patches: Medical-grade silicone patches can be applied to the décolletage to hydrate the skin and reduce the appearance of wrinkles. Products like Wrinkles Schminkles have gained popularity for their effectiveness in smoothing chest wrinkles. Incorporating these preventive measures and treatments can help maintain the youthful appearance of the décolletage .

Chapter 37: The Hand Rejuvenation

Ageing hands often reveal a person's age just as much if not more than the face. Over time, the skin on the hands becomes thinner, veins and tendons become more prominent, and volume loss creates a bony appearance. The natural ageing process, combined with sun exposure and environmental factors, leads to a loss of collagen, elasticity, and hydration, making the hands look fragile and wrinkled.

Fortunately, advancements in aesthetic medicine offer several effective treatments to rejuvenate ageing hands, restoring volume, improving skin quality, and enhancing overall appearance.

2 treatments of 1.5ml of Radiesse. 1 month apart

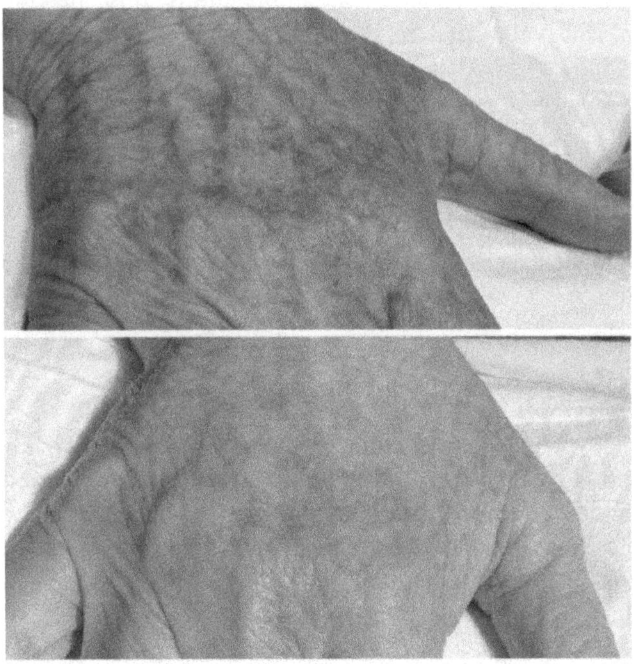

Before and after pic . 6 months post treatment

Platelet-Rich Plasma (PRP) therapy is a natural approach to hand rejuvenation. By using the patient's own blood, PRP harnesses growth factors to stimulate collagen production, improve skin texture, and enhance hydration. The regenerative properties of PRP can reduce crepiness and improve overall skin resilience, making it a great option for those seeking a natural, gradual improvement.

Dermal Fillers: Restoring Volume

Injectable fillers provide an immediate solution to volume loss in the hands.

By replenishing lost fullness, fillers help smooth the skeletal appearance, reducing the visibility of veins and tendons.

Hyaluronic acid fillers, calcium hydroxylapatite (Radiesse), and poly-L-lactic acid (Sculptra) are commonly used for this purpose. Each has unique benefits:

Hyaluronic Acid Fillers: Provide instant hydration and volume, though results may be temporary.

Sculptra: Works gradually by stimulating collagen production, creating a more natural, long-term improvement.

Radiesse: My personal favourite for hand rejuvenation. Unlike other fillers, Radiesse not only stimulates collagen but also has an opaque quality, making it excellent for disguising prominent veins and tendons. It offers both immediate and long-term benefits, giving hands a smoother, more youthful appearance.

Skin Boosters: Hydration and Glow

For those with crepey, thin skin, skin boosters such as polynucleotides or micro-injections of hyaluronic acid can deeply hydrate the skin, improving elasticity and texture. These treatments work well in combination with fillers to enhance overall hand rejuvenation.

Choosing the Right Treatment

The best approach to hand rejuvenation often involves a combination of treatments tailored to the individual's needs. While PRP and skin boosters improve skin quality over time, fillers like Radiesse provide immediate structural support and collagen stimulation. Protecting the hands with sunscreen, moisturizers, and a good skincare routine further enhances the results.

Ageing hands no longer have to be a telltale sign of age. With the right combination of treatments, hands can remain as youthful and elegant as the rest of you.

Chapter 38: Ageing and Thinning Hair. Understanding Causes and Exploring Treatments

Hair plays a significant role in personal identity and self-esteem. As individuals age, it is common to experience hair thinning and loss. Understanding the structure of hair, the reasons behind its thinning, and the available treatments can aid in manageing and potentially mitigating these changes.

Structure of Hair

Each hair strand comprises two main parts:

1. **Hair Shaft**: The visible part above the skin's surface.

2. **Hair Root**: Located beneath the skin, housed within the hair follicle.

The hair shaft consists of three layers:

Cuticle: The outermost layer made of overlapping cells, protecting the inner layers.

Cortex: The middle layer containing keratin, providing strength, colour, and texture.

Medulla: The innermost layer, present in thicker hair strands, whose function is not fully understood.

Causes of Hair Thinning with Age

Several factors contribute to hair thinning as individuals age:

Hormonal Changes: Decreased estrogen levels in women during menopause and increased sensitivity to dihydrotestosterone (DHT) in both genders can lead to hair follicle miniaturization.

Genetics: A family history of hair loss increases the likelihood of experiencing similar patterns.

Thyroid Disorders: Both hyperthyroidism and hypothyroidism can disrupt the hair growth cycle, leading to thinning.

Reduced Blood Supply: Ageing can lead to decreased circulation to hair follicles, impairing nutrient delivery and hair growth.

Nutritional Deficiencies: Lack of essential nutrients like iron, zinc, and vitamins can weaken hair structure.

Mechanical Stress: Hairstyles that pull hair tightly can cause traction alopecia, leading to receding hairlines.

Treatment Options

Various treatments are available to address hair thinning:

1. Platelet-Rich Plasma (PRP) Therapy

PRP involves injecting concentrated platelets from the patient's blood into the scalp to stimulate hair growth.

Procedure: Blood is drawn, processed to concentrate platelets, and injected into thinning areas.

Benefits: May promote hair growth and increase hair density.

Considerations: Multiple sessions are often required; results vary among individuals.

2. Mesotherapy

This technique involves injecting a mixture of vitamins, minerals, and medications into the scalp.

Procedure: Microinjections deliver nutrients directly to hair follicles.

Benefits: Aims to improve scalp health and stimulate hair growth.

Considerations: Effectiveness varies; multiple treatments may be necessary.

3. Exosome Therapy

A novel treatment using exosomes (small vesicles) to promote hair regeneration.

Procedure: Exosomes are injected into the scalp to encourage hair follicle activity.

Benefits: Potential to stimulate hair growth at the cellular level.

Considerations: Still under research; availability may be limited.

4. Low-Level Laser Therapy (LLLT) Caps

Devices that emit low-level lasers to stimulate hair follicles.

Procedure: Wearing a laser-emitting cap for a specified duration regularly.

Benefits: Non-invasive method to promote hair growth.

Considerations: Requires consistent use over time; results vary.

5. Scalp Micropigmentation (SMP)

A cosmetic tattooing technique to create the illusion of fuller hair.

Procedure: Pigment is applied to the scalp to mimic hair follicles.

Benefits: Provides the appearance of density in thinning areas.

Considerations: Does not promote hair growth; primarily aesthetic.

6. Topical Home Care

Incorporating specific products into daily routines can support hair health.

Options: Topical minoxidil, specialized shampoos, and conditioners.

Benefits: May slow hair loss and promote regrowth.

Considerations: Consistency is key; results may take months to appear.

Consulting with a dermatologist or hair specialist is essential to determine the most appropriate treatment based on individual needs and the underlying causes of hair thinning.

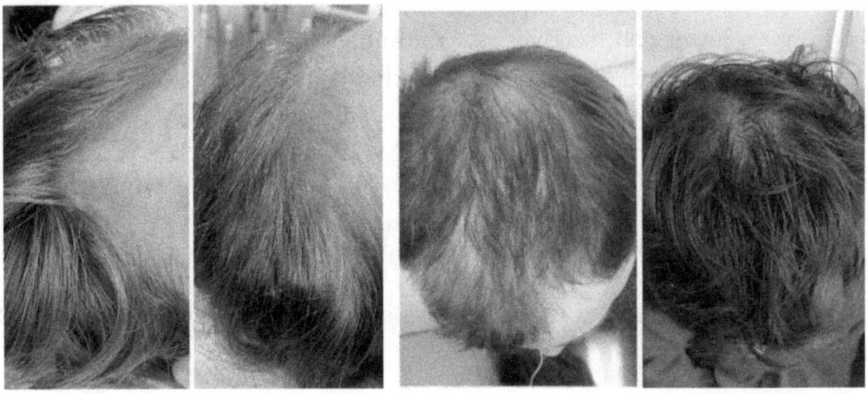

3 monthly sessions of PRP , after 6 months post last treatment.

Chapter 39: Body Skin "How It Differs from Facial Skin & Effective Treatments for Rejuvenation and Tightening"

Understanding the Structural Differences Between Facial and Body Skin

While the skin functions as a protective barrier throughout the body, its structure varies depending on location. The body's skin differs significantly from facial skin, influencing how it ages, heals, and responds to treatments.

1. Thickness

Body skin is generally thicker than facial skin, except in delicate areas like the eyelids.

The dermis on the body is denser, containing thicker collagen fibers, making it more resistant to external factors but slower to regenerate.

2. Collagen and Elasticity

Body skin has a lower cell turnover rate, meaning it renews more slowly than facial skin. It contains fewer sebaceous glands, making it more prone to dryness and laxity over time.

3. Fat Distribution and Cellulite Formation

Facial fat is evenly distributed, maintaining smooth contours.

Body fat is compartmentalized within fibrous septae (connective tissue bands), which contribute to cellulite formation.

4. Healing and Regeneration

Facial skin heals faster due to its higher vascularization.

Body skin, especially in areas like the thighs and abdomen, has poorer circulation, leading to slower healing and collagen remodeling.

Cellulite : What Causes It?

Cellulite affects up to 90% of women and is caused by a combination of:

Fibrous septae pulling the skin downward, creating dimples.

Fat pushing between these bands, leading to a lumpy appearance.

Weakening of skin structure due to collagen loss and poor circulation.

Hormonal factors, especially estrogen, which influences fat storage and skin integrity.

Genetics, which determine skin thickness, elasticity, and fat distribution.

Because cellulite is not just a fat issue but a structural problem, traditional weight loss methods do not always help. Effective treatments must target the connective tissue, skin quality, and circulation to achieve visible improvement.

Advanced Treatments for Body Skin Rejuvenation and Tightening

Improving skin laxity, volume loss, and cellulite requires injectables, energy-based devices, regenerative treatments, and mechanical techniques.

1. Subcision for Cellulite Releasing Fibrous Septae with a Cannula

How it Works: A blunt-tip cannula is used to manually break the fibrous septae responsible for cellulite dimpling.

Why it's Important: Once released, the skin can smooth out naturally, reducing visible dimples.

Best for:

Deep, tethered cellulite

Prepping the skin for biostimulatory fillers like Sculptra

Combining with PRP to speed healing and collagen stimulation

2. Sculptra® Hyperdiluted Collagen Biostimulation

How it Works: Sculptra (poly-L-lactic acid) is a collagen stimulator that, when hyperdiluted, spreads over a large area to enhance skin thickness, elasticity, and volume.

Best for:

Crepey skin on arms, abdomen, thighs, and buttocks

Skin laxity and cellulite improvement

Combining with subcision to fill areas of volume loss

3. Radiesse® Hyperdiluted Immediate & Long-Term Tightening

How it Works: Radiesse (calcium hydroxylapatite) stimulates collagen while providing an immediate lifting effect. When hyperdiluted, it improves skin texture, hydration, and firmness.

Best for:

Décolletage rejuvenation

Knees, arms, and abdominal skin tightening

Smoothing skin after cellulite treatments

4. PRP (Platelet-Rich Plasma) : Regenerative Therapy

How it Works: PRP contains growth factors that stimulate collagen and elastin, improving skin renewal and tissue repair.

Best for:

Stretch marks and scarring

Post-subcision healing and enhanced skin tightening

Combination with microneedling or radiofrequency for deeper skin remodelling

5. Radiofrequency (RF) Thermal Skin Tightening

How it Works: RF energy heats the dermis, stimulating collagen contraction and gradual remodelling over time.

Best for:

Post-pregnancy skin tightening

Moderate laxity on the abdomen, arms, and thighs

Cellulite reduction (when paired with lymphatic drainage)

Popular RF Devices: Thermage®, Exilis®, Venus Legacy®

6. Ultherapy® Ultrasound-Based Deep Lifting

How it Works: Ultherapy delivers micro-focused ultrasound energy to stimulate collagen production at the SMAS layer (deep connective tissue).

Best for:

Tightening loose skin on arms, stomach, knees, and buttocks

Patients wanting a non-invasive lifting effect

7. Morpheus®: RF Micro needling for Deep Tissue Remodelling

How it Works: A combination of micro needling and RF energy penetrates deep into the skin and tightens underlying tissue.

Best for:

Crepey skin and mild volume loss on arms, abdomen, and thighs

Cellulite dimpling improvement

Long-term skin firming and collagen regeneration

Other Skin Tightening & Cellulite Reduction Technologies

Emsculpt Neo® Uses RF heating and high-intensity focused electromagnetic (HIFEM) stimulation to tighten skin and tone muscles. Ideal for abdomen, buttocks, and arms.

Velashape® A combination of infrared light, RF, and vacuum suction to improve cellulite and skin tone.

Carboxytherapy: Injecting CO2 gas under the skin to increase circulation and collagen production, improving cellulite and elasticity.

Endermologie® A mechanical massage therapy that enhances lymphatic drainage and stimulates fibroblasts to reduce cellulite.

Combining Treatments for Optimal Results

The best outcomes for body skin rejuvenation and cellulite reduction come from combining multiple treatments:

Subcision + Sculptra/Radiesse Breaking down fibrous bands, then adding collagen stimulation and volume.

Morpheus8 + PRP Combining microneedling, RF, and regenerative therapy for long-term firming.

Ultherapy + RF treatments Deep collagen activation paired with surface tightening.

Muscle stimulation (Emsculpt Neo) + skin tightening Enhancing underlying structure for better skin support.

Conclusion

Body skin differs from facial skin in its thickness, collagen structure, fat distribution, and ability to heal. These differences require specialized treatments to improve laxity, volume loss, and cellulite.

By incorporating a combination of injectables, regenerative therapies, and energy-based treatments, practitioners can offer their patients highly effective, long-lasting solutions for firmer, smoother, and more youthful-looking skin.

With the right approach, non-surgical skin tightening and cellulite reduction can deliver remarkable, natural-looking result helping patients achieve renewed confidence in their bodies.

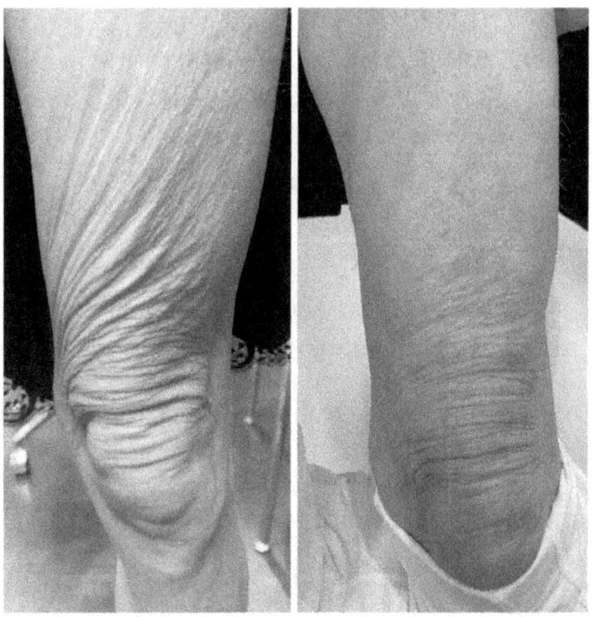

3 Monthly Sessions of PRP with cannula

Part 4- Understanding Injectables & Regenerative Aesthetics

Chapter 40: Beauty Through the Ages

The Original Quest for Youth

Sometimes patients ask me whether the desire to look younger is a modern obsession. I always smile when I hear that question.

The truth is that people have been searching for beauty, youth and vitality for thousands of years.

Long before cosmetic clinics, injectables and skin boosters existed, women and men were experimenting with treatments designed to improve their appearance. They may not have understood collagen, elastin, antioxidants or cellular regeneration, but they understood something very important:

Looking good made them feel good.
When we look back through history, it becomes clear that today's aesthetic treatments are simply the latest chapter in a very old story.
The products may have changed, but human nature has not.

Cleopatra's Famous Milk Baths
Perhaps the most famous beauty icon in history is Cleopatra.
Legend tells us she bathed in donkey's milk to keep her skin youthful, soft and radiant.
At first glance it sounds like little more than an extravagant royal ritual.
Yet modern science suggests there was some wisdom behind it.
Milk contains lactic acid, a naturally occurring alpha hydroxy acid that gently exfoliates the skin.
In other words, Cleopatra may have been enjoying one of the world's earliest chemical peels.
Thousands of years later, we are still using the same principle in aesthetic medicine.
The packaging has changed. The science has improved. The goal remains exactly the same.

The Egyptians Were Skincare Pioneers
Ancient Egyptians were remarkably advanced when it came to beauty and skincare.

They understood the importance of protecting the skin from the harsh desert environment and created preparations using natural oils, plant extracts and minerals.
Both men and women lined their eyes with black kohl.
While it created the dramatic look we associate with ancient Egypt, it also helped reduce glare from the sun and may have offered protection against eye infections.
Beauty and medicine have always shared a close relationship.
Many of the ingredients used by the Egyptians contained antibacterial and anti-inflammatory properties long before science understood why they worked.

The Greeks and the Pursuit of Harmony
The ancient Greeks viewed beauty differently.
For them, beauty was not simply about appearance.

It reflected balance, symmetry and harmony.
They believed the most attractive faces possessed proportion and structure.
Sound familiar?

Much of modern facial assessment is still based on these same principles.
Facial thirds. Facial fifths. Symmetry. Proportion.

Even the famous Golden Ratio, often discussed in aesthetics today, can be traced back to ideas that fascinated Greek mathematicians and philosophers thousands of years ago. While fashions come and go, our appreciation of facial balance has remained remarkably consistent.

Roman Beauty Rituals

The Romans inherited many of the beauty traditions of the Greeks and Egyptians and added a few of their own.
Roman women used sour wine, fermented fruit extracts and grape residues as skin treatments.
Without realising it, they were applying natural fruit acids to their skin.
Today we call them chemical peels.
Back then they simply called them beauty treatments.

It is fascinating to think that some of the most advanced cosmetic procedures offered in modern clinics are based on principles discovered centuries ago.

Honey: Nature's Original Skin Treatment

Long before pharmaceutical companies existed, honey was one of nature's most prized remedies.
The Egyptians used it to treat wounds.
The Greeks used it for skin health.
Many ancient cultures recognised its healing properties.
Today we know honey possesses antibacterial, anti-inflammatory and wound-healing benefits. Modern medicine has simply confirmed what our ancestors discovered through observation.
Sometimes the oldest treatments still have value.

Beauty Wasn't Always Safe

Not every beauty trend throughout history deserves a comeback.
In fact, some were downright dangerous.
Ancient Greek and Roman women often used lead-based powders to create pale skin, which was considered fashionable and a sign of wealth.
Centuries later, Victorian women continued the practice.
Unfortunately, the consequences included hair loss, skin damage, neurological problems and lead poisoning.
The pursuit of beauty has occasionally come at a very high price.
It serves as a reminder that just because something is fashionable does not mean it is safe.

Rice Water and Ancient Wisdom

For centuries, women in China and Japan washed their hair and skin with fermented rice water. Rich in amino acids, minerals and antioxidants, rice water is still found in many skincare products today.

Modern laboratories continue to study ingredients that traditional cultures were using hundreds of years ago. Sometimes innovation is not about discovering something new. Sometimes it is about rediscovering something old.

The First Injectable Disaster

As fascinating as ancient beauty treatments were, perhaps one of the most important lessons in aesthetic history came much later.

In the late nineteenth and early twentieth centuries, paraffin wax was injected into the face in an attempt to restore volume and smooth wrinkles.

Initially the results looked promising. Patients loved the immediate improvement.
Unfortunately, the complications that followed were devastating.
The paraffin migrated. Lumps formed. Chronic inflammation developed. Faces became distorted.
What initially appeared to be a miracle treatment eventually became a cautionary tale.

The lesson remains relevant today.
Just because a treatment creates volume does not mean it belongs in the face.

What History Teaches Us

When we look back through thousands of years of beauty rituals, one thing becomes clear.
People have always wanted the same things.
Healthy skin.A youthful appearance. Confidence. Vitality.
A reflection in the mirror that matches how they feel inside.
The methods have changed dramatically.
We have moved from milk baths to skin boosters.
From honey masks to growth factors.
From paraffin injections to biofillers.
Yet the desire remains the same.
The story of aesthetic medicine is not really the story of beauty.
It is the story of humanity's endless search for wellbeing, confidence and self-expression

And as we continue to explore regenerative medicine, biofillers and cellular therapies, we are simply writing the next chapter in a story that began thousands of years ago.

Beauty trends come and go. Products come and go. Technology continues to evolve.
But one thing never changes.
People want to look like the healthiest, happiest version of themselves.
That has been true for thousands of years, and I suspect it always will be.

.

Chapter 41: The Evolution of Cosmetic Injectables

From Collagen to Regeneation

A Brief Timeline of Injectable Milestones

- **1980s–1990s:** Bovine collagen fillers such as Zyderm and Zyplast introduce non-surgical volume restoration.
- **1990s:** Silicone and semi-permanent fillers like Artecoll gain popularity, highlighting the challenges of long-lasting products.
- **Late 1990s–2000s:** Hyaluronic acid fillers, including Restylane and Juvederm, transform aesthetic medicine.
- **2000s:** Botulinum toxin becomes a mainstream cosmetic treatment for dynamic wrinkles.
- **2000s–2010s:** Collagen stimulators such as Sculptra and Radiesse shift the focus toward tissue regeneration.
- **2010s:** PRP and other autologous therapies expand regenerative treatment options.
- **2020s:** Biofillers, polynucleotides and advanced regenerative therapies place tissue health and repair at the centre of aesthetic practice.

When I first entered aesthetic medicine, the treatments available looked very different from what we have today.

In many ways, the industry has undergone a complete transformation.

New injectors entering the profession today have access to products, technology and training that simply did not exist when I began. They can choose from dozens of filler ranges, collagen stimulators, skin boosters, polynucleotides, biofillers and regenerative treatments.

It wasn't always that way.

The journey from the early days of cosmetic injectables to the regenerative medicine era has been fascinating to witness. Looking back, it is remarkable how far we have come.

In the beginning, we were largely replacing volume.

Today, we are trying to regenerate tissue.

The philosophy has changed just as much as the products.

The Collagen Years

Long before hyaluronic acid fillers became household names, collagen was the injectable of choice.

The most widely used products were Zyderm and Zyplast, both derived from bovine collagen.

At the time they were revolutionary.

For the first time, practitioners could soften lines and restore volume without surgery.

Patients loved the immediate results, but the products had limitations.

Because they were derived from cow collagen, allergy testing was required before treatment. Patients often needed to return for skin testing and then wait before proceeding with treatment.

The results were relatively short-lived, often lasting only a few months.

Even so, for many patients these products represented the beginning of non-surgical facial rejuvenation.

Today, many younger injectors have never heard of Zyderm or Zyplast, yet these products paved the way for everything that followed.

Silicone: The Permanent Solution That Wasn't

There was also a period when liquid silicone was promoted as a permanent filler.

The idea was attractive. One treatment. Permanent results. No need for ongoing maintenance.

Unfortunately, the reality was often very different.

While some patients experienced satisfactory outcomes, others developed complications years later. Migration, chronic inflammation, nodules and deformities became increasingly recognised.

The problem with permanent products is simple.

Faces change. Ageing continues.

What looks appropriate at forty may not look appropriate at sixty.

The industry gradually moved away from permanent fillers in favour of products that could be adjusted, refined or dissolved if necessary.

It was an important lesson.

Sometimes permanence is not an advantage.

Artecoll and the Rise of Semi-Permanent Fillers

Artecoll was one of the first products to bridge the gap between temporary and permanent correction.

It combined bovine collagen with tiny polymethylmethacrylate (PMMA) microspheres.

The collagen provided immediate correction while the microspheres remained behind to stimulate a longer-lasting result.

For many patients it worked well.

However, as with all semi-permanent and permanent products, complications could be difficult to reverse.

The lesson remained the same.

The longer a product stays in the face, the more important injector skill and patient selection become.

The Hyaluronic Acid Revolution

Everything changed when hyaluronic acid fillers arrived.

Restylane was one of the first products to gain widespread popularity and it transformed the industry almost overnight.

Unlike collagen, allergy testing was no longer required.

The results were more predictable. Longevity improved. The safety profile was excellent.

Most importantly, the product integrated naturally into tissue.

For the first time, injectors had a filler that was versatile, reliable and relatively forgiving.

Soon after came Juvederm.

While Restylane and Juvederm were both hyaluronic acid fillers, they offered different rheological properties and treatment characteristics.

The arrival of these products sparked a boom in non-surgical cosmetic treatments.

Lips became fuller. Cheeks became more defined. Nasolabial folds softened.

The injectable industry exploded.

At the time, it felt revolutionary.

Looking back now, it was only the beginning.

Botox Changes Everything

Around the same period, another product was quietly changing aesthetic medicine forever.

Botulinum toxin.

Originally used for medical conditions such as strabismus, blepharospasm and muscle disorders, practitioners soon recognised its cosmetic potential.

For the first time, dynamic wrinkles could be softened without surgery.

Foreheads became smoother. Frown lines softened. Crow's feet faded.

Patients loved the results because they looked refreshed without appearing dramatically different.

Today Botox has become so familiar that many people forget how revolutionary it once was.

It fundamentally changed how society viewed ageing.

The Age of Collagen Stimulation

As the years passed, injectors began asking a new question.

What if we could stimulate the body to rebuild itself?

This led to the rise of biostimulators. Sculptra was one of the first major products in this category.

Rather than filling tissue directly, Poly-L-Lactic Acid stimulated the body's own collagen production.

Results developed gradually and naturally.

Patients were not buying filler. They were investing in collagen.

Radiesse followed with a different mechanism.

Its calcium hydroxyapatite microspheres provided immediate support while also stimulating collagen production over time.

For many injectors, this represented a shift in thinking.

We were no longer simply replacing lost volume.

We were encouraging the body to regenerate.

The Platelet Revolution

Then came Platelet Rich Plasma.

PRP fascinated both practitioners and patients because the treatment used the patient's own blood.

No synthetic filler. No foreign material.

Just growth factors and regenerative potential harvested from the body's own healing mechanisms.

Initially PRP was viewed with some scepticism.

Today it is widely used for facial rejuvenation, hair restoration, scar treatment and tissue regeneration.

PRP opened the door to an entirely new way of thinking about aesthetics.

Instead of asking what product could be added, practitioners began asking how the body's natural repair systems could be activated.

Biofillers and Autologous Treatments

One of the most exciting developments in recent years has been the emergence of biofillers.

Using platelet-rich fibrin and processed plasma proteins, practitioners can now create volume using the patient's own biological material.

For many patients this is an appealing concept.

Their own tissue becomes the treatment.

It represents a move away from synthetic materials and towards personalised regenerative medicine.

It is also a reminder that some of the most exciting innovations in aesthetics may come from the patient themselves.

Polynucleotides and the Regenerative Era

If the collagen era was about replacing volume and the biostimulator era was about building collagen, the current era is increasingly focused on tissue health.

Polynucleotides have emerged as one of the most exciting regenerative treatments available.

Rather than creating volume, they work at a cellular level to support repair, hydration and tissue quality.

The focus is no longer simply how a face looks.

It is how the tissue functions.

This represents a significant philosophical shift in aesthetic medicine.

Patients today are increasingly asking for healthier skin rather than bigger cheeks.

They want glow rather than volume.

Quality rather than quantity.

Regeneration rather than camouflage.

Looking Ahead

The future of aesthetics is likely to become even more regenerative.

Biofillers, Polynucleotides, Exosomes, Cell signalling therapies, Tissue engineering, Longevity medicine, Artificial intelligence.

Many of the treatments that seem cutting-edge today will eventually become routine.

Just as Zyderm and Zyplast once seemed revolutionary.

What remains unchanged is the patient sitting in the chair.

They still want to look like themselves. They still want natural results. They still want to age well.

The products will continue to evolve. The technology will continue to evolve.

But the art of listening, assessing and treating the whole person will always remain at the heart of aesthetic medicine.

Nita's Clinical Pearl

When I look back at the evolution of cosmetic injectables, one thing stands out.

The industry has moved from filling faces to restoring tissue.

From correction to regeneration.

And in my opinion, that is exactly where the future belongs.

Chapter 42: Aesthetic Myths, Misconceptions and Social Media Misinformation

Separating Fact From Fiction

Never before have people had access to so much information about cosmetic treatments.

Unfortunately, never before have they been exposed to so much misinformation.

Every week I hear patients repeat things they have read online, seen on TikTok or heard from a friend who heard it from someone else.

Some myths are harmless. Others create unnecessary fear.

A few can prevent people from receiving treatments that may genuinely help them.

As injectors, one of our responsibilities is education.

Let's separate some of the most common myths from reality.

Myth #1: Botox Is a Toxin So It Must Be Dangerous

This is probably the most common misconception of all.

Yes, Botulinum Toxin is derived from a naturally occurring bacterium.

However, the doses used in aesthetic medicine are extremely small and have been extensively studied for decades.

Botox has one of the largest safety databases in aesthetic medicine.

Like any medication, it must be used appropriately and by trained practitioners.

The word toxin sounds frightening. The science is far less dramatic.

Myth #2: Botox Makes Everyone Look Frozen

Not true.

Poor Botox creates frozen faces. Good Botox creates relaxed faces.

The goal is not to eliminate every movement.

The goal is to soften excessive muscle activity while maintaining natural expression.

When patients tell me they are afraid of looking frozen, I often explain that most people never notice good Botox.

They simply think the person looks refreshed.

Myth #3: Dermal Fillers Stretch The Skin Forever

This myth refuses to die.

Patients often worry that if they stop having filler their skin will stretch and sag.

In reality, ageing continues whether we have filler or not.

Appropriately placed filler can support tissue and improve facial proportions.

If the filler gradually dissolves, the patient simply returns to their natural ageing process.

The exception is repeated overfilling over many years, which can alter tissue behaviour and facial appearance.

The problem is not filler. The problem is too much filler.

Myth #4: All Filler Migrates

Migration has become one of the most overused words in aesthetics.

Can filler migrate? Yes.

Does all filler migrate? Absolutely not.

Most properly placed filler remains remarkably stable.

Migration is more likely when excessive volumes are placed, incorrect products are used, or treatments are repeated too frequently.

Social media has created the impression that every filler treatment eventually migrates. The reality is far more nuanced.

Myth #5: Bigger Lips Are Better Lips

One of the greatest misconceptions of the social media era.

Beautiful lips are not defined by volume.

They are defined by proportion. Balance, Shape And suitability to the individual's face.

A small, naturally shaped lip often looks far more attractive than a large lip that overwhelms facial harmony.

The best lip enhancement is usually the one nobody notices.

Myth #6: Botox Causes Addiction

Botox is not physically addictive.

However, many patients enjoy the way they look and feel after treatment and choose to continue.

This is very different from addiction.

Most patients simply prefer the softened lines and refreshed appearance.

If they stop treatment, the muscles gradually return to their normal activity.

Nothing dramatic happens. The ageing process simply continues.

Myth #7: Sculptra Causes Granulomas

This myth has persisted for years.

As discussed in an earlier chapter, many of the lumps historically attributed to Sculptra were not true granulomas.

In the early days, lower dilution protocols and less refined injection techniques occasionally resulted in product clustering and localised collagen accumulation.

Modern dilution techniques, improved training and better understanding of the product have dramatically reduced these complications.

True granulomas remain uncommon.

Myth #8: PRP Is Just a Vampire Facial

Thank you, Hollywood.

PRP became famous after celebrity photographs showing blood-covered faces appeared online.

The media quickly labelled it the "Vampire Facial."

While the name attracted attention, it completely missed the science.

PRP is a regenerative treatment that uses the patient's own platelets and growth factors to stimulate healing and tissue repair.

It is far more sophisticated than the nickname suggests.

Myth #9: If It's Natural, It's Safe

This is one of the most dangerous myths in healthcare.

Natural does not automatically mean safe.

Poison ivy is natural. Snake venom is natural.

Many natural substances can cause allergic reactions, infections or serious complications.

Safety depends on evidence, appropriate use and clinical judgement, not whether something comes from nature.

Myth #10: Cosmetic Treatments Are Only For Vanity

This myth says far more about society than it does about patients.

Most people do not seek treatment because they want to become someone else.

They want their appearance to better reflect how they feel.

The woman who looks permanently tired despite feeling energetic.

The man whose frown lines make him appear angry.

The cancer survivor rebuilding confidence after treatment.

The menopausal woman navigating enormous physical changes.

Aesthetic medicine is often less about vanity and more about confidence, self-expression and wellbeing.

Myth #11: More Product Equals Better Results

This is perhaps the most expensive myth in aesthetics.

The most attractive faces are rarely the faces with the most product.

The best results often come from restraint.

A small amount of product in the right place can create far more improvement than large volumes placed indiscriminately.

The goal is not to look injected. The goal is to look well.

Myth #12: Ageing Is Something To Fight

This may be the biggest myth of all.

Ageing is not a disease. It is a privilege.

The purpose of aesthetic medicine is not to stop ageing. That is impossible. The purpose is to help people age well.

To look healthy, To look vibrant, To feel confident, To remain recognisably themselves.

The best aesthetic work never tries to erase age. It simply softens its impact.

Nita's Clinical Pearl

One of the most valuable things an injector can offer a patient is not a treatment.

It is education. A patient who understands their face, their options and realistic outcomes will almost always be happier than a patient who arrives with unrealistic expectations created by social media.

Trends come and go. Myths come and go. Good clinical judgement never goes out of fashion.

Chapter 43: Botulinum Toxin Type A What It Is, Manufacturing, Safety, and Variants

What Is Botulinum Toxin Type A?

Botulinum toxin type A is a purified neurotoxin derived from the Clostridium botulinum bacterium. It is important to note that Botox is NOT the bacterium itself rather, it is a highly refined neurotoxin that is carefully extracted, purified, and diluted to ensure safe medical and cosmetic use.

Botulinum Toxin vs. Clostridium Botulinum Bacteria

Clostridium botulinum is a naturally occurring bacterium found in soil, lakes, and forests.

This bacterium can produce botulinum toxin under certain conditions, such as low-oxygen environments. The toxin is one of the most potent biological substances, capable of blocking nerve signals and causing paralysis in high doses. In medicine, only a purified and controlled amount of botulinum toxin type A is used making it safe when administered correctly.

How Was Botulinum Toxin Discovered?

The first therapeutic use of botulinum toxin was pioneered in the 1970s by ophthalmologists Dr. Jean and Dr. Alastair Carruthers while treating eye muscle disorders (e.g., strabismus, blepharospasm). They observed that patients developed smoother skin in treated areas, leading to the cosmetic use of botulinum toxin. In 1991, the first botulinum toxin treatment for wrinkles was documented, and Botox® was officially approved for cosmetic use.

How Is Botox Manufactured?

The production of Botox (OnabotulinumtoxinA) involves a highly controlled, multi-step purification and testing process to ensure its safety and efficacy. The manufacturing process includes:

1. Culturing the Bacteria

The process begins with the controlled growth of Clostridium botulinum in a secure laboratory environment.

The bacterium is grown under strict conditions to allow it to naturally produce botulinum toxin type A.

2. Harvesting the Toxin

Once enough toxin is produced, the bacteria are removed, leaving only the botulinum toxin. The toxin is carefully extracted and separated from other bacterial components.

3. Purification Process

The extracted botulinum toxin undergoes multiple purification steps to remove any unwanted proteins or contaminants. This process ensures that only the pure, active botulinum toxin type A remains. The purified toxin is then stabilized using human albumin, a protein that helps maintain its structure and effectiveness.

4. Dilution & Standardization

The purified botulinum toxin is diluted to an exact concentration to create the final medical-grade Botox product. Each batch is rigorously tested to ensure potency, consistency, and safety. The product is then packaged into vials and stored under strict temperature-controlled conditions to preserve its activity.

Why Is Botox Safe for Medical Use?

Although botulinum toxin in its natural form is highly toxic, the controlled doses used in Botox treatments are small, purified, and carefully measured for safety.

Extremely Low Doses: The amount of botulinum toxin used in medical treatments is millions of times lower than what would cause toxicity.

Purified & Stabilized: The purification process removes unnecessary bacterial components, ensuring only the active neurotoxin is present.

FDA & TGA Approved: Botox has been extensively studied and approved by regulatory agencies such as the U.S. FDA (Food and Drug Administration) and Australia's TGA (Therapeutic Goods Administration) for both medical and cosmetic use.

Injected in Targeted Areas: Unlike botulism (which affects the whole body), Botox is administered in small, precise doses to specific muscles making it a safe and effective localized treatment.

Different Types of Botulinum Toxin Type A & Their Differences

There are now many different brands of botulinum toxin available worldwide, each with different formulations, carrier proteins, diffusion properties, and unit measurements.

Common FDA/TGA-Approved Brands and Their Differences

Brand	Protein Composition	Carrier/Base	Key Differences
Botox (OnabotulinumtoxinA)	Has complexing proteins	Human albumin & saline	Most well-known, stable diffusion, predictable effects
Xeomin (IncobotulinumtoxinA)	No accessory proteins (pure toxin)	Human albumin & saline	No complexing proteins = reduced risk of resistance
Dysport (AbobotulinumtoxinA)	Has complexing proteins	Human albumin & lactose	Spreads more than Botox, good for larger areas
Jeuveau (PrabotulinumtoxinA)	Has complexing proteins	Human albumin & saline	Marketed as #Newtox in the U.S.
Revance Daxxify (DaxxibotulinumtoxinA -lanm)	Peptide-stabilized (no human albumin)	Peptide-based carrier	Potentially longer-lasting results
Lytebo (Botulinum Toxin Type A, China-based)	Has complexing proteins	Glucose & gelatin	Newer product, limited international experience

Understanding units in Botulinum Toxin

A unit measures the toxin biological activity (its ability to block nerve signals).

However, units are NOT interchangeable between brands because each company uses a different potency assay.

Brand	Unit Conversion	Key Differences
Botox & Xeomin	1 Botox unit = 1 Xeomin unit	Direct unit-to-unit conversion
Dysport	2.5 Dysport units = 1 Botox unit	Dysport diffuses more, requiring more units for an equivalent effect
Jeuveau/Nuceiva	1:1 with Botox	Considered equivalent to Botox in dosing
Lytebo	Similar to Botox (research ongoing)	Limited data outside China
Daxxify	1:1 with Botox	Early studies suggest longer duration

WARNING: Counterfeit & Illegal Botulinum Toxin Products

Dangers of Fake or Unapproved Botulinum Toxin

Recent Incident in Sydney:

Three people were hospitalized with botulism poisoning after receiving botulinum toxin injections from an unlicensed backyard injector who bought fake products from the internet. Symptoms included severe muscle paralysis, difficulty breathing, and hospitalization.

How to Avoid Counterfeit Toxins

Only receive treatments from licensed medical professionals (doctors, registered nurses, trained aesthetic practitioners).

Ensure the clinic uses FDA- or TGA-approved brands. Avoid discount offers from non-reputable sources (e.g., home-based injectors, overseas imports). Check the packageing legitimate toxins come with lot numbers, expiration dates, and secure labeling. Do not buy toxins online,only licensed professionals can legally obtain these medications.

Conclusion

Botox is NOT the bacterium it is a purified, controlled form of botulinum toxin type A.

It is produced through a strict manufacturing process, ensuring safety, purity, and effectiveness. There are now many different brands on the market, each with unique properties, diffusion rates, and unit conversions.FDA/TGA-approved toxins include Botox, Xeomin, Dysport, Jeuveau, Lytebo, and Daxxify. Counterfeit and illegally imported toxins pose serious health risks, including botulism poisoning.

Always seek treatment from a reputable clinic that uses licensed and approved botulinum toxin brands.

Understanding the manufacturing, purification, and regulatory approval of Botox helps dispel myths and reinforces why choosing a qualified provider is essential for both safety and results.

Relfydess™: The New Tox on the Block

What is Relfydess™

Relfydess™ (RelabotulinumtoxinA) is a new botulinum toxin introduced by Galderma as an alternative to established brands like Botox®, Dysport®, Xeomin®, and Jeuveau®. It stands out due to its ready-to-use liquid formulation, a different botulinum strain, and potentially longer-lasting effects. Designed for facial wrinkle treatment, it offers fast-acting, consistent results while simplifying the preparation process for practitioners.

Key Differences of Relfydess™

1. Different Botulinum Strain

• Most neuromodulators (Botox, Dysport, Xeomin, Jeuveau) are derived from the Hall strain of Clostridium botulinum.

Relfydess™ comes from a different botulinum strain, which may contribute to variations in diffusion, longevity, and resistance development.

2. Unit Measurement and Volume

Relfydess™ uses the same unit measurement as Dysport®, meaning that the dose conversion will align with Dysport protocols.

However, its injection volume matches Botox®, making it easier to transition for practitioners familiar with Botox's dilution and handling.

3. Ready-to-Use Liquid Formula

Unlike Botox, Dysport, and Jeuveau, which come as a powder that requires reconstitution, Relfydess™ is pre-mixed in liquid form.

This eliminates potential dilution errors, ensures consistent dosing, and streamlines the preparation process.

4. Potential for Faster Onset

Botox and Xeomin typically take 3–5 days for visible results.

Dysport has a faster onset (2–3 days) but diffuses more widely.

Clinical studies suggest Relfydess™ may start working as early as Day 1 for some patients, making it one of the quickest-acting options available.

5. Duration of Effects

Botox, Dysport, Xeomin, and Jeuveau generally last 3–4 months before retreatment is needed.

Early data indicates Relfydess™ may last up to 6 months in some patients, potentially offering extended effectiveness.

Considerations for Practitioners and Patients

For injectors, the pre-mixed formulation can reduce preparation time and improve consistency. However, those accustomed to Botox or Dysport may need to adjust unit conversions.

For patients, Relfydess™ may offer a faster onset and longer duration, but individual results can vary.

Since Relfydess™ uses a different botulinum strain, it may be an option for those who have developed resistance to other toxins.

How Relfydess™ Compares to Other Toxins.

Feature	**Relfydess™**	**Botox® (OnabotulinumtoxinA)**	**Dysport® (AbobotulinumtoxinA)**	**Xeomin® (IncobotulinumtoxinA)**	**Jeuveau® (PrabotulinumtoxinA)**
Botulinum Strain	Unique strain	*Hall strain	Hall strain	Hall strain (purified)	Hall strain
Formulation	Pre-mixed liquid	Powder (requires mixing)	Powder (requires mixing)	Powder (no complexing proteins)	Powder (requires mixing)
Onset of Action	As early as 1 day	3–5 days	2–3 days (faster spread)	3–4 days	3–4 days
Longevity	Up to 6 months	3–4 months	3–4 months	3–4 months	3–4 months
Spread/Diffusion	Balanced	Precise	More diffusion	Precise	Similar to Botox
Resistance Risk	Lower (unique strain)	Can develop resistance	Can develop resistance	Lower (no complexing proteins)	Can develop resistance
Unit Measurement	Same as Dysport	Botox units	Dysport units	Botox units	Botox units

** OnabotulinumtoxinA • The "Hall strain" is the original strain used by Dr. Edward J. Schantz in the 1940s for medical research and is still used in the production of Botox today.*

Aesthetic Areas Treated and Injection Considerations with Botulinum Toxin A:

1. Forehead (Frontalis)

Goal: Smooth horizontal lines while maintaining brow position.

Care: Avoid injecting too low or too deep laterally — may drop brows or cause heavy eyelids. Use light dosing across upper frontalis to preserve natural movement and lift.

2. Frown Lines (Glabellar Complex – Procerus & Corrugators)

Goal: Soften vertical "11" lines.

Care: Avoid injecting too deep into the central glabella near the supraorbital foramen — can affect levator palpebrae superioris, causing ptosis.

3. Crow's Feet (Orbicularis Oculi)

Goal: Soften lateral eye wrinkles. Care: Avoid deep or low injection near zygomatic arch — may cause cheek shelving or heavy nasolabial folds.

4. Bunny Lines (Nasalis)

Goal: Reduce nasal scrunch lines. Care: Avoid diffusion toward the levator labii superioris alaeque nasi — may drop the upper lip.

5. Lip Lines (Perioral)

Goal: Soften vertical lip lines. Care: Over-treatment may elongate the top lip, distort smile or affect lip competence. Use microdoses.

6. DAO (Depressor Anguli Oris)

Goal: Upturn marionette area/downturned mouth corners. Care: Avoid diffusion to depressor labii inferioris (DLI) — may cause crooked smile or lip drop.

7. Masseter Muscle

Goal: Facial slimming, treat bruxism or clenching. Care: Avoid superior and anterior spread to risorius muscle — may impair smiling or cause flat expression.

8. Nose

Tip Lift: Microdose into depressor septi nasi to lift tip.

Narrowing: Target nasalis for gentle narrowing.

Hay Fever Relief: Intranasal injection may reduce symptoms (off-label).

9. Nefertiti Lift

Target: Lower face/jawline — platysma.

Goal: Sharpen jawline, reduce jowls. Care: Correct dosing avoids weakening neck support.

10. Platysma Bands

Goal: Soften neck bands, improve neck profile. Care: Over-treatment may affect swallowing or lifting the head.

11. Eyebrow Lifts

Medial Lift: Relax depressor supercilii (DSS).

Lateral Lift: Inject into lateral orbicularis or temporalis to elevate tail of brow.

12. Hyperhidrosis

Areas: Axillae, palms, soles, scalp. Care: Treat one hand at a time to avoid bilateral weakness.

13. Trapezius Muscles

Goal: Slim upper shoulders for a more elegant neck profile.

14. Calf Slimming (Popular in Asia)

Target: Gastrocnemius. Care: High doses required; avoid weakness in gait.

15. Mesotherapy (Micro-Botox)

Use: Superficial injections to reduce pore size, oil, and acne activity.

16. Bell's Palsy

Goal: Relax unaffected side to create facial symmetry. Care: Requires expert anatomical precision and custom dosing.

Expected Results of Botulinum Toxin A Injection:

Onset: 3–5 days. Peak Effect: 10–14 days

Duration: 3–4 months on average (masseters and hyperhydrosis 7-9 months.)

Chapter 44: Understanding Dermal Fillers: Composition, Manufacturing, and Rheology

What Are Dermal Fillers?

Dermal fillers are gel-like substances injected beneath the skin to restore volume, smooth wrinkles, enhance facial contours, and hydrate the skin. Most modern dermal fillers are composed of hyaluronic acid (HA), a naturally occurring substance in the human body that retains moisture and adds plumpness to the skin. Unlike botulinum toxin (which relaxes muscles), fillers work by physically adding volume to areas that have lost structure due to ageing or other factors.

Where Do Fillers Come From?

Modern HA fillers are made in laboratories through a process called bacterial fermentation. Special strains of Streptococcus bacteria are used to produce hyaluronic acid, which is then purified, cross-linked (to make it last longer in the skin), and turned into a smooth injectable gel.

Discovery of Dermal Fillers: Early fillers included collagen-based products derived from bovine (cow) sources, requiring allergy testing. In the late 1990s, scientists developed hyaluronic acid (HA) fillers, which were safer, more biocompatible, and longer-lasting. Today, HA fillers are the most commonly used fillers worldwide due to their natural integration with human tissue and reversibility using the enzyme hyaluronidase.

Hyaluronic Acid in the Body

HA is a sugar molecule (glycosaminoglycan) found naturally in skin, joints, and connective tissues. It can hold up to 1,000 times its weight in water, making it a key molecule for skin hydration and volume retention. Our body naturally produces and degrades HA daily, with enzymes like hyaluronidase breaking it down within hours to days.

Why Do HA Fillers Last Longer?

Since natural HA degrades quickly, scientists developed synthetic modifications to make HA fillers last longer in the skin.

How Are HA Fillers Made?

The Manufacturing Process of HA Fillers

1. **Fermentation**: HA is synthesized through bacterial fermentation (typically using Streptococcus bacteria). The HA is then purified and processed into a gel-like form.

2. **Crosslinking with BDDE**: To increase longevity, HA molecules are chemically crosslinked using 1,4-butanediol diglycidyl ether (BDDE).. BDDE acts as a binding agent, linking HA molecules together, preventing rapid degradation, and extending the fillers durability.

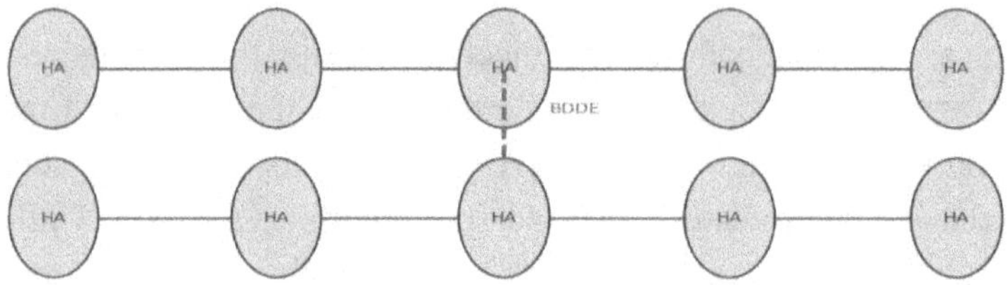

Chains of HA crosslinked with BDDE to increase longevity

3. **Customization of HA Fillers**: Different fillers are created by modifying the level of crosslinking, particle size, and gel consistency, producing different types suited for various treatments.

What Is BDDE?

BDDE (1,4-Butanediol Diglycidyl Ether) is a crosslinking agent used to stabilize HA in dermal fillers. Without BDDE, HA fillers would break down within days. The amount of BDDE and the crosslinking method determine how firm, elastic, and long-lasting the filler will be.

How Does Crosslinking Affect Longevity & Thickness?

The more crosslinking, the longer-lasting and firmer the filler:

Crosslinking Level	Filler Properties	Best Use Cases
Low Crosslinking	More fluid, hydrating, integrates easily	Skin boosters, superficial fine lines
Moderate Crosslinking	Balance of flexibility and structure	Lips, tear troughs, mid-face volume
High Crosslinking	Thick, firm, long-lasting	Cheeks, jawline, deep structural support

Different HA Filler Technologies & How They Work

PEG vs. BDDE Cross-Linking in Dermal Fillers: What's the Difference?

Most dermal fillers use hyaluronic acid (HA), but to make them last longer in the skin, the HA needs to be stabilized using a chemical cross-linking process. The traditional method uses BDDE (1,4-Butanediol Diglycidyl Ether), while a newer alternative is PEG (Polyethylene Glycol) cross-linking.

BDDE has been the standard for years and is safe for most people, but tiny traces of the chemical may remain in the filler after manufacturing. In rare cases, BDDE-based fillers can trigger inflammatory reactions or delayed nodules, especially in sensitive individuals.

PEG, on the other hand, is a medical-grade polymer known for its biocompatibility and low immune response. PEG-crosslinked fillers, such as Neauvia's range, have been designed to be BDDE-free, meaning they contain no epoxy-based crosslinkers. PEG-based fillers are reported to cause less swelling, lower risk of immune reactions, and smoother integration into the skin. They also have a more elastic and flexible texture, making them ideal for natural-looking volume and movement.

Both BDDE and PEG fillers are safe and effective, but PEG cross-linking offers a purer, more advanced alternative with a lower risk of long-term complications.

Various filler brands have proprietary crosslinking technologies that influence their consistency, longevity, and integration.

PEG Cross-Linking in Dermal Fillers: Another HA Linking technology

Polyethylene Glycol (PEG) cross-linking is a modern advancement in dermal fillers, offering longer-lasting, more hydrating, and biocompatible results compared to traditional BDDE (1,4-butanediol diglycidyl ether) cross-linking. This technology creates a smooth, natural look with reduced risk of swelling or inflammation, making it ideal for delicate areas like under-eyes, lips, and hands.

Why Choose PEG Fillers?

Longer-Lasting – PEG stabilizes hyaluronic acid (HA) more effectively, slowing breakdown.

Superior Hydration – PEG fillers retain more water, improving skin plumpness.

Low Inflammation Risk – PEG is highly biocompatible, reducing sensitivity or swelling.

Soft, Natural Integration – Especially useful for areas requiring smooth transitions.

Fillers That Use PEG Technology

• **Neauvia Intense & Neauvia Stimulate** – Provides volume and stimulates collagen production.

• **Matex Lab HA Hydrogels** – A range of hydration-focused fillers for different facial areas.

• **Novel PEGDE-HA 24** – Specifically designed for natural lip enhancement with minimal swelling.

Filler Technologies Explained

When it comes to dermal fillers, not all hyaluronic acid (HA) gels are created equal. The way the HA is crosslinked and structured affects how the filler behaves — its softness, longevity, lift capacity, and integration into tissue. Here's a breakdown of some of the most widely used proprietary technologies in today's top fillers:

1. Vycross Technology (Allergan – Juvederm Voluma, Volbella, Volift, etc.)

• What it is: A blend of low and high molecular weight HA, crosslinked together using BDDE.

• Why it matters: The low-weight HA allows for tighter crosslinking, making the gel smoother and longer-lasting.

• Designed to integrate well with tissue and give natural volume with minimal swelling.

• Voluma is firmer for cheeks and structure, while Volbella is softer for lips and fine lines.

• Bonus: High moldability and durability with fewer lumps.

2. Hyalocross Technology (Allergan – Juvederm Ultra and Ultra Plus)

• What it is: An earlier generation technology that uses only high molecular weight HA, crosslinked with BDDE.

• Why it matters: Gives a more gel-like consistency, slightly more water-attracting (hydrophilic), so more swelling than Vycross.

• Good for volumizing lips or nasolabial folds, but doesn't last as long as Vycross fillers.

• Still widely used due to its proven performance and affordability.

3. RHA (Resilient Hyaluronic Acid – Teoxane RHA 1–4)

• What it is: HA that is minimally crosslinked and processed gently to preserve its natural long-chain structure.

• Why it matters: Moves dynamically with facial expressions, making it ideal for lips, perioral lines, and dynamic areas.

• Designed to mimic natural HA more closely, offering a soft, elastic feel.

• RHA 4 is great for structure, while RHA 1 and 2 are better for fine lines and lips.

4. CPM (Cohesive Polydensified Matrix – Belotero by Merz)

• What it is: A unique crosslinking process that creates zones of varying density within the filler gel.

• Why it matters: Allows the filler to integrate seamlessly into tissue, minimizing the risk of lumps or Tyndall effect.

• Belotero Balance is so fine it can be used in the superficial dermis.

• Excellent for tear troughs, fine lines, and blending into delicate areas.

5. OBT (Optimal Balance Technology – Restylane Refyne, Defyne, etc. by Galderma)

• What it is: A crosslinking technique balancing HA size, flexibility, and support for natural facial movement.

• Why it matters: Designed to offer flexibility in motion while still lifting and contouring.

• Refyne is softer and better for moderate lines, while Defyne gives more structure for deeper folds.

• The structure allows strong support with stretch, making it ideal for smile lines and mobile areas.

6. NASHA® (Non-Animal Stabilized Hyaluronic Acid) was the first hyaluronic acid (HA) filler technology used in aesthetics. Developed for the Restylane® range, it uses a unique sieving process that filters the gel into uniform particle sizes, creating a structured, cohesive gel.

This makes it ideal for precise placement, contouring, and lifting—perfect for areas like the nasolabial folds, cheeks, and lips. Fillers made with NASHA® include Restylane® Classic, Restylane® Lyft, and Restylane® Vital.

Unlike other technologies that offer soft, flexible gels for dynamic movement (like OBT/XpresHAn or RHA®), NASHA® fillers are firmer and hold their shape.

This structure gives greater control for sculpting and definition, making them a go-to for injectors seeking predictable, long-lasting results with minimal migration.

Common HA Filler Technologies

Technology	Manufacturer	Properties	Best Used For
Vycross®	Juvederm (Allergan)	Small and large HA molecules mixed for smooth integration	Lips, under-eye, cheeks
Hylacross®	Juvederm (Allergan)	Larger, more structured HA chains	Nasolabial folds, volumization
Resilient Hyaluronic Acid (RHA®)	Teoxane	More elastic, moves with facial expressions	Dynamic areas (lips, nasolabial folds)
Cohesive Polydensified Matrix	Belotero (Merz)	Highlyadaptable, integrates well	Fine lines, tear troughs
OBT (Optimal Balance Technology)	Restylane (Galderma)	Balanced crosslinking, adaptable texture	Mid-face, lips, contouring
Nasha	Restylane (Galderma)	Structured, firm, mouldable precise	Chin, jaw, cheeks, lips
Cold X (Cold cross linking)	Hugal	Low temp cross linking for purity and homogeneity	Cheeks, lips, perioral area
Ultra High Flexibility	QT Fillers/ BioPlus	Very elastic HA gel for high mobility areas	Perioral area, lips, tear troughs
Ariessence (Advanced HA technology)	Koru Pharmaceuticals	Lightweight gel with high moldability , balanced elasticity and cohesiveness	Lips, tear troughs,

Each brand modifies its crosslinking and particle size to create fillers tailored to different facial areas.

Rheology: Understanding the Properties of Fillers

Why Rheology Matters in Filler Selection

Rheology is the study of how a filler behaves under pressure and movement. It helps clinicians choose the right filler for the right area.

Key Rheological Properties of Fillers

Property	Meaning	Importance in Treatment
(Gel Elasticity or Stiffness)	Higher G= firmer filler, lower G = softer filler	High G cheeks, jawline; Low G = lips, under-eye
Viscosity	How thick or fluid the filler is	Higher viscosity = better volume support
Cohesivity	How well the filler holds together	High cohesivity = better lift, low cohesivity = smooth integration
Elasticity (Stretchability)	Ability to move with facial expressions	High elasticity = ideal for dynamic areas like lips

Example:

Cheekbone augmentation needs a filler with high G prime (firm structure) like Restylane Lyft or Juvederm Voluma

Lips require a softer, more flexible filler with moderate elasticity, like RHA 2 or Juvederm Volbella.

Skin Boosters: Hydration Without Structure

Unlike dermal fillers used for volume, skin boosters have minimal crosslinking, allowing them to spread easily and deeply hydrate the skin.

What Makes Skin Boosters Different?

Instead of lifting or contouring, skin boosters improve hydration, elasticity, and skin texture.

They are microinjected into the dermis, not deep like traditional fillers.

Skin boosters stimulate collagen production and moisture retention, creating glowing, plump skin.

Popular Skin Boosters:

Profhilo® (NAHYCO® technology hybrid HA molecules)

Juvederm Volite, Restylane Skinboosters, Teosyal Redensity

Choosing the Right Filler for Each Area

A skilled injector must select the correct filler based on:

The treatment area (e.g., deep structure vs. superficial hydration)

The patient's skin type and movement dynamics

The desired longevity and integration

Area	Recommended Filler Type
Cheeks & Jawline	High G prime (firm, lifting) Allergan Voluma, Volux Restylane Lyft Teoxane Ultra Deep
Tear Troughs (Under Eyes)	Low G prime™ (soft, hydrating) Belotero Balance, Teoxane Redensity 2
Lips	Moderate elasticity Teoxane RHA 2, Allergan Juvederm Volbella are for a natural look. Higher G prime is chosen for more defined fuller lips.
Nasolabial Folds	Medium viscosity Restylane Defyne, or Volyme. Juvederm Ultra
Skin Hydration (No Volume)	Skin boosters Profhilo, Volite

Conclusion

Dermal fillers are primarily made of hyaluronic acid (HA), a natural substance in the body. HA is broken down quickly, so crosslinking with BDDE is used to extend its longevity.

The more crosslinking, the thicker and longer-lasting the filler. Different brands use proprietary crosslinking technologies to modify filler behavior.

Rheology determines which filler is best suited for specific facial areas. Skin boosters, with minimal crosslinking, are designed for hydration rather than volume.

By understanding filler properties, technology, and rheology, clinicians can achieve safe, natural-looking, and long-lasting results tailored to each patient's needs.

FILLER VOLUME: SMALL AMOUNTS, BIG IMPACT

It's amazing how such tiny volumes of filler can create beautiful, natural-looking results.

1 SYRINGE = 1 ML OF FILLER

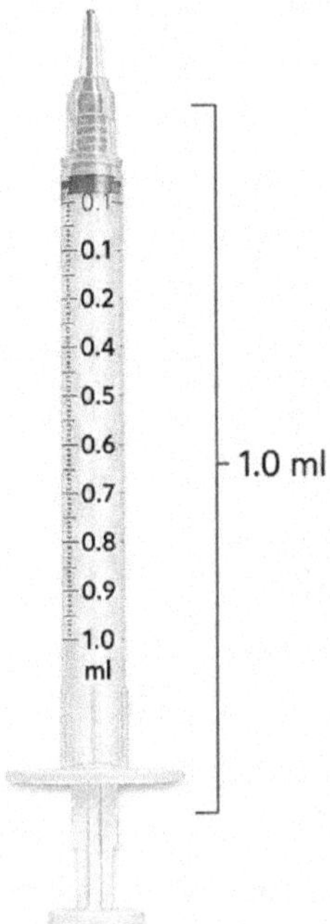

1 TABLESPOON (TBSP) = 10 ML

Visualizing filler volumes in a 10 ml tablespoon

1 ML (0.1 TBSP)	2 ML (0.2 TBSP)	3 ML (0.3 TBSP)	5 ML (0.5 TBSP)	6 ML (0.6 TBSP)

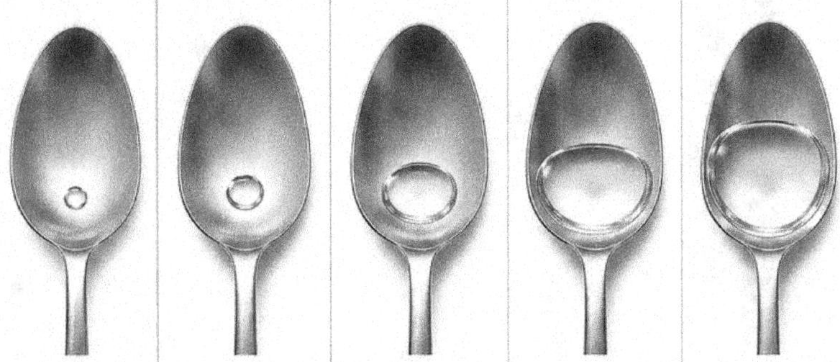

Very small amount	Tiny amount	Small amount	Half a tablespoon	More than half

7 ML (0.7 TBSP)	8 ML (0.8 TBSP)	9 ML (0.9 TBSP)	10 ML (1.0 TBSP)

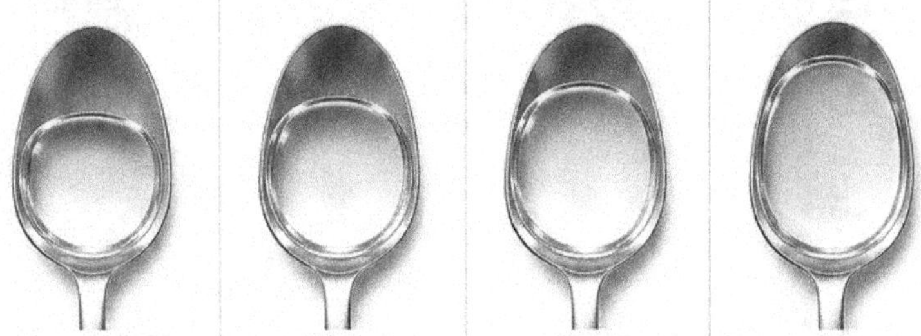

Approaching full	Nearly there	Almost a full tbsp	1 Full Tablespoon

DID YOU KNOW?

HOW MUCH DO YOU NEED TO SEE A RESULT?

While every face is unique, most people will need **at least 3 mls** of filler to see a noticeable result.

Smaller amounts (1–2 mls) may be used for subtle refinements, but 3 mls or more is often the starting point for visible, natural-looking improvement.

Your provider will create a personalized plan based on your goals, facial anatomy, and the areas treated.

COMMON GUIDELINES

Lips: 1–2 ml
Under Eyes: 1–2 ml
Cheeks: 2–4 ml per side
Nasolabial Folds: 1–2 ml
Chin: 1–2 ml
Jawline: 2–4 ml
Full Face: 6–10+ ml

Remember: *It*'s not just about the amount,
it's about the right placement, the right product, and the right technique.
Subtle, natural results are always the goal.

Nita's Filler Preference Guide for Specific Areas

Area	Method	Juvederm®	Restylane®	Teoxane®	Belotero®	Stylage®	Artefiller
Forehead	Deep injection or cannula	Volift	Refyne	RHA 3	Balance	S, M	Fine Lines
Temple	Deep injection or cannula	Voluma	Volume	Ultra Deep	Volume	M, L, XL	Volume
Zygoma	Deep injection	Volux or Voluma	Defyne, Volume	Ultra Deep	Intense	L, XL, XXL	Volume
Pre-Auricular	Cannula	Voluma or Volift	Volume	RHA 4	Volume	M, L	Volume
Malar	Deep injection	Volift or Voluma	Volume	RHA 4	Volume	L, XL	Volume
Nasolabial Folds	Cannula	Voluma or Ultra Plus	Volume	RHA 4 or Ultra Deep	Volume	L, XL	Universal
Piriform Fossa	Deep injection	Voluma or Volux	Defyne	Ultra Deep	Intense	XL, XXL	Volume
Nose	Deep bridge injection or cannula	Ultra Plus	Lyft	Ultra Deep	Intense	XL	Volume
Lips	Cannula or injection above muscle	Ultra Plus, Ultra, Volift, Volbella	Refyne, Volyme	RHA 3, RHA Kiss	Shape, Contour, Balance	S, M, L	Soft Lips
Marionette	Cannula or needle	Voluma, Ultra Plus, Volift	Volyme	RHA 4	Volume	L, XL	Universal
Upper Lip Lines	Cannula or needle	Volift, Volbella	Refyne	RHA 3, Redensity® II	Balance	S	Soft
Chin	Cannula or deep injection	Voluma, Volux	Defyne, Lyft	Ultra Deep	Intense	XL, XXL	Volume
Jaw	Cannula	Volux	Defyne, Lyft	Ultra Deep	Intense	XXL	Volume
Pre-Jowl Sulcus	Deep injection	Voluma, Volux, Ultra Plus	Volume, Defyne, Lyft	Ultra Deep	Volume	XL, XXL	Volume
Tear Troughs	Cannula	Volbella	Refyne, Lyft (deep)	Redensity® II	Balance or Soft	S, M	—
Fine Lines & Wrinkles	Superficial Injection	Volbella	Refyne	Redensity® II	Balance or Soft	S	Fine Lines
Hands	Cannula or needle injection	Volite, Ultra	Skinboosters	Redensity® I	Balance	L	—

METHOD KEY

Deep Injection = Supraperiosteal or deep fat compartment placement
Cannula = Blunt-tip cannula technique
Needle = Sharp needle placement
Superficial Injection = Dermal placement for fine lines and skin quality

Chapter 45: Filler Brands and There Ranges

Restylane® (Galderma)

Restylane® is one of the world's most established and extensively researched dermal filler brands, manufactured by Galderma. It was the first hyaluronic acid (HA) filler to receive FDA approval and has been used globally for over two decades.

What sets Restylane apart is its diverse product portfolio, designed to treat different facial layers, movement patterns, and aesthetic concerns — from deep structural support to delicate skin quality improvement.

Restylane® Technologies Explained

Understanding the technology behind the gel is essential, as it determines how the filler behaves once injected.

1. NASHA™ Technology

(Non-Animal Stabilized Hyaluronic Acid)

- Produces firmer, more particulate gels, Minimal swelling
- Excellent lifting capacity and projection
- Best suited to structural support and deep injections

Key Characteristics

- High G' (firmness), Sharp definition, Stable shape over time
- Lower water attraction → less post-treatment swelling

2. OBT™ / XpresHAn™ Technology

(Optimal Balance Technology)

- Designed to move naturally with facial expressions
- Softer, more elastic gels
- Ideal for dynamic areas of the face

Key Characteristics

- Balanced firmness and flexibility, Adapts to facial movement
- Smooth integration into tissue, Natural-looking results at rest and in motion

The Complete Restylane® Range

Products, Technology & Indications

Restylane Lyft®

Technology: NASHA™

Indications

- Cheek augmentation, Midface volume restoration, Jawline contouring
- Structural support, Age-related volume loss

Key Features

- Firm, lifting gel
- Excellent for deep supraperiosteal placement, Provides strong projection and contour

Best for: Patients with significant volume loss or needing strong foundational support.

Restylane Defyne®

Technology: XpresHAn™

Indications

- Nasolabial folds, Marionette lines, Chin shaping, Lower face support with movement

Key Features

- Supports facial expressions without stiffness
- Excellent balance of strength and flexibility

Best for: Patients with expressive faces who need structure without rigidity.

Restylane Refyne®

Technology: XpresHAn™

Indications

- Mild to moderate nasolabial folds, Perioral lines, Smile lines

Key Features

- Softer than Defyne, Allows subtle correction
- Maintains natural animation

Best for: Early ageing or patients seeking subtle refinement.

Restylane Volyme®

Technology: NASHA™

Indications

- Cheek volumisation, Facial contouring, Structural midface support

Key Features

- High lifting power, Long-lasting volume, Excellent cheek projection

Best for: Midface rejuvenation and contour enhancement.

Restylane Kysse®

Technology: XpresHAn™

Indications

- Lip augmentation, Lip definition, Lip hydration, Perioral lines

Key Features

- Designed specifically for lips
- Soft, flexible, kissable texture, Maintains natural lip movement

Best for: Patients wanting natural, expressive lips without stiffness.

Restylane Silk®

Technology: NASHA™

Indications

- Fine perioral lines, Smoker's lines, Subtle lip enhancement, Tear troughs (experienced injectors only)

Key Features

- Very fine particle size, Smooth integration in delicate areas

Best for: Fine line correction and precision work.

Restylane Eyelight®

Technology: NASHA™

Indications

- Tear trough correction, Under-eye hollows

Key Features

- Specifically designed for the infraorbital region, Low swelling profile

- High safety margin when used correctly

Best for: Patients with under-eye volume loss and hollowing.

Restylane Skinboosters™

(Vital & Vital Light)

Technology: NASHA™

Indications

- Skin hydration, Texture improvement, Fine lines, Crepey skin

Key Features

- Micro-droplet placement, Improves skin quality rather than volume, Enhances glow and elasticity

Best for: Patients seeking skin rejuvenation without altering facial shape.

Restylane Volyme + Lidocaine

Same indications as Volyme with enhanced comfort.

Clinical Considerations

- All Restylane products use non-animal HA. HA is fully reversible with hyaluronidase. Products vary in G', elasticity, and particle size
- Correct product selection + anatomical knowledge is critical to safety and results

Summary Table

Product	Technology	Primary Use
Lyft	NASHA	Structural lift, cheeks, jawline
Volyme	NASHA	Midface volume
Defyne	XpresHAn	Deep folds with movement
Refyne	XpresHAn	Moderate folds
Kysse	XpresHAn	Lips
Silk	NASHA	Fine lines
Eyelight	NASHA	Tear trough
Skinboosters	NASHA	Skin quality

Allergan Aesthetics – JUVÉDERM® Collection

Allergan Aesthetics, an AbbVie company, is one of the most recognised global leaders in medical aesthetics. The JUVÉDERM® range is among the most widely used hyaluronic acid (HA) fillers worldwide and is known for its smooth gel consistency, longevity, and predictable outcomes.

Juvederm fillers are designed to address volume loss, contouring, facial shaping, and skin quality, with different products tailored to specific facial depths and aesthetic goals.

Juvederm® Technologies Explained

All Juvederm fillers are based on proprietary cross-linking technologies that determine how the gel behaves in tissue.

1. Hylacross™ Technology

- Earlier Juvederm technology
- Uses highly cross-linked HA chains of uniform molecular weight
- Produces a smooth, cohesive gel, High water affinity → more hydration and volume

Key Characteristics

- Smooth consistency, Strong volumising effect
- Softer lift compared to Vycross, Slightly higher swelling potential

Best suited for: Lips, superficial to mid-dermal volume correction, soft contouring.

2. Vycross™ Technology

- Advanced Allergan technology, Combines low- and high-molecular-weight HA
- Requires less HA to achieve structure, Results in longer-lasting, more efficient gels

Key Characteristics

- Greater longevity, Less post-treatment swelling, Smooth tissue integration
- Strong lift with natural contours

Best suited for: Structural support, contouring, deep and mid-face volumisation, jawline and chin.

The Juvederm® Range

Products, Technology & Indications

Juvederm Voluma® XC

Technology: Vycross™

Indications

- Cheek augmentation, Midface volume loss, Chin projection, Structural facial contouring

Key Features

- High lifting capacity, Excellent projection, Long duration (up to 18–24 months in some patients)

Best for: Foundational support and facial reshaping.

Juvederm Volift® XC

(Also known as Juvederm Vollure® in some markets)

Technology: Vycross™

Indications

- Nasolabial folds, Marionette lines, Cheeks, Jawline refinement

Key Features

- Balance of lift and flexibility, Softer than Voluma
- Integrates well in dynamic areas

Best for: Moderate volume loss where movement matters.

Juvederm Volbella® XC

Technology: Vycross™

Indications

- Lips (subtle enhancement), Perioral lines, Tear troughs (experienced injectors only)

Key Features

- Low G', Soft, spreadable gel, Minimal swelling, Excellent for delicate areas

Best for: Refinement rather than volume.

Juvederm Ultra® Range

(Ultra 2, 3, 4)

Technology: Hylacross™

Indications

- Lips, Nasolabial folds, Marionette lines, Moderate volume replacement

Key Features

- Smooth, hydrating gels, Softer feel, Shorter longevity than Vycross range

Best for: Patients wanting softness, hydration, and flexibility.

Juvederm Ultra Plus®

Technology: Hylacross™

Indications

- Deeper folds, Volume replacement, Facial contouring

Key Features

- More robust than Ultra, Higher lifting capacity
- Noticeable volumising effect

Best for: Moderate to deeper wrinkles with volume loss.

Juvederm Volux®

Technology: Vycross™

Indications

- Jawline definition, Chin enhancement, Lower face contouring

Key Features

- Highest G' in the Juvederm range, Strong structural support, Excellent shape retention

Best for: Lower face sculpting and definition.

Juvederm Volite®

Technology: Vycross™

Indications

- Skin hydration, Texture improvement, Fine lines, Crepey skin

Key Features

- Skin booster, not a volumiser, Micro-droplet technique, Improves elasticity, glow, and smoothness
- Long-lasting skin quality improvement (up to 9 months)

Best for: Patients seeking skin rejuvenation without changing facial shape.

Clinical Considerations

- Juvederm fillers have high HA concentration, Strong water-binding capacity → excellent hydration, All products are reversible with hyaluronidase
- Product choice must consider:
    - Facial movement, Tissue depth, Desired lift vs softness
    - Risk areas (especially tear troughs and lips)

Summary Table

Product	Technology	Primary Use
Voluma	Vycross	Cheeks, chin, structure
Volift / Vollure	Vycross	Folds, cheeks, jawline
Volbella	Vycross	Lips, tear trough, fine lines
Volux	Vycross	Jawline, chin
Ultra	Hylacross	Lips, folds
Ultra Plus	Hylacross	Deeper folds
Volite	Vycross	Skin quality.

TEOSYAL® (Teoxane Laboratories, Switzerland)

TEOSYAL® is a premium Swiss hyaluronic acid (HA) dermal filler range developed by Teoxane Laboratories, a company known for its strong focus on rheology, safety, and tissue integration.

Teosyal fillers are widely respected for their purity, predictability, and broad product selection, allowing injectors to tailor treatments precisely to facial anatomy, movement, and skin quality.

Teosyal® Technologies Explained

Teosyal fillers are produced using proprietary cross-linking technologies that influence firmness, elasticity, and integration into tissue.

1. RHA® Technology

(Resilient Hyaluronic Acid)

- Designed to adapt to facial movement

- Mimics the natural behaviour of HA in youthful skin, Maintains softness while providing structure

Key Characteristics

- High stretch and resilience, Natural expression at rest and in motion
- Excellent integration in dynamic areas, Reduced stiffness during facial animation

Best suited for: Dynamic facial areas where movement and expression are critical.

2. Preserved Network Technology

- Maintains the long-chain HA structure
- Results in smooth, cohesive gels, Minimal chemical modification of HA

Key Characteristics

- High purity, Predictable behaviour
- Good longevity, Excellent safety profile

Best suited for: Structural support, volume restoration, and contouring.

The TEOSYAL® Range

Products, Technology & Indications

Teosyal RHA® 1

Technology: RHA®

Indications

- Fine lines, Perioral lines, Superficial wrinkles, Skin texture refinement

Key Features

- Very soft and flexible, Maintains natural facial expressions

Best for: Early ageing and subtle corrections.

Teosyal RHA® 2

Technology: RHA®

Indications

- Moderate wrinkles, Nasolabial folds, Marionette lines

Key Features

- Balance of softness and support, Adapts well to movement

Best for: Dynamic mid-face wrinkles.

Teosyal RHA® 3

Technology: RHA®

Indications

- Deeper wrinkles, Nasolabial folds, Facial contouring

Key Features

- Greater lifting capacity, Still flexible during expression

Best for: Advanced folds in expressive faces.

Teosyal RHA® 4

Technology: RHA®

Indications

- Cheek volume restoration, Jawline support, Facial contouring

Key Features

- Highest firmness in RHA range
- Strong structural support with movement adaptability

Best for: Dynamic contouring and volumisation.

Teosyal Ultra Deep®

Technology: Preserved Network

Indications

- Cheeks, Chin projection, Jawline sculpting, Deep volume restoration

Key Features

- Very high G', Strong lifting and projection, Excellent shape retention

Best for: Structural foundation and facial framework.

Teosyal Global Action®

Technology: Preserved Network

Indications

- Moderate to deep wrinkles, Nasolabial folds, Marionette lines

Key Features

- Balanced firmness, Good durability, Smooth tissue integration

Best for: Classic wrinkle correction.

Teosyal Kiss®

Technology: Preserved Network

Indications

- Lip augmentation, Lip definition, Perioral lines

Key Features

- Soft yet structured, Natural lip movement, Smooth feel

Best for: Natural lip enhancement.

Teosyal Redensity I®

Technology: Preserved Network + Dermal Redensification Complex

Indications

- Skin hydration, Texture improvement, Fine lines, Dull skin

Key Features

- HA combined with amino acids, antioxidants, minerals, and vitamins
- Improves skin quality without volume

Best for: Skin revitalisation and glow.

Teosyal Redensity II®

Technology: Preserved Network

Indications

- Tear trough correction, Under-eye hollows

Key Features

- Low swelling formulation, Designed specifically for the infraorbital area
- Excellent safety profile when used correctly

Best for: Delicate under-eye rejuvenation.

Clinical Considerations

- Teosyal fillers are high-purity, non-animal HA. All products are reversible with hyaluronidase

- RHA range is ideal for highly expressive patients

Product choice should consider:

  - Facial movement, Tissue depth, Desired projection vs flexibility, Risk zones (tear trough, lips)

Summary Table

Product	Technology	Primary Use
RHA 1	RHA	Fine lines
RHA 2	RHA	Moderate wrinkles
RHA 3	RHA	Deep folds
RHA 4	RHA	Dynamic contouring
Ultra Deep	Preserved Network	Structural volume
Global Action	Preserved Network	Wrinkle correction
Kiss	Preserved Network	Lips
Redensity I	PN + Dermal Complex	Skin quality
Redensity II	PN	Tear trough

NEAUVIA® (Matex Lab, Switzerland / Italy

NEAUVIA® is a next-generation hyaluronic acid (HA) dermal filler range developed by Matex Lab, combining Swiss precision with Italian innovation. What distinguishes Neauvia from many traditional fillers is its PEG-crosslinking technology and the inclusion of amino acids in selected products, positioning it at the intersection of structural filler and biostimulation.

Neauvia fillers are designed to provide strong structural support, excellent tissue integration, reduced inflammatory response, and long-term skin quality improvement.

Neauvia® Technologies Explained

1. PEG Cross-Linking Technology

(Polyethylene Glycol)

Unlike traditional BDDE cross-linking, Neauvia uses PEG, a biocompatible polymer widely used in medical devices.

Key Advantages

- High biocompatibility, Lower inflammatory response, Increased gel stability
- Improved longevity, Reduced risk of delayed hypersensitivity reactions

Clinical Benefit: PEG creates a strong yet flexible HA network that integrates smoothly into tissue while maintaining structural integrity.

2. Amino Acid Enrichment

(Specific products only)

Certain Neauvia fillers are enriched with glycine and L-proline, essential building blocks for collagen synthesis.

Key Advantages

- Supports fibroblast activity, Encourages collagen production
- Provides a biostimulatory effect beyond volume

Clinical Benefit: Improves skin quality, elasticity, and firmness over time.

The NEAUVIA® Range

Products, Technology & Indications

Neauvia Intense®

Technology: PEG-crosslinked HA

Indications

- Cheek volumisation, Jawline contouring, Chin projection, Deep structural support

Key Features

- Very high G’
- Strong lifting and projection, Excellent shape retention

Best for: Foundational facial framework and contouring.

Neauvia Intense Lips®

Technology: PEG-crosslinked HA

Indications

- Lip augmentation, Lip contouring, Lip hydration

Key Features

- Soft yet supportive gel, Natural lip movement, Reduced swelling profile

Best for: Natural-looking lips with definition and softness.

Neauvia Intense Rheology®

Technology: PEG-crosslinked HA

Indications

- Midface volume restoration, Nasolabial folds, Facial contouring

Key Features

- Optimised balance of elasticity and firmness
- Adapts well to dynamic areas

Best for: Areas requiring both support and movement.

Neauvia Stimulate®

Technology: PEG-crosslinked HA + Amino Acids

Indications

- Facial volume loss, Skin laxity , Collagen depletion

Key Features

- Biostimulatory filler, Supports collagen production
- Gradual skin quality improvement

Best for: Patients with ageing skin needing structure plus regeneration.

Neauvia Hydro Deluxe®

Technology: PEG-crosslinked HA + Amino Acids

Indications

- Skin hydration, Texture improvement, Fine lines, Crepey skin

Key Features

- Skin booster, not a volumiser, Improves elasticity and glow, Long-lasting hydration

Best for: Skin rejuvenation without volume change.

Neauvia Flux®

Technology: PEG-crosslinked HA

Indications

- Superficial wrinkles, Fine lines, Tear troughs (experienced injectors only)

Key Features

- Low G', Smooth, spreadable gel, Minimal swelling

Best for: Delicate areas and fine corrections.

Neauvia Organic Intense®

Technology: PEG-crosslinked HA (High purity, organic origin)

Indications

- Structural volumisation, Facial contouring

Key Features

- Extremely high purity HA, Strong lifting capacity, Excellent tissue integration

Best for: Patients requiring robust support with excellent tolerability.

Clinical Considerations

- PEG technology offers enhanced biocompatibility. Reduced inflammatory and oedema profile. All Neauvia fillers are reversible with hyaluronidase
- Amino-acid enriched products provide added biostimulation
- Ideal for patients concerned about: Longevity, Tissue tolerance, Skin quality improvement alongside volume

Summary Table

Product	Technology	Primary Use
Intense	PEG	Structural volume
Intense Lips	PEG	Lip enhancement
Intense Rheology	PEG	Dynamic contouring
Stimulate	PEG + Amino Acids	Biostimulation
Hydro Deluxe	PEG + Amino Acids	Skin quality
Flux	PEG	Fine lines
Organic Intense	PEG	High-strength

Merz Aesthetics – Belotero® & Radiesse®

Merz Aesthetics is a global medical aesthetics company headquartered in Germany, known for its science-driven, anatomy-respecting approach to facial rejuvenation. Unlike some companies that focus solely on hyaluronic acid (HA) fillers, Merz offers both HA fillers and biostimulatory fillers, allowing practitioners to address volume, contour, structure, and collagen stimulation.

Merz's injectable portfolio centres around two flagship ranges:

- Belotero® – Hyaluronic acid fillers
- Radiesse® – Calcium hydroxylapatite (CaHA) biostimulatory filler

Merz® Technologies Explained

CPM® Technology

(Cohesive Polydensified Matrix)

Used in the Belotero® HA range

CPM technology creates a homogeneous, cohesive HA gel with varying densities within the same syringe.

Key Characteristics

- Smooth, uniform integration. Minimal palpability
- Reduced risk of Tyndall effect, Excellent tissue spread

Clinical Benefit: Allows fillers to integrate seamlessly into superficial and mid-dermal layers, producing soft, natural results, especially in delicate areas.

CaHA Microsphere Technology

Used in Radiesse®

Radiesse is composed of calcium hydroxylapatite microspheres suspended in a gel carrier.

Key Characteristics

- Immediate structural support
- Long-term collagen stimulation, Biostimulatory rather than hydrophilic
- Non-HA filler (not reversible with hyaluronidase)

Clinical Benefit: Improves skin firmness, thickness, and elasticity over time while providing immediate contouring.

The BELOTERO® Range

Hyaluronic Acid Fillers

Belotero Balance®

Technology: CPM®

Indications

- Fine to moderate lines, Perioral lines, Tear troughs (experienced injectors only), Superficial wrinkles

Key Features

- Soft, smooth gel, Excellent superficial integration
- Minimal Tyndall risk

Best for: Delicate areas and fine line correction.

Belotero Intense®

Technology: CPM®

Indications

- Nasolabial folds, Marionette lines, Moderate to deep wrinkles

Key Features

- Greater lifting capacity than Balance, Maintains smooth tissue integration

Best for: Wrinkle correction requiring more support without stiffness.

Belotero Volume®

Technology: CPM®

Indications

- Cheek volumisation, Midface volume loss, Facial contouring

Key Features

- Higher G', Strong yet smooth projection, Natural contouring

Best for: Midface rejuvenation and volume restoration.

Belotero Lips®

Technology: CPM®

Indications

- Lip augmentation, Lip definition, Perioral lines

Key Features

- Designed specifically for lips. Soft, flexible, natural feel, Good hydration

Best for: Natural, soft lip enhancement.

Belotero Revive®

Technology: CPM® + Glycerol

Indications

- Skin hydration, Texture improvement, Fine lines

Key Features

- Skin booster rather than volumiser, Improves elasticity and glow. Enhances skin quality without altering facial shape

Best for: Patients seeking skin rejuvenation rather than volume.

The RADIESSE® Range

Biostimulatory Fillers

Radiesse®

Composition: Calcium Hydroxylapatite (CaHA)

Indications

- Jawline contouring, Cheek support, Chin projection, Lower face lifting, Hand rejuvenation

Key Features

- Immediate lift and contour, Long-term collagen stimulation
- Improves skin thickness and firmness, Results may last 12–18 months or longer

Best for: Structural support and collagen regeneration.

Radiesse® (+)

(With lidocaine)

Same indications as Radiesse®, with improved patient comfort.

Diluted / Hyperdiluted Radiesse®

(Advanced injector technique)

Indications

- Skin laxity, Crepey skin, Neck, décolletage, Arms, abdomen, knees, buttocks

Key Features

- Acts as a pure biostimulator, Improves skin quality and firmness
- No volumisation when diluted appropriately

Best for: Skin tightening and collagen stimulation.

Clinical Considerations

- Belotero products are HA and reversible, Radiesse is non-HA and not reversible. Radiesse should not be used in lips or tear troughs
- Product selection must consider:
  - Desired volume vs stimulation
  - Reversibility, Skin thickness and laxity, Anatomical risk zones

Summary Tables

Belotero®

Product	Technology	Primary Use
Balance	CPM	Fine lines
Intense	CPM	Moderate–deep wrinkles
Volume	CPM	Cheek volume
Lips	CPM	Lips
Revive	CPM + Glycerol	Skin quality

Radiesse®

Product	Composition	Primary Use
Radiesse	CaHA	Structure & collagen
Radiesse (+)	CaHA + Lidocaine	Structure with comfort
Hyperdiluted Radiesse	CaHA	Skin tightening

QT® Fillers (South Korea)

QT® Fillers are a Korean hyaluronic acid (HA) dermal filler range developed to deliver reliable lifting capacity, smooth tissue integration, and clear product differentiation. Like many high-quality Korean fillers, QT focuses on high purity HA, consistent rheology, and cost-effective performance, making the range popular in markets where value, predictability, and versatility are important.

QT fillers are designed with a layered approach to facial rejuvenation, offering different gel strengths for superficial lines, mid-dermal correction, and deep structural support.

QT® Technology Explained

HCCL™ Cross-Linking Technology

(High Concentration Cross-Linked Hyaluronic Acid)

QT fillers are manufactured using HCCL™ technology, which creates a stable, cohesive HA gel network with controlled elasticity and lifting capacity.

Key Characteristics

- High-purity, non-animal HA, Uniform gel consistency
- Good balance between firmness and spreadability. Reliable shape retention, Smooth extrusion and handling

Clinical Benefit: Predictable results with good longevity and controlled tissue integration.

Advanced Purification Process

- Low residual BDDE
- Reduced endotoxin levels, Improved tolerability

Clinical Benefit: Lower inflammatory response and good safety profile when used appropriately.

The QT® Filler Range

Products, Technology & Indications

QT fillers are often grouped by depth and firmness, allowing straightforward product selection.

QT Hard

Technology: HCCL™

Indications

- Jawline definition, Chin projection, Structural facial contouring

- Deep supraperiosteal placement

Key Features

- Highest G' in the QT range, Strong lifting and projection
- Excellent shape retention

Best for: Lower-face sculpting and foundational support.

QT Sub-Q

Technology: HCCL™

Indications

- Cheek volumisation, Midface volume loss, Facial contouring

Key Features

- High firmness, Good lifting capacity, Stable integration in deep planes

Best for: Deep volume restoration and facial framework.

QT Deep

Technology: HCCL™

Indications

- Nasolabial folds, Marionette lines, Moderate to deep wrinkles

Key Features

- Medium-high G', Balanced lift and flexibility

Best for: Classic wrinkle correction with support.

QT Soft

Technology: HCCL™

Indications

- Lips, Perioral lines, Superficial wrinkles

Key Features

- Softer gel texture, Smooth spreadability, Natural movement

Best for: Subtle lip enhancement and surface refinement.

QT Fine

Technology: HCCL™

Indications

- Fine lines, Superficial wrinkles, Tear troughs (experienced injectors only)

Key Features

- Low G', Minimal swelling profile, Precise placement

Best for: Delicate areas and fine corrections.

QT Volume

Technology: HCCL™

Indications

- General volumisation, Facial contouring, Mild to moderate volume loss

Key Features

- Balanced firmness, Versatile mid-to-deep placement

Best for: All-round volumisation where extreme firmness is not required

Clinical Considerations

- QT fillers use non-animal hyaluronic acid. All QT fillers are reversible with hyaluronidase. Clear firmness gradation assists safe product selection
- Suitable for:
    - Budget-conscious patients, Clinics seeking reliable, predictable fillers
    - Structured, stepwise facial rejuvenation

Summary Table

Product	Technology	Primary Use
QT Hard	HCCL	Jawline, chin, structure
QT Sub-Q	HCCL	Deep cheek volume
QT Deep	HCCL	Moderate–deep folds
QT Volume	HCCL	General volumisation
QT Soft	HCCL	Lips, superficial lines
QT Fine	HCCL	Fine lines, delicate areas

EPTQ® (Jetema Co. Ltd, South Korea)

EPTQ® is a premium Korean hyaluronic acid (HA) dermal filler range manufactured by Jetema, a globally recognised medical aesthetics company. EPTQ has gained strong international traction due to its high purity HA, advanced cross-linking technology, predictable rheology, and excellent value, while still meeting stringent global manufacturing standards.

The EPTQ range is designed to provide clear differentiation between lifting, contouring, and softer volumisation, making product selection intuitive for injectors and results consistent for patients.

EPTQ® Technology Explained

HET™ Technology (High Elasticity Technology)

EPTQ fillers are produced using HET™ cross-linking, which creates a uniform, highly elastic gel structure with minimal residual BDDE.

Key Characteristics

- High purity HA, Consistent particle size. Strong elasticity with smooth extrusion, Low endotoxin levels, Excellent tissue integration

Clinical Benefit: Predictable lift, smooth placement, and reduced inflammatory response.

Low Residual BDDE Process

- Enhanced purification process, Reduced risk of irritation and inflammation, Improved safety profile

Clinical Benefit: Improved tolerability and suitability for a wide range of patients.

The EPTQ® Range

Products, Technology & Indications

EPTQ fillers are clearly categorised into Classic, S-Line, and E-Line, making selection based on firmness and indication straightforward.

EPTQ S 500

Technology: HET™

Indications

- Cheek augmentation, Jawline contouring, Chin projection, Structural facial support

Key Features

- Highest G' in the EPTQ range, Strong lifting and projection, Excellent shape retention

Best for: Foundational structure and facial framework.

EPTQ S 300

Technology: HET™

Indications

- Midface volumisation, Nasolabial folds, Marionette lines

Key Features

- Balanced firmness and elasticity, Smooth tissue integration

Best for: Moderate volume loss and contouring.

EPTQ S 100

Technology: HET™

Indications

- Fine lines, Superficial wrinkles, Tear troughs (experienced injectors only)

Key Features

- Lower G', Smooth spreadability, Minimal swelling

Best for: Delicate areas and superficial corrections.

EPTQ E 400

Technology: HET™

Indications

- Cheek volume, Facial contouring, Structural support

Key Features

- Firm, cohesive gel, High lifting power

Best for: Structural contouring with controlled projection.

EPTQ E 200

Technology: HET™

Indications

- Moderate wrinkles, Nasolabial folds, Marionette lines

Key Features

- Medium firmness, Natural integration

Best for: Classic wrinkle correction.

EPTQ E 100

Technology: HET™

Indications

- Fine lines, Superficial wrinkles, Perioral lines

Key Features

- Soft gel consistency, Smooth finish

Best for: Surface refinement and subtle correction.

EPTQ KISS

Technology: HET™

Indications

- Lip augmentation, Lip contouring, Lip hydration

Key Features

- Designed specifically for lips, Soft, elastic texture, Maintains natural lip movement

Best for: Natural-looking lip enhancement

EPTQ SENSE

Technology: HET™

Indications

- Skin hydration, Texture improvement, Fine lines

Key Features

- Skin booster rather than volumiser, Micro-droplet technique, Improves elasticity and glow

Best for: Skin rejuvenation without altering facial shape.

Clinical Considerations

- EPTQ fillers use non-animal HA. High purity and low endotoxin levels

- All products are reversible with hyaluronidase. Clear G' differentiation simplifies product choice. Particularly popular where value, predictability, and versatility are important

Summary Table

Product	Technology	Primary Use
S 500	HET	Structural support
S 300	HET	Volume & contour
S 100	HET	Fine lines
E 400	HET	Contouring
E 200	HET	Moderate wrinkles
E 100	HET	Superficial lines
KISS	HET	Lips
SENSE	HET	Skin quality

HUGEL® (South Korea)

HUGEL® is a major South Korean pharmaceutical and medical aesthetics company with a rapidly expanding global footprint. While best known internationally for its neuromodulators, Hugel has also developed a high-quality hyaluronic acid (HA) dermal filler range, reflecting the Korean aesthetic philosophy of natural enhancement, smooth tissue integration, and skin quality preservation.

As Korean fillers gain increasing acceptance worldwide, Hugel represents a brand that is well positioned for current and future expansion into markets such as Australia, pending regulatory approvals.

HUGEL® Filler Technologies Explained

Advanced HA Cross-Linking & Purification Technology

Hugel fillers are manufactured using high-purity, non-animal hyaluronic acid, with a focus on:

- Uniform particle size, Controlled cross-linking
- Low residual BDDE, Low endotoxin levels

Key Characteristics

- Smooth, cohesive gel structure

- Good elasticity and lifting capacity
- Predictable handling and extrusion, Reliable tissue integration

Clinical Benefit: Balanced performance across superficial, mid-dermal, and deep planes, with a focus on natural, harmonious results.

Korean Aesthetic Philosophy

Korean filler development traditionally prioritises:

- Soft tissue integration over exaggerated projection
- Skin hydration and quality alongside volume
- Gradual, natural-looking enhancement

Clinical Benefit: Fillers that are well suited to subtle contouring, refinement, and layered facial rejuvenation.

The HUGEL® Filler Range

Products, Technology & Indications

(Product naming and availability may vary by market)

HUGEL Volume

Technology: Cross-linked HA

Indications

- Cheek volumisation, Midface volume loss, Facial contouring

Key Features

- High G', Good lifting and projection
- Stable shape retention

Best for: Structural midface support and volume restoration.

HUGEL Deep

Technology: Cross-linked HA

Indications

- Nasolabial folds, Marionette lines, Moderate to deep wrinkles

Key Features

- Balanced firmness and elasticity
- Smooth integration in mid-dermal planes

Best for: Classic wrinkle correction with support.

HUGEL Fine

Technology: Cross-linked HA

Indications

- Fine lines, Superficial wrinkles, Perioral lines, Tear troughs (experienced injectors only)

Key Features

- Low G', Smooth spreadability, Minimal swelling profile

Best for: Delicate areas and surface refinement.

HUGEL Lips

Technology: Cross-linked HA

Indications

- Lip augmentation, Lip definition, Lip hydration

Key Features

- Soft, elastic gel, Maintains natural lip movement, Smooth finish

Best for: Natural, hydrated, expressive lips.

HUGEL Skin Booster

Technology: Lightly cross-linked HA

Indications

- Skin hydration, Texture improvement, Fine lines, Dull or crepey skin

Key Features

- Micro-droplet technique
- Improves glow and elasticity, Does not add volume

Best for: skin rejuvenation without altering facial shape.

Clinical Considerations

- Hugel fillers use non-animal hyaluronic acid, Designed for smooth, controlled integration, All HA fillers are reversible with hyaluronidase
- Product selection should consider:
    - Desired lift vs softness

- Facial movement, Skin thickness, Cultural aesthetic preferences

Summary Table

Product	Technology	Primary Use
Hugel Volume	Cross-linked HA	Structural volume
Hugel Deep	Cross-linked HA	Moderate–deep folds
Hugel Fine	Cross-linked HA	Fine lines
Hugel Lips	Cross-linked HA	Lips
Hugel Skin Booster	Lightly cross-linked HA	Skin quality

Evolysse® (Evolus / Symatese)

Evolysse® is a next-generation hyaluronic acid (HA) filler line that represents one of the most recent technological advancements in the dermal filler category. Developed by Evolus in collaboration with Symatese, Evolysse uses an innovative Cold-X™ Technology manufacturing process to better preserve the natural structure of HA for smoother, more natural-looking results.

Unlike many traditional HA fillers made at higher temperatures, Cold-X™ technology processes HA at very low, near-freezing temperatures, which helps maintain longer HA chains and reduces the need for excessive cross-linking. This approach aims to produce a gel that integrates seamlessly into tissue, moves naturally with facial expressions, and may require less product for equivalent correction.

Evolysse® Technology Explained

Cold-X™ Technology

This proprietary manufacturing process is the defining feature of Evolysse fillers.

Key Advantages

- Preserves HA's natural structure: Low-temperature processing reduces fragmentation of the HA molecule.
- Natural tissue integration: The resulting gel integrates smoothly into facial tissue with minimal stiffness.
- Versatile performance: Designed to be injected at different levels depending on the area treated.
- Reduced hydrophilicity: Early clinical impressions suggest less unwanted swelling compared with some other HA fillers.

Clinical Benefit: Evolysse delivers a natural look and feel with effective correction of dynamic lines and facial volume loss, without the "overfilled" appearance that concerns many patients.

The Evolysse® Range

Products, Technology & Indications

As of 2025, the Evolysse line comprises two FDA-approved HA fillers, each formulated with Cold-X technology for specific treatment goals.

Evolysse Form

Technology: Cold-X™

Indications

- Moderate to deep smile lines and laugh lines (e.g., nasolabial folds). Facial contouring and volume restoration in deeper planes, Structural support for areas requiring lift and definition

Key Features

- Firmer gel with cohesive structure, Designed for deeper injection planes, Provides lift as well as softening of folds

Best for: Patients needing substantial correction and support in deeper folds and facial contours.

Evolysse Smooth

Technology: Cold-X™

Indications

- Fine lines and superficial wrinkles, Perioral lines, Gentle contouring and refinement, Subtle volume enhancement

Key Features

- Softer gel texture than Form, Easier spreadability in more superficial planes. Natural, subtle enhancement

Best for: Delicate areas such as around the mouth, mild folds, or early ageing signs where a softer touch is preferred.

Clinical Notes

- Both Evolysse Form and Evolysse Smooth are FDA-approved for correction of moderate-to-severe dynamic facial wrinkles and folds such as nasolabial folds in adults. Results typically last up to 12 months in many patients, though duration varies with treatment area, individual factors, and injector technique.

- Like other HA fillers, Evolysse gels are reversible with hyaluronidase if needed.
- The Cold-X™ process aims to minimize fragmentation and improve natural movement, potentially reducing the likelihood of stiffness or "puffy" results.

Summary Table

Product	Technology	Primary Use
Evolysse Form	Cold-X™	Deep volume, structural support, moderate–severe folds
Evolysse Smooth	Cold-X™	Superficial lines, fine wrinkle refinement, subtle enhancement.

STYLAGE® (Vivacy Laboratories, France)

STYLAGE® is a premium French hyaluronic acid (HA) dermal filler range developed by Laboratoires Vivacy. The brand is well known for integrating antioxidant technology into its fillers, positioning Stylage not only as a volumising and contouring solution, but also as a product range designed to protect skin from oxidative stress and premature ageing.

Stylage fillers are recognised for their smooth texture, versatility, and refined aesthetic outcomes, making them suitable for both structural work and delicate, superficial corrections.

Stylage® Technologies Explained

IPN-Like® Technology

(InterPenetrated Network-Like Technology)

Stylage fillers are manufactured using IPN-Like cross-linking, which creates a three-dimensional HA network that balances firmness with flexibility.

Key Characteristics

- Strong gel cohesion, Smooth tissue integration, Good elasticity
- Controlled projection and spread

Clinical Benefit: Predictable lift with natural facial movement and good longevity.

Antioxidant Enrichment (Mannitol or Sorbitol)

A defining feature of Stylage is the inclusion of antioxidants within many products.

Why this matters

- Antioxidants help reduce oxidative degradation of HA
- May prolong filler longevity
- Can reduce post-injection inflammation and swelling

Clinical Benefit: Improved tolerance, smoother healing, and enhanced durability of results.

The STYLAGE® Range

Products, Technology & Indications

Stylage fillers are grouped clearly by depth, firmness, and indication, making selection intuitive.

Stylage XXL

Technology: IPN-Like + Mannitol

Indications

- Cheek volumisation, Jawline contouring, Chin projection, Structural facial support

Key Features

- Very high G', Strong lifting and projection, Excellent shape retention

Best for: Deep structural support and facial framework.

Stylage XL

Technology: IPN-Like + Mannitol

Indications

- Midface volume restoration, Facial contouring, Deep nasolabial folds

Key Features

- High firmness, Smooth integration

Best for: Volume restoration with contour control.

Stylage L

Technology: IPN-Like + Mannitol

Indications

- Moderate to deep wrinkles, Nasolabial folds, Marionette lines

Key Features

- Balanced lift and flexibility, Good longevity

Best for: Classic wrinkle correction with support.

Stylage M

Technology: IPN-Like + Mannitol

Indications

- Moderate wrinkles, Perioral lines, Facial refinement

Key Features

- Medium G', Natural movement

Best for: Dynamic areas requiring softness with support.

Stylage S

Technology: IPN-Like + Sorbitol

Indications

- Fine lines, Superficial wrinkles, Perioral lines

Key Features

- Soft gel consistency, Precise placement, Minimal swelling

Best for: Surface refinement and fine line correction.

Stylage Special Lips®

Technology: IPN-Like + Mannitol

Indications

- Lip augmentation, Lip contouring, Lip hydration

Key Features

- Designed specifically for lips
- Soft, flexible texture, Maintains natural lip movement

Best for: Natural, expressive lip enhancement.

Stylage Hydro® / HydroMax®

Technology: IPN-Like + Sorbitol

Indications

- Skin hydration, Texture improvement, Fine lines, Crepey skin

Key Features

- Skin booster, not a volumiser
- Improves elasticity and glow, HydroMax offers enhanced hydration and longevity

Best for: Skin quality improvement without volume change.

Clinical Considerations

- Stylage fillers use non-animal HA, Many products include lidocaine for comfort. Antioxidant content may reduce swelling and HA breakdown
- All Stylage fillers are reversible with hyaluronidase
- Suitable for:
    - Patients prone to swelling, Refinement and natural aesthetics, Structured yet flexible facial rejuvenation

Summary Table

Product	Technology	Primary Use
XXL	IPN-Like + Mannitol	Structural volume
XL	IPN-Like + Mannitol	Deep volume
L	IPN-Like + Mannitol	Deep wrinkles
M	IPN-Like + Mannitol	Moderate wrinkles
S	IPN-Like + Sorbitol	Fine lines
Special Lips	IPN-Like + Mannitol	Lips
Hydro / HydroMax	IPN-Like + Sorbitol	Skin quality

CHROMA® (Croma-Pharma GmbH, Austria)

CHROMA® is an Austrian pharmaceutical company with a strong European reputation for medical-grade injectables, including hyaluronic acid (HA) dermal fillers, skin boosters, and regenerative products. Croma is particularly known for its strict manufacturing standards, pharmaceutical-level purity, and safety-first design philosophy.

CHROMA fillers are developed to provide predictable rheology, smooth tissue integration, and a broad portfolio that allows injectors to treat everything from delicate superficial lines to deep structural volume.

CHROMA® Technologies Explained

Monophasic Cross-Linked HA Technology

CHROMA fillers are produced as homogeneous monophasic gels, meaning the HA particles are evenly distributed throughout the gel.

Key Characteristics

• Smooth, cohesive consistency, Uniform extrusion force

• Reduced lumpiness and palpability, Predictable tissue behaviour

Clinical Benefit: Even integration into tissue with controlled spread and reliable aesthetic outcomes.

High-Purity Manufacturing Standards

• Non-animal sourced hyaluronic acid, Low residual BDDE

• Low endotoxin levels, Pharmaceutical-grade quality control

Clinical Benefit: Excellent tolerability and safety profile, particularly important in delicate facial areas.

The CHROMA® Filler Range

Products, Technology & Indications

(Product names may vary slightly by market)

CHROMA Volume

Technology: Monophasic cross-linked HA

Indications

• Cheek volumisation, Midface volume loss, Facial contouring, Structural support

Key Features

• High G', Strong lifting and projection, Stable shape retention

Best for: Foundational volume and facial framework.

CHROMA Deep

Technology: Monophasic cross-linked HA

Indications

• Nasolabial folds, Marionette lines, Moderate to deep wrinkles

Key Features

• Balanced firmness and elasticity, Smooth mid-dermal integration

Best for: Classic wrinkle correction with support.

CHROMA Derm

Technology: Monophasic cross-linked HA

Indications

• Moderate wrinkles, Facial refinement, Dynamic areas requiring flexibility

Key Features

• Medium G', Natural movement

Best for: Areas where expression needs to be preserved.

CHROMA Fine

Technology: Monophasic cross-linked HA

Indications

• Fine lines, Superficial wrinkles, Perioral lines, Tear troughs *(experienced injectors only)*

Key Features

• Low G', Smooth spreadability, Minimal swelling profile

Best for: Delicate areas and fine corrections.

CHROMA Lips

Technology: Monophasic cross-linked HA

Indications

• Lip augmentation, Lip definition, Lip hydration

Key Features

• Soft, elastic gel, Maintains natural lip movement, Smooth finish

Best for: Natural-looking, hydrated lips.

CHROMA Skin Booster

Technology: Lightly cross-linked HA

Indications

• Skin hydration, Texture improvement, Fine lines, Dull or crepey skin

Key Features

• Micro-droplet technique

• Improves elasticity and glow, No volumisation

Best for: Skin rejuvenation without changing facial shape.

Clinical Considerations

CHROMA fillers are HA-based and reversible with hyaluronidase

Designed for smooth, predictable integration

Suitable for: Refinement and natural aesthetics, Layered facial rejuvenation, Patients prioritising safety and tolerance

Fillmed — A Scientific Aesthetic Medicine Brand

Laboratoires FILLMED is a French aesthetic medicine company founded in 1978 by Dr. Michel Tordjman, a pioneer in combining clinical science with anti-ageing treatments for dermatologists, plastic surgeons and trained aesthetic medicine professionals. The brand has a long track record in developing medical-grade solutions for skin rejuvenation, tissue quality improvement and age-related volume loss.

Fillmed products are designed to correct signs of ageing, revitalise skin and enhance facial structure, using biocompatible hyaluronic acid and advanced formulations. The company's portfolio spans injectable fillers, mesotherapy solutions, peels and professional skin-quality boosters — all aimed at delivering reliable, natural-looking results backed by science.

Core Philosophy & Technology

Tri-Hyal® Technology

A hallmark of Fillmed's dermal fillers, Tri-Hyal® technology combines three different molecular weights of hyaluronic acid (free, long chains and very long chains) in a balanced formula. This enables gradual integration into tissue, better hydration, improved elasticity, and a smoother, more natural outcome compared with single-weight HA fillers.

Non-Animal Hyaluronic Acid

Fillmed's products are made of non-animal origin HA, reducing the risk of allergic reactions and improving biocompatibility — a standard in modern medical aesthetics.

The Art Filler Range — Dermal Fillers for Different Aesthetic Goals

Fillmed's Art Filler® collection is its flagship range of injectable dermal fillers, each tailored to specific treatment needs within facial rejuvenation:

1. Art Filler Fine Lines

- Target: Superficial or fine wrinkles (e.g., around eyes, mouth and forehead).
- Profile: Softer, smoother gel designed for delicate areas.
- Benefits: Subtle wrinkle smoothing with natural integration.
- With Lidocaine: Often includes a small percentage of lidocaine to improve comfort during injection.

2. Art Filler Universal

- Target: Versatile, medium-to-deep wrinkles and general facial contouring.
- Use: Can be used for smoothing folds (e.g., nasolabial lines), restoring mid-facial volume and light lip contouring.
- Composition: Balanced level of HA with lidocaine for comfort and hydration.
- Notes: A go-to filler when a practitioner wants one product that performs well in multiple areas of the face.

3. Art Filler Volume

- Target: Deep volume restoration — cheeks, chin, jawline and temples.
- Profile: Higher cohesivity and cross-linking to support deeper tissue structure and volume replacement.
- Benefits: Adds lift and shape to areas with age-related volume loss.

4. Art Filler Lips & Lips Soft

- Art Filler Lips: Designed for more pronounced lip volume and projection.
- Art Filler Lips Soft: A gentler formulation for natural lip enhancement, contour and hydration.

- Both include Lidocaine: For greater comfort during lip injections.
- Indications: Lip augmentation, border definition, smoothing perioral lines.

Other Hyaluronic Acid-Based Solutions

Beyond the classic Art Filler line, Fillmed also offers HA-based mesotherapy and hydration boosters such as:

M-HA 10

- A pure, non-crosslinked hyaluronic acid solution used in mesotherapy to replenish hydration, improve skin tone and elasticity, and soften fine lines.
- Ideal for superficial rejuvenation on areas like face, neck, décolletage and hands.

How Fillmed Fits Into the Aesthetic Medicine Landscape

Fillmed stands out for:

- Its medical-science foundation and long heritage since the late 1970s.
- The Tri-Hyal® approach that emphasises skin biology and tissue integration.
- A broad range that spans fine lines, volume replacement and skin hydration, giving practitioners flexibility across treatment plans.

Summary : Filler Brands and Their Ranges

Dermal fillers are not interchangeable products. Each brand and range has been developed with specific technologies, gel properties, and clinical purposes in mind. Understanding these differences is essential for achieving safe, natural, and long-lasting results.

This chapter has explored the major global filler brands — European, Korean, American, and emerging technologies — highlighting how rheology, cross-linking, and formulation influence how a filler behaves in the face.

Key Points for Patients

1. One Face, Many Filler Types

There is no single “best filler.” Different areas of the face require fillers that:

- Lift and support (cheeks, jawline, chin), Move naturally (smile lines, lips)
- Blend seamlessly (under-eyes, fine lines), Improve skin quality (hydration, elasticity)

Your injector chooses the filler based on your anatomy and goals, not brand popularity.

2. Technology Matters

Fillers differ in:

- Firmness (G'), Flexibility and stretch, Water attraction and swelling potential, Longevity, How they integrate into tissue

These differences determine whether a filler lifts, softens, hydrates, or stimulates collagen.

3. Natural Results Are Designed, Not Injected

The most natural outcomes come from:

- Using the correct filler in the correct layer, Restoring structure rather than overfilling, Respecting facial movement and proportions

Good filler work should enhance how you already look — not change who you are.

4. Safety Comes Before Aesthetics

All dermal fillers are medical devices. Safe treatment depends on:

- Injector training and anatomical knowledge, Appropriate product selection, Conservative dosing
- Understanding reversibility and risk zones

Choosing an experienced injector is more important than choosing a brand.

5. Longevity Is Individual

How long fillers last varies depending on:

- Product type, Area treated, Facial movement, Individual metabolism

Longer-lasting is not always better — adjustability and safety are key.

Key Points for Injectors

1. Brand Ranges Exist for a Reason

Each filler range offers:

- A spectrum of firmness and elasticity, Products designed for different facial depths, Specific behaviour in static vs dynamic areas

Mastering a range allows precision, predictability, and layered treatment planning.

2. Choose Fillers Based on Tissue, Not Habit

Clinical decision-making should be guided by: Skin thickness, Degree of volume loss, Movement patterns, Treatment depth, Patient age and hormonal status

Different tissues require different gel behaviours.

3. Reversibility and Risk Management Are Core Skills

- HA fillers allow reversibility and flexibility, Non-HA fillers require advanced training, Product choice must reflect injector experience and patient risk profile

Safety planning is part of artistry.

4. Modern Aesthetics Go Beyond Volume

Today's best outcomes combine:

- Structural HA fillers, Flexible fillers for movement, Skin boosters, Biostimulators for collagen support

A multimodal approach delivers long-term facial health, not just short-term correction.

5. Confidence Comes from Understanding

Injectors who understand:

- Filler technologies, Rheology, Brand differences, Anatomical application

achieve better results with less product and fewer complications.

Dermal fillers are tools — not trends.

The success of any treatment depends on:

- The right filler, In the right place
- At the right depth, For the right patient
- Used by the right injector

When filler brands and ranges are understood and respected, outcomes become natural, safe, and sustainable.

Chapter 46: The Hybrids

Where hyaluronic acid meets regeneration

There has been a noticeable shift happening in aesthetics over the past few years. We are no longer simply filling faces. Patients today are asking for healthier skin, better quality tissue, firmness, glow, and longevity. They want to look refreshed, not altered. Softer, not puffier. More rested, not "done."

This changing philosophy is where hybrid injectables have emerged.

Hybrids sit somewhere between traditional dermal fillers and regenerative medicine. They combine the immediate benefits of hyaluronic acid with ingredients that stimulate the skin to regenerate itself over time. In simple terms, they aim to give patients something they can see early, while also encouraging long-term improvement beneath the surface.

Traditional hyaluronic acid fillers were designed primarily to replace volume. They attract water, create softness, and can restore contour very effectively. However, on their own, they do little to improve the actual behaviour of ageing skin. Over time, repeated filling without regeneration can sometimes lead to heaviness, puffiness, and loss of natural facial movement.

Biostimulants changed that conversation.

Products containing ingredients such as calcium hydroxyapatite, poly-L-lactic acid, amino acids, polynucleotides, and other regenerative molecules began focusing less on volume and more on collagen stimulation, tissue quality, and skin integrity. The challenge, however, was that many biostimulators worked slowly. Patients often had to wait weeks or months to see visible improvement.

Hybrids bridge that gap beautifully.

They combine the immediate softness and hydration of HA with the delayed regenerative effect of collagen stimulation. The result is a treatment that not only improves appearance today, but also works quietly in the background to strengthen the skin over time.

What I personally find most exciting about hybrids is that they represent a move toward more intelligent aesthetics. The goal is no longer to simply add more product. The goal is to improve the quality and function of the tissue itself.

This makes hybrids ideal for patients who are beginning to age but do not yet need large amounts of volume. They work beautifully for skin laxity, crepey skin, thinning tissue, or patients who have previously been overfilled and now want a softer, more natural approach.

One of the most important developments in this space has been the evolution of calcium hydroxyapatite combined with hyaluronic acid technology.

Calcium hydroxyapatite has long been respected for its ability to stimulate collagen and improve dermal thickness. Traditionally, it was used on its own or diluted to create a softer regenerative effect. The newer hybrid direction combines the regenerative strength of CaHA with the softness and spreadability of HA, creating treatments that feel more natural in the tissue while still stimulating collagen production over time.

Merz Aesthetics has led much of the early work in this area. These newer approaches allow practitioners to achieve immediate soft support while progressively improving firmness, elasticity, and skin quality. I find these treatments particularly useful in the lower face, neck, jawline, and areas where tissue quality matters more than projection.

Poly-L-lactic acid has also evolved within the hybrid conversation.

PLLA is a powerful collagen stimulator that works by triggering a controlled inflammatory response within the skin. Historically, it required careful preparation and patience, with results gradually appearing over months. The idea of combining PLLA with hyaluronic acid is to soften the delivery and create more predictable, elegant outcomes. Patients receive early hydration and subtle improvement while collagen stimulation develops slowly underneath. This reflects where aesthetics is heading overall — softer treatments with regenerative intent.

One of the earliest and most established hybrid concepts involved combining hyaluronic acid with amino acids. Amino acids support fibroblast activity and collagen synthesis, making them ideal partners for HA. Rather than creating obvious volume, these treatments improve skin density, hydration, elasticity, and fine lines.

Sunekos is probably one of the best-known examples in this category. I have always found these treatments particularly beautiful around delicate areas such as the eyes, where heavy filler can easily create puffiness or distortion. Instead of forcing volume into fragile tissue, the skin is encouraged to behave more youthfully itself.

Polynucleotides and regenerative cellular molecules are now expanding this field even further.

These treatments focus heavily on tissue repair, hydration, cellular signalling, and reducing inflammation. Combined with HA, they create a strong skin-conditioning effect rather than structural augmentation. They are ideal for fragile skin, post-procedure recovery, crepey tissue, and patients wanting a subtle regenerative approach rather than traditional filling. This is where the industry is clearly moving — toward regeneration over replacement.

Even Allergan, historically associated with hyaluronic acid technology and structural fillers, is now moving toward this regenerative philosophy. Their newer research and product development reflect a major shift in thinking within aesthetics.

The focus is no longer simply on how much volume a filler creates, but how the product behaves within the tissue over time.

There is increasing emphasis on tissue integration, collagen stimulation, skin quality, longevity, and maintaining natural movement. Allergan's newer regenerative filler concepts and biofiller technologies are designed to work more harmoniously with the skin rather than simply occupying space within it.

This represents an important evolution in aesthetics.

One of the most interesting hybrid developments to emerge in recent years is HArmonyCa™, developed by Allergan Aesthetics, now part of AbbVie. The technology originally came from an Israeli company called Luminera, which Allergan acquired as part of its move toward regenerative aesthetics and hybrid injectable technology.

HArmonyCa reflects the changing direction of the industry. Rather than simply creating volume, the focus is now shifting toward improving tissue quality, collagen support, and natural facial ageing. The product combines hyaluronic acid for immediate hydration and soft support with calcium hydroxyapatite microspheres, which stimulate collagen production gradually over time.

What makes HArmonyCa different from traditional fillers is that it sits between a filler and a biostimulator. The HA component provides an early visible improvement, while the calcium hydroxyapatite works more slowly beneath the surface to improve firmness, elasticity, and skin quality. The aim is not simply to "fill" the face, but to encourage healthier tissue behaviour over time.

This reflects a much broader movement within aesthetics away from overfilled faces and toward regenerative medicine. Patients increasingly want natural movement, better skin quality, and subtle rejuvenation rather than exaggerated volume. Treatments such as HArmonyCa represent this evolution beautifully because they focus not only on how the face looks immediately after treatment, but also on how the tissue ages and behaves long term.

Clinically, these treatments are particularly useful in areas where skin laxity and collagen depletion are more important than pure volume loss, such as the lower face, jawline, lateral cheeks, and neck. The results are usually softer, more integrated, and more natural appearing than heavily volumising filler treatments.

In many ways, HArmonyCa represents the bridge between traditional filler medicine and the future of regenerative aesthetics.

The future is not about larger cheeks or exaggerated volume. It is about restoring healthy tissue behaviour while maintaining natural anatomy and facial expression.

Neauvia was one of the early innovators to recognise this direction. Their philosophy centred around regeneration, biocompatibility, and tissue integration long before these concepts became mainstream. Their work combining HA with calcium hydroxyapatite reflected the understanding that the future of aesthetics would depend on improving skin quality rather than simply replacing volume.

Biofillers also sit beautifully within this regenerative category, even though they are not manufactured hybrids in the traditional sense.

In many ways, they behave like one.

Biofillers are created using the patient's own blood-derived components, processed into a soft injectable material that provides both subtle volume and regenerative stimulation. They offer immediate soft tissue improvement while growth factors continue working over time to support collagen production and tissue repair.

One of the greatest advantages of biofillers is their biocompatibility.

Because the material comes from the patient themselves, there is minimal risk of allergic reaction or foreign body response. For patients with sensitivities, autoimmune concerns, or those wanting a more natural option, biofillers are often one of the most elegant choices available.

Clinically, they create very soft, natural results. They improve hydration, skin quality, and crepey texture beautifully, particularly around delicate areas such as the tear troughs or fine lines. They do not behave like traditional structural fillers and are not designed to create dramatic lift or contour. Instead, they integrate gently and almost invisibly into the tissue.

The result is often difficult to detect — which in aesthetics is usually the highest compliment.

Of course, it is important to understand the limitations of hybrids and biofillers. They do not replace surgery where significant laxity exists, nor do they replace structural fillers when major volume loss is present. Their strength lies in regeneration, subtlety, and tissue quality.

This regenerative movement is also extending into the concept of longevity medicine.

Products such as Longeva reflect this broader direction. The emphasis is shifting toward cellular health, skin longevity, tissue function, and supporting the biology of ageing itself rather than simply masking its appearance.

In the coming years, I believe we will see injectables that influence cellular metabolism, inflammation, mitochondrial function, and even genetic signalling pathways involved in ageing.

The pipeline is expanding rapidly.

We are already seeing developments involving HA combined with exosomes, growth factors, peptides, and advanced bioactive molecules. Future injectables may target multiple layers of the skin simultaneously, improving not only volume and hydration but also the actual behaviour and lifespan of skin cells.

To me, this is one of the most exciting eras aesthetics has entered.

The future is becoming less about changing faces and more about restoring tissue health, preserving natural beauty, and ageing intelligently.

Chapter 47: Skin Boosters

One of the biggest shifts in aesthetic medicine over the past decade has been the move away from simply filling lines and replacing volume. Today's patients are asking for healthier skin, improved texture, luminosity, elasticity, and prevention.

This is where skin boosters shine.

Unlike traditional dermal fillers, skin boosters are designed to improve skin quality rather than create volume. Most are injected superficially into the dermis using microdroplets, where they hydrate the skin and stimulate fibroblasts to produce collagen and elastin.

The ideal skin booster depends on the patient's age, skin quality, lifestyle, and treatment goals.

1. Skinvive®

Manufacturer: Allergan Aesthetics

Composition

- Microdroplets of hyaluronic acid (HA)
- Cross-linked HA technology, No volumising effect

How It Is Injected

- Tiny intradermal microdroplets, 32G needle, Multiple injection points
- Usually cheeks only

Treatment Series

- Single treatment, Maintenance every 6–9 months

Best Areas

- Cheeks, Lower face, Early ageing skin

Results

- Improved hydration, Increased luminosity, Better skin smoothness
- Improved skin texture, Natural glow without added volume

2. Restylane Skinboosters™

Manufacturer Galderma

Products

- Restylane Vital, Restylane Vital Light

Composition

- Stabilised hyaluronic acid (NASHA technology)

How It Is Injected

- Intradermal microdroplets, Needle or cannula
- Usually performed over large treatment areas

Treatment Series

- Three treatments, Four weeks apart, Maintenance every 6 months

Best Areas

- Face, Neck, Décolletage, Hands

Results

- Deep hydration, Improved elasticity
- Improved skin texture, Softening of fine lines, Improved radiance

3. Teosyal Redensity 1®

Manufacturer Teoxane

Composition

- Hyaluronic acid, 8 amino acids, 3 antioxidants, Zinc, Copper, Vitamin B6

How It Is Injected

- Intradermal microdroplets, Needle or cannula

Treatment Series

- Three treatments, Three weeks apart
- Maintenance every 4–6 months

Best Areas

- Face, Neck, Décolletage, Hands

Results

- Deep hydration, Improved skin quality, Increased radiance
- Softening of fine lines, Cellular repair support

Redensity 1 is often considered one of the most sophisticated skin boosters because it combines hydration with nutrients that support fibroblast function and skin repair.

4. Jalupro®

Manufacturer Professional Dietetics

Products

- Jalupro Classic, Jalupro HMW, Jalupro Super Hydro

Composition

Jalupro Classic

- Hyaluronic acid, Amino acid complex

Jalupro HMW

- Higher molecular weight hyaluronic acid, Amino acids

Jalupro Super Hydro

- Hyaluronic acid, Amino acids, Peptides

How It Is Injected

- Intradermal microdroplets, Dermal injections, Strategic lifting points with Super Hydro

Treatment Series

Classic: Four sessions, 7–10 days apart

HMW: Three sessions, Monthly

Super Hydro: Two to three treatments, Monthly

Best Areas

- Face, Neck, Under-eye region, Hands

Results

- Fibroblast stimulation, Collagen support, Improved hydration
- Improved elasticity, Better skin quality

5. Neauvia Hydro Deluxe®

Manufacturer Matex Lab

Composition

- Hyaluronic acid, Calcium Hydroxyapatite (CaHA), Glycine, L-Proline

How It Is Injected

- Intradermal microdroplets, Needle technique

Treatment Series

- Three sessions, Four weeks apart

Best Areas

- Face, Neck, Hands

Results

- Hydration, Collagen stimulation
- Improved elasticity, Improved skin density, Improved firmness

Neauvia Hydro Deluxe is unique because it combines hyaluronic acid with calcium hydroxyapatite and amino acids, providing both hydration and collagen stimulation.

6. Belotero Revive®

Manufacturer Merz Aesthetics

Composition

- Hyaluronic acid, Glycerol

How It Is Injected

- Superficial intradermal microdroplets, Fine needle technique

Treatment Series

- Two to three sessions, Four weeks apart

Best Areas

- Face, Early ageing skin

Results

- Long-lasting hydration, Improved elasticity
- Increased luminosity, Smoother skin texture

The addition of glycerol improves water retention, creating prolonged hydration.

7. Viscoderm®

Manufacturer IBSA

Composition

- Hyaluronic acid

How It Is Injected

- Intradermal injections, Microdroplet technique

Treatment Series

- Three sessions, Every 2–4 weeks

Best Areas

- Face, Neck, Hands

Results

- Improved hydration, Softer skin, Increased luminosity
- Fine line reduction

Viscoderm is one of Europe's longest-established injectable skin hydration treatments.

8. NCTF 135 HA®

Manufacturer Filorga

Composition

- Hyaluronic acid, 59 active ingredients, Vitamins, Minerals, Coenzymes
- Amino acids, Nucleic acids, Antioxidants

How It Is Injected

- Mesotherapy technique, Microdroplets
- Dermapen infusion, Mesogun delivery

Treatment Series

- Three to five treatments, Two weeks apart

Best Areas

- Face, Neck, Décolletage, Hands

Results

- Deep hydration, Improved radiance, Skin revitalisation, Enhanced skin quality
- Reduced fatigue appearance

NCTF is often called a "skin multivitamin" because of its impressive blend of nutrients.

9. Seventy Hyal 2000®

Manufacturer VIVACY

Composition

- High molecular weight hyaluronic acid

How It Is Injected

- BAP (Bio Aesthetic Points), Cannula, Microdroplet technique

Treatment Series

- Two treatments, Four weeks apart

Best Areas

- Face, Neck, Hands

Results

- Intense hydration, Improved glow, Improved elasticity, Smoother skin texture

10. Profhilo

Manufacturer IBSA Derma

Composition: Profhilo contains one of the highest concentrations of pure hyaluronic acid (64 mg/2 ml) without any chemical cross-linking agents.

Injection Technique: Administered using the Bio-Aesthetic Points (BAP) technique, which involves injecting small amounts into specific points on the face to ensure even distribution and optimal results.

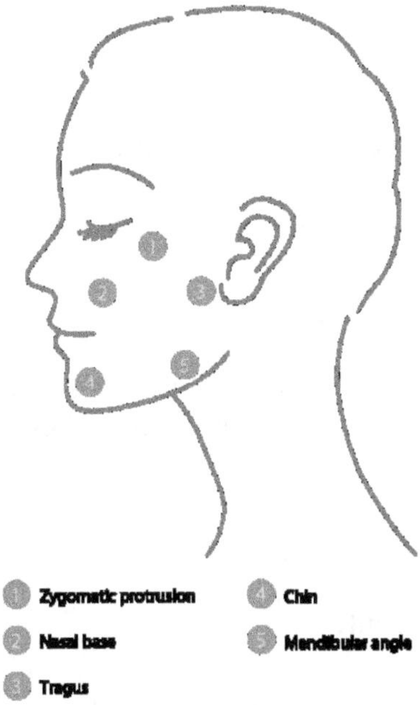

Profhilo with Needle to face

Results: Patients often notice improved skin hydration, elasticity, and a subtle lifting effect within a few weeks. A typical protocol involves two sessions spaced four weeks apart.

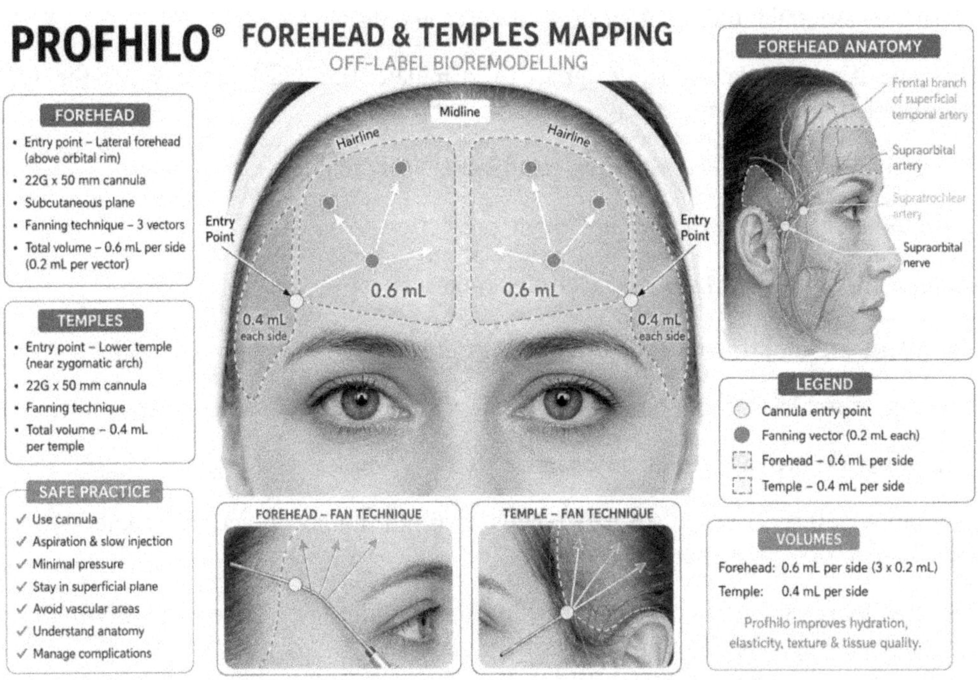

Profhilo with Canula to forehead and temples

11. Sunekos

Manufacturer Professional Dietetics

Regenerative Skin Support Without Volume

Sunekos is often grouped under the term "skin booster," but that description is incomplete.

It is not simply a hydrating injectable.

Sunekos is a regenerative treatment designed to support fibroblast function and improve the extracellular matrix — without adding volume.

That distinction is critical.

It does not inflate tissue. It strengthens it.

What Makes Sunekos Different?

Traditional skin boosters typically contain hyaluronic acid alone. Their primary effect is hydration and temporary plumping.

Sunekos combines: Hyaluronic acid

A patented amino acid complex

The amino acids include: Glycine, L-Proline, L-Lysine, L-Alanine, L-Valine

These are essential building blocks for collagen and elastin synthesis.

This specific formulation is designed to stimulate fibroblast activity — the cells responsible for producing: Collagen, Elastin, Fibronectin

Rather than filling the face, Sunekos improves dermal biology.

It supports regeneration. It does not create projection.

Understanding Fibroblasts and Cellular Senescence

Fibroblasts are the structural cells within the dermis.

With age, fibroblasts: Slow down, Produce less collagen, Become less responsive

Enter a state known as cellular senescence

Cellular senescence refers to aged cells that no longer function efficiently and contribute to tissue degeneration.

Sunekos helps support fibroblast function by providing the biochemical environment needed for collagen production and dermal repair.

It supports the structure of the skin — without volumising it.

Sunekos Performa

Sunekos Performa contains: Low molecular weight hyaluronic acid

The amino acid complex described above

It is designed for delicate areas and early ageing.

Ideal areas: Under-eye region, Upper eyelids (carefully selected cases), Neck, Décolletage, Fine lines

Performa improves: Skin thickness, Elasticity, Crepiness, Fine lines

It does not fill hollows. It improves the quality of the skin covering them.

Sunekos 1200

Sunekos 1200 contains: Higher molecular weight hyaluronic acid

The same amino acid complex

The higher molecular weight component provides greater dermal support and tissue reinforcement.

It is better suited to areas with more advanced dermal depletion.

Common areas: Midface skin quality, Lower face, Jawline region

Areas of collagen loss

Sunekos 1200 does not act as filler.

It does not lift or sculpt. It strengthens and supports dermal integrity.

Can Sunekos Be Used Under the Eyes?

Yes — and this is one of its most valuable applications.

Under-eye ageing is often due to: Skin thinning, Reduced elasticity, Early collagen decline, Mild hollowing

Using filler alone in thin under-eye skin can create heaviness.

Sunekos Performa improves: Dermal thickness, Fine crepiness, Elasticity, Brightness

It enhances tissue quality without adding weight.

How Is Sunekos Injected?

Sunekos is typically administered using:

Small micro-deposits, Linear threading techniques, Strategic dermal placement.

It is injected into the dermis to stimulate fibroblast activity.

It is not placed as a bolus for projection.

A typical course includes: Three to four sessions, Two weeks apart

Results develop gradually as collagen production improves.

What Sunekos Does and Does Not Do

Sunekos can: Improve skin elasticity, Enhance hydration

Support collagen production, Improve dermal thickness, Reduce fine lines, Support fibroblast function

Sunekos does not: Add facial projection, Replace dermal filler, Lift cheeks, Reshape contours, Create jawline definition

It is regenerative support, not volumisation.

When Not to Use Sunekos

Understanding its limits is essential.

Sunekos is not appropriate when:

Significant structural volume loss is present

Advanced cheek collapse requires projection

Deep tear trough hollowing needs structural correction

Severe lower face heaviness requires lifting strategies

It is not suitable for patients seeking: Immediate dramatic results, Facial sculpting, Projection or contour enhancement

Sunekos improves skin quality. It does not replace filler where structure is missing.

It should not be used in areas of: Active infection, Active herpes outbreak, Inflamed skin

Known hypersensitivity to ingredients

The Balanced Approach

The most common mistake in aesthetics is treating lines before structure.

The second most common mistake is adding volume without improving skin quality.

Sunekos works best when integrated into a long-term strategy:

Structure when needed, Regeneration always, Maintenance consistently

It represents a shift in modern aesthetics:

From filling, To regenerating

From inflating, To strengthening

From chasing lines, To supporting biology

That is responsible rejuvenation.

Choosing the Right Skin Booster

Not all skin boosters are created equal.

For pure hydration

- Skinvive, Viscoderm, Restylane Skinboosters, Seventy Hyal

For hydration plus skin nutrition

- Redensity 1, NCTF 135 HA, Jalupro

For hydration plus collagen stimulation

- Neauvia Hydro Deluxe, Jalupro Super Hydro

For early ageing and prevention

- Belotero Revive, Skinvive, Seventy Hyal

For mature, crepey skin

- Redensity 1, NCTF 135 HA, Jalupro HMW, Neauvia Hydro Deluxe

The future of aesthetics is not about making faces bigger. It is about creating healthier skin. Skin boosters occupy a unique space between skincare and injectables, helping patients achieve fresher, more radiant skin while still looking completely natural.

12. Tesoro Collagen

Tesoro Collagen is an injectable skin booster designed to improve skin quality by supporting collagen regeneration rather than adding volume. It belongs to the newer generation of regenerative aesthetic treatments that focus on skin health, texture, and resilience.

What Makes Tesoro Collagen Different

Tesoro Collagen is formulated with recombinant human-like collagen (RHLC). This collagen is laboratory-engineered to closely replicate the structure of natural human collagen, unlike older collagen products derived from animal sources. Because it mimics the body's own collagen, it integrates well into the dermis and is associated with a lower risk of allergic reactions or inflammatory responses.

Rather than acting as a traditional filler, Tesoro Collagen works by supporting the extracellular matrix, encourageing fibroblast activity and improving the skin's natural regenerative processes.

How It Works in the Skin

When injected into the dermis, Tesoro Collagen helps to:

- Improve skin firmness and elasticity, Enhance hydration and skin texture

- Support collagen synthesis over time, Improve skin quality rather than alter facial shape

Results develop gradually, as the skin responds biologically to stimulation, making this treatment ideal for patients seeking natural, subtle rejuvenation.

Areas Commonly Treated

Tesoro Collagen is particularly well suited to delicate and thin-skinned areas, including:

- Under-eye region, Face (fine lines and crepey skin), Neck and décolletage, Hands

It may also be used to improve overall skin quality in patients with early signs of ageing or loss of dermal density.

Treatment Protocol

A typical treatment course involves:

- A series of three sessions, spaced approximately four weeks apart
- Gradual improvement seen after the second session
- Maintenance treatments every six to twelve months, depending on skin condition and ageing factors

Because this is a regenerative treatment, results are progressive rather than immediate.

Key Ingredients and Skin Benefits

In addition to recombinant human-like collagen, Tesoro Collagen formulations often include:

- Sodium hyaluronate for hydration, Amino acids essential for collagen synthesis
- Peptides that support skin repair and renewal, Supporting ingredients that enhance skin tone and vitality

This combination targets both hydration and structural support within the dermis.

Who Is It Best Suited For

Tesoro Collagen is suitable for patients who:

- Want skin rejuvenation without added volume, Prefer gradual, natural-looking results
- Have early to moderate signs of skin ageing
- Are concerned about skin thinning, fine lines, or loss of elasticity

It is not a replacement for dermal fillers, but rather a complementary treatment within a comprehensive skin rejuvenation plan.

Clinical Considerations

Tesoro Collagen should only be administered by trained medical professionals. As with all injectable treatments, patient selection, correct injection depth, and appropriate technique are essential to achieve optimal outcomes and minimise risk.

Expected Results

Patients can anticipate the following outcomes from skin booster treatments:

Immediate Hydration: Skin appears more hydrated and plump shortly after treatment.

Improved Texture and Elasticity: Over subsequent weeks, the skin becomes smoother and more elastic.

Reduction in Fine Lines: Fine lines and superficial wrinkles diminish, leading to a more youthful appearance.

Enhanced Radiance: Overall skin tone appears more even and luminous.

Results vary based on the specific product used, individual skin conditions, and adherence to the recommended treatment protocol.

In summary, skin boosters offer a versatile and effective solution for individuals seeking to enhance their skin's hydration, texture, and overall vitality.

Sunekos® vs Profhilo® – Understanding the Science of Regenerative Skin Rejuvenation

One of the most common questions patients and injectors ask is:

"Which is better, Profhilo or Sunekos?"

The answer is not quite as simple as choosing a winner. Both products represent an evolution away from traditional fillers and towards regenerative aesthetics. However, they take very different pathways to achieve skin rejuvenation.

Understanding these differences helps us appreciate why each product has a place in modern aesthetic practice.

The Evolution of Regenerative Aesthetics

For many years aesthetic medicine focused on replacing lost volume.

We filled folds. We filled cheeks. We filled lips.

Today, patients are increasingly asking for something different.

They want:

- Better skin quality, Improved elasticity
- Firmer tissue, Natural rejuvenation, Long-term skin health

This shift has led to the emergence of bio-remodelling and extracellular matrix (ECM) regeneration.

Profhilo and Sunekos both sit within this category.

What Is Profhilo?

Profhilo was one of the first products to challenge the traditional filler model.

Rather than creating volume, Profhilo uses highly purified, non-crosslinked hyaluronic acid that spreads through tissue and acts as a biological signalling molecule.

It is often described as a **bio-remodeller**.

Profhilo's strengths include:

- Excellent hydration, Tissue quality improvement
- Strong safety profile, Extensive post-marketing data, Ease of treatment

More than 40,000 patients have been included in published safety evaluations, demonstrating a very low complication rate.

Profhilo stimulates fibroblasts through hyaluronic acid receptor signalling, encouraging collagen production and tissue remodelling.

It was genuinely innovative and changed the way many practitioners viewed skin rejuvenation.

What Is Sunekos?

Sunekos takes regenerative medicine a step further.

Like Profhilo, it contains hyaluronic acid.

However, it also contains a patented blend of six amino acids known as HY6AA:

- Glycine, Proline, Lysine, Leucine, Valine, Alanine

These amino acids are the actual building blocks required to manufacture collagen and elastin.

Rather than simply sending a signal to fibroblasts, Sunekos attempts to provide both the signal and the raw materials needed for regeneration.

This distinction forms the foundation of the Sunekos philosophy.

The House-Building Analogy

The easiest way to understand the difference is to imagine building a house.

Profhilo provides the architectural plans. It tells the builder what to construct.

Sunekos provides the plans and delivers the bricks, timber, and cement needed to complete the project.

Both products stimulate fibroblasts.

Only one supplies the amino acid substrates needed to manufacture collagen and elastin.

Why Hyaluronic Acid Matters

Many people think hyaluronic acid simply hydrates the skin.

In reality, HA is an active signalling molecule.

It communicates with specialised receptors including:

CD44

Responsible for: Tissue homeostasis, ECM maintenance, Cell migration, Anti-inflammatory signalling

RHAMM (CD168)

Associated with: Cell proliferation, Fibroblast activation, Tissue regeneration

TLR Receptors

Can influence inflammatory pathways.

The molecular weight of hyaluronic acid determines which receptors are preferentially activated and therefore which biological response occurs.

Is More Hyaluronic Acid Better?

Marketing often focuses on HA concentration.

However, biology does not always reward "more."

Once cellular receptors become saturated, increasing the HA concentration may not significantly increase biological activity.

The key question is not: *"How much hyaluronic acid was injected?"*

The more important question is: *"Did the skin produce healthier collagen, elastin, and extracellular matrix?"*

The Importance of Amino Acids

Collagen and elastin are proteins.

Proteins cannot be manufactured without amino acids. This concept seems obvious, yet it is often overlooked.

The six amino acids contained in Sunekos each perform specific functions:

Glycine: The backbone of collagen and elastin.

Proline: Provides collagen stability and strength.

Lysine: Required for collagen cross-linking and maturation.

Leucine: Stimulates protein synthesis.

Valine: Essential for elastin formation.

Alanine: Supports elastin assembly and extracellular matrix organisation.

Research suggests that the correct ratio of these amino acids is necessary to achieve simultaneous collagen and elastin production.

The Role of Lysine

Among the six amino acids, lysine deserves special attention.

Lysine contributes to:

Collagen Maturation: Without lysine, collagen fibres remain immature and mechanically weak.

Elastin Formation: Lysine is involved in elastin cross-linking, which allows skin to maintain elasticity.

Tissue Strength

Lysyl oxidase uses lysine to create stronger connective tissue networks.

Some Sunekos research also suggests lysine may help reduce hyaluronidase activity, potentially slowing HA breakdown and extending the biological signalling period.

Receptor-Clean Signalling

One of the unique concepts behind Sunekos is receptor separation.

Instead of combining different molecular weights of HA into one syringe, Sunekos separates them into two products.

Sunekos 1200

Uses high molecular weight HA. Designed for deeper tissue layers.

Aims to stimulate:

- CD44 signalling, Anti-inflammatory pathways
- Deep fibroblasts, Endogenous HA production

Sunekos Performa

Uses lower molecular weight HA. Designed for superficial tissues.

Aims to stimulate:

- RHAMM signalling, Fibroblast proliferation
- Elastin production, Fibronectin synthesis

The theory is that each receptor pathway can be activated without interference from competing molecular weights.

Extracellular Matrix Regeneration

The extracellular matrix contains: Collagen, Elastin, Fibronectin, Hyaluronic acid, Structural proteins

Published Sunekos data suggests stimulation of:

- Collagen I, Collagen III, Collagen IV, Collagen VII, Elastin, Fibronectin

Profhilo also stimulates collagen production, but much of its published evidence centres around hyaluronic acid receptor signalling rather than amino acid substrate delivery.

Areas Where Sunekos Excels

Clinically, Sunekos is particularly useful for:

Under Eyes: Thin skin, Fine lines, Crepey texture

Forehead: Static wrinkles, Skin quality improvement

Neck: Crepiness, Horizontal lines

Décolletage: Sun damage, Fine wrinkling

Hands: Thinning skin, Texture changes

These are areas where volume is often less important than tissue quality.

Safety

Both products have excellent safety profiles.

Advantages include: Non-crosslinked HA, No BDDE cross-linking agents, Minimal granuloma risk, Biocompatible ingredients, Reversible with hyaluronidase

Common side effects include: Redness, Swelling, Bruising, Tenderness

These are generally mild and temporary.

Australian Considerations

In Australia, Profhilo is registered with a specific intended use involving the malar and sub-malar cheek regions for contour redefinition and laxity remodelling.

As healthcare professionals, it is important that practitioners remain aware of TGA advertising regulations and approved indications when discussing treatment options with patients.

My Clinical Thoughts

I do not see Profhilo and Sunekos as direct competitors. I see them as different tools.

Profhilo was a groundbreaking product that helped move aesthetic medicine away from simple filling and toward bio-remodelling.

Sunekos builds upon that concept by introducing amino acid substrate delivery and a more focused extracellular matrix regeneration strategy.

If I had to summarise the difference in one sentence, it would be this:

Profhilo tells the fibroblast what to do.

Sunekos tells the fibroblast what to do, provides the building materials to do it, and may extend the time available for the work to be completed.

Whether one is superior will continue to be debated as more research emerges.

What is certain is that both products reflect the future direction of aesthetics.

The future is not simply about replacing lost volume. It is about improving the health of the tissue itself. And that is where regenerative medicine is taking us.

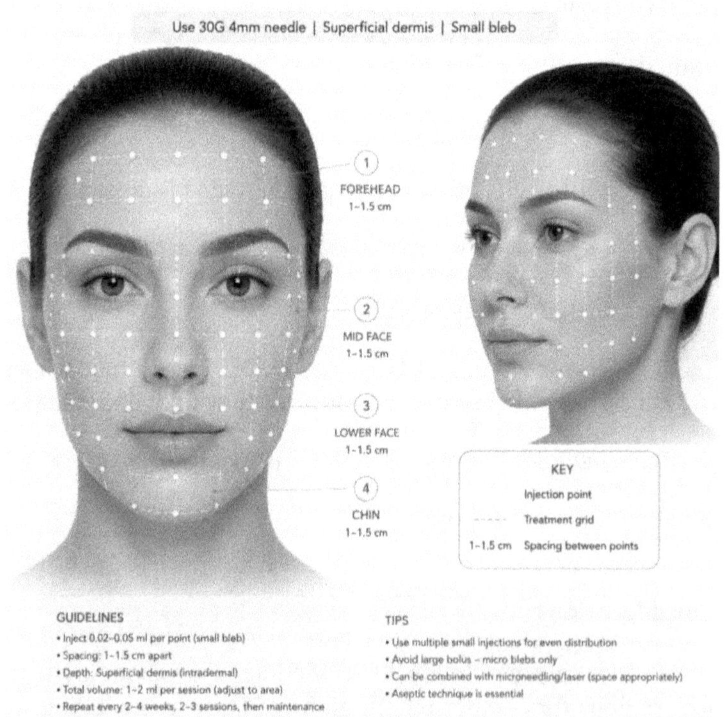

Choosing the Right Skin Booster

Not all skin boosters are created equal.

FOR PURE HYDRATION

Skinvive

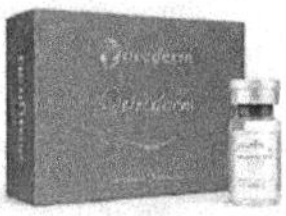

- Improves hydration
- Improves smoothness
- Enhances luminosity
- Supports skin quality

Viscoderm

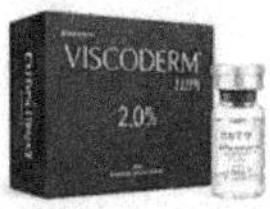

- Hydrates skin
- Improves texture
- Softens fine lines
- Restores skin luminosity

Restylane Skinboosters

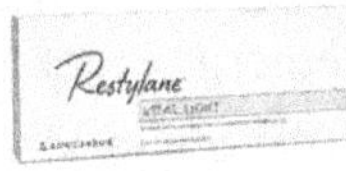

- Deep hydration
- Improves elasticity
- Improves skin texture
- Softens fine lines

Seventy Hyal

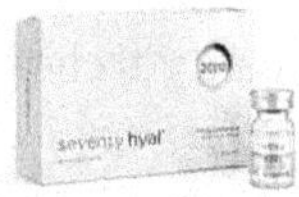

- Deep hydration
- Improves elasticity
- Improves skin texture
- Softens fine lines

Profhilo

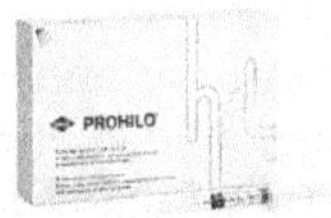

- Intense hydration
- Improves skin laxity
- Remodelling & bio-stimulation
- Improves overall skin quality

FOR HYDRATION PLUS SKIN NUTRITION

Redensity 1

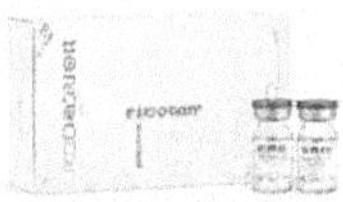

- Improves hydration
- Improves radiance
- Improves skin quality
- Softens fine lines
- Supports microcirculation and microdroplets

NCTF 135 HA

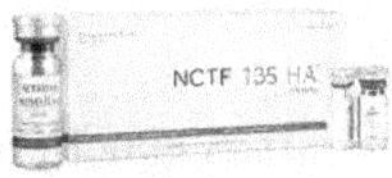

- Deep hydration
- Revitalises skin
- Improves tone & radiance
- Antioxidant protection
- Improves elasticity

Jalupro

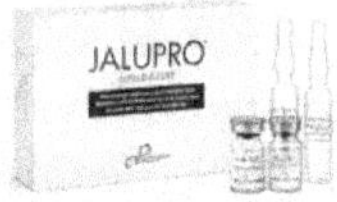

- Deep hydration
- Collagen stimulation
- Improves elasticity
- Improves skin density
- Improves firmness

Sunekos 1200

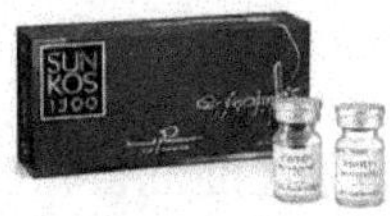

- Hydration
- Skin nutrition
- Improves elasticity
- Brightens dark circles
- Improves skin quality

FOR HYDRATION PLUS COLLAGEN STIMULATION

Neauvia Hydro Deluxe

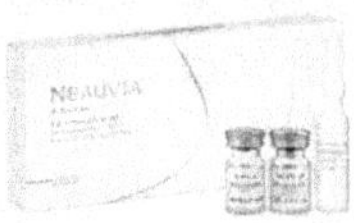

- Deep hydration
- Collagen stimulation
- Improves elasticity
- Improves elasticity
- Improves skin density
- Improves firmness

Jalupro Super Hydro

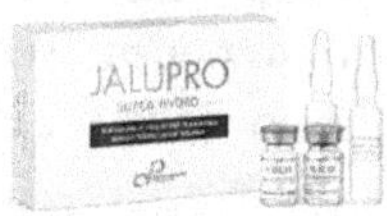

- Improves hydration
- Improves elasticity
- Improves luminosity
- Improves skin smoothness

Sunekos 200

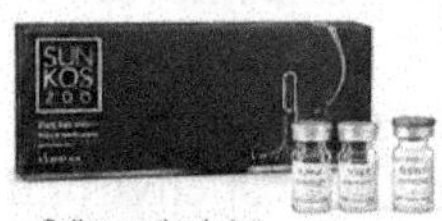

- Collagen stimulation
- Improves elasticity
- Improves firmness
- Reduces fine lines
- Overall skin rejuvenation

FOR EARLY AGEING AND PREVENTION

Belotero Revive

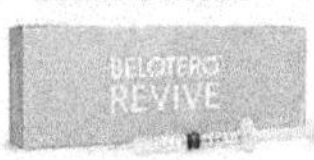

- Improves hydration
- Improves skin smoothness
- Enhances luminosity
- Creates a healthy glow

Skinvive

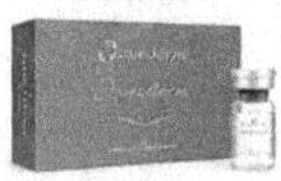

- Improves hydration
- Improves smoothness
- Enhances luminosity
- Supports skin quality

Seventy Hyal

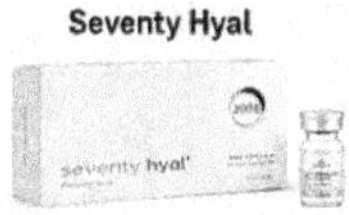

- Deep hydration
- Improves elasticity
- Improves skin texture
- Softens fine lines

Profhilo

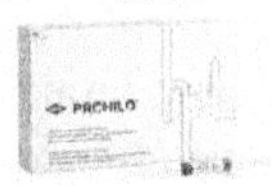

- Intense hydration
- Improves skin laxity
- Remodelling & bio-stimulation
- Improves overall skin quality

FOR MATURE, CREPEY SKIN

Redensity 1

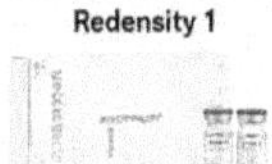

- Improves hydration
- Improves radiance
- Improves skin quality
- Softens fine lines
- Supports microcirculation and microdroplets

NCTF 135 HA

- Deep hydration
- Revitalises skin
- Improves tone & radiance
- Antioxidant protection
- Improves elasticity

Jalupro HMW

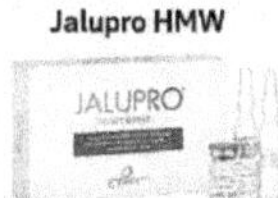

- Improves hydration
- Improves elasticity
- Improves luminosity
- Improves skin smoothness

Neauvia Hydro Deluxe

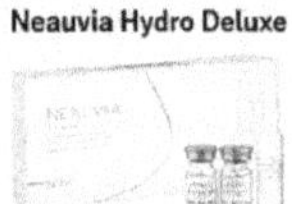

- Deep hydration
- Collagen stimulation
- Improves elasticity
- Improves skin density
- Improves firmness

Profhilo

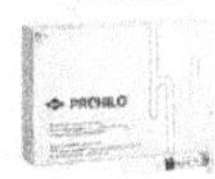

- Intense hydration
- Improves skin laxity
- Remodelling & bio-stimulation
- Improves overall skin quality

Chapter 48: Glass Skin

What is Glass Skin?

One of the biggest beauty trends to emerge from South Korea is the concept of **Glass Skin**. Unlike traditional beauty ideals that focus on covering imperfections with makeup, glass skin is about creating skin that is so healthy, hydrated, smooth, and luminous that it appears almost transparent—like a sheet of polished glass.

Glass skin is not a treatment. It is a skin condition and a goal.

The hallmark features of glass skin include:

- Even skin tone, Refined pores, Deep hydration
- Smooth texture, Minimal inflammation
- A natural reflective glow, Healthy skin barrier function

When light hits glass skin, it reflects evenly across the surface because the skin is well hydrated and smooth. In contrast, dehydrated, rough, or damaged skin scatters light unevenly, making the complexion appear dull and tired.

The Science Behind Glass Skin

Glass skin is achieved by optimizing the health of the epidermis, particularly the outermost layer known as the **stratum corneum**. When this layer contains adequate moisture and intact lipids, it functions as an effective barrier, preventing water loss and protecting against environmental damage.

Hydrated skin cells become plumper and smoother, allowing light to reflect more uniformly. This creates the characteristic dewy appearance associated with glass skin.

Collagen and elastin within the dermis also play an important role. Healthy collagen supports skin firmness, while elastin allows the skin to rebound and maintain a youthful appearance.

How to Achieve Glass Skin

The Korean approach focuses on consistency rather than aggressive treatments.

The key principles are:

Gentle Cleansing

The skin should be clean but never stripped of its natural oils.

Hydration

Multiple layers of hydrating products are often used rather than a single heavy cream.

Barrier Repair

Ingredients such as ceramides, hyaluronic acid, glycerin, and peptides help strengthen the skin barrier.

Sun Protection

Daily sunscreen is non-negotiable. UV damage is one of the fastest ways to lose skin clarity and luminosity.

Regular Exfoliation

Gentle exfoliation removes dead surface cells and allows fresh skin to reflect light more effectively.

Professional Treatments That Support Glass Skin

Many aesthetic treatments can accelerate the glass skin effect.

These include:

- Skin boosters, Mesotherapy, PRP and PRF, Biofiller
- Polynucleotides, Sunekos, Profhilo
- Microneedling, PRX-T33, Light chemical peels, LED phototherapy

These treatments improve hydration, collagen production, and skin quality rather than simply adding volume.

The Glass Skin Routine

Morning
Cleanse → Antioxidant serum → Hydrating serum → Moisturiser → SPF

Evening
Cleanse → Active treatment (retinoid, peptides, or pigment corrector) → Hydrating serum → Moisturiser

My Thoughts

As an aesthetic nurse, I believe the future of beauty is moving away from simply filling faces and toward improving skin quality. Patients today are less interested in looking "done" and more interested in looking healthy, rested, and naturally radiant.

Glass skin represents this shift perfectly. It is not about changing your face. It is about creating the healthiest version of your skin possible.

When skin is healthy, hydrated, and functioning well, it reflects light beautifully. And that glow is something no amount of makeup can truly replicate. For me, that is the essence of modern aesthetics.

Chapter 49: Bio-Stimulants: How They Work & Why They're Game-Changers in Aesthetic Medicine

What Are Bio-Stimulants?

Bio-stimulants are injectable treatments that stimulate the body's natural collagen production rather than simply adding volume like traditional hyaluronic acid (HA) fillers. They work by triggering a wound-healing response, leading to gradual and long-lasting skin rejuvenation and structural support.

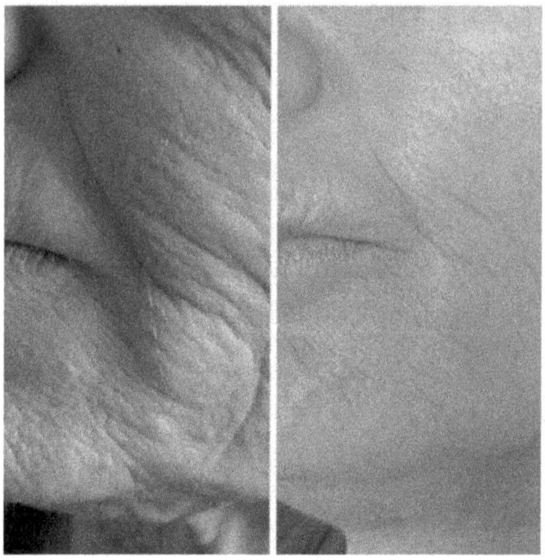

Two of the most well-known bio-stimulants in aesthetic medicine are Sculptra (poly-L-lactic acid) and Radiesse (calcium hydroxylapatite, CaHA).

How Do Sculptra & Radiesse Work?

Bio-Stimulant	Primary Component	Mechanism of Action	Collagen Type Stimulated
Sculptra	Poly-L-lactic acid (PLLA)	Stimulates fibroblasts to increase collagen production over time	Primarily Type I Collagen (strong structural collagen)
Radiesse	Calcium hydroxylapatite (CaHA) microspheres	Provides immediate volume while stimulating fibroblasts for long-term collagen production	Primarily Type I & Type III Collagen (Type III is found in youthful skin)

Sculptra (PLLA) Long-Lasting, Natural Rejuvenation

Works gradually by stimulating fibroblasts to produce Type I collagen, which supports the skin's structure and firmness.

Results appear over 3-6 months after a series of three sessions, spaced one month apart.

Lasts up to two years, but annual maintenance is recommended due to ongoing fat and bone volume loss (especially for patients on weight loss medications like Ozempic).

Injectors can target deeper layers even down to the bone for profound rejuvenation.

Radiesse (CaHA) Instant & Long-Term Lifting Power

Provides immediate volume due to its thick, opaque gel carrier, making it ideal for hand rejuvenation and deep facial volumization.

Over time, stimulates both Type I and Type III collagen, enhancing skin elasticity and firmness.

Can be used undiluted for deep structural support (cheeks, jawline) or hyperdiluted for skin rejuvenation (decolletage, neck, arms, abdomen).

Indications for Use: Where Do Bio-Stimulants Work Best?

Sculptra :Best for Gradual, Natural Full-Face Rejuvenation

Cheeks, temples, jawline (treats deeper fat and bone loss).

Pre-jowl sulcus & marionette lines (restores structural integrity).

Decolletage arms, knees (firms and thickens ageing skin).

Buttocks and hip dips (for non-surgical body contouring).

Radiesse Best for Instant Lift & Targeted Rejuvenation

Hands (its opacity hides vein prominence and volume loss).

Jawline and chin (provides immediate contouring).

Hyperdiluted for skin rejuvenation on neck, arms, thighs, and abdomen.

Hyperdiluted Sculptra & Radiesse for Skin Rejuvenation

Hyperdiluted versions of Sculptra and Radiesse are fantastic for improving skin quality, texture, and elasticity.

When diluted with saline and lidocaine, they can be injected more superficially to treat crepey, sagging skin.

Best for neck, décolletage, arms, and knees, where traditional fillers may not be suitable.

Why Sculptra Is My Favorite Bio-Stimulant (After PRP)

Sculptra provides gradual, natural volume restoration , patients look like a better version of themselves, not overfilled.

It's a long-term collagen stimulator, meaning the results continue improving over time.

The ability to target deep fat pads and bone allows for profound facial rejuvenation.

A must-have treatment for patients experiencing facial volume loss due to ageing or weight loss (e.g., Ozempic users).

Conclusion: Bio-Stimulants Are the Future of Aesthetic Medicine

Sculptra (PLLA) and Radiesse (CaHA) stimulate collagen for long-term rejuvenation.

Sculptra boosts Type I collagen, while Radiesse enhances both Type I and Type III collagen.

Treatment areas include the face, hands, neck, and even body contouring (buttocks, arms, knees).

Hyperdiluted versions improve skin laxity and texture without adding bulk.

For optimal results, patients should complete a series of treatments and maintain yearly top-ups.

With bio-stimulants, we are shifting from simply filling lines to rebuilding the skin's foundation, allowing for natural, long-lasting rejuvenation.

JULÄINE

The New Generation of PLLA Biostimulation

As aesthetic medicine evolves, there has been a major movement away from simply filling the face toward treatments that stimulate the skin to regenerate itself naturally.

Patients today are increasingly asking for:

- Better skin quality, Firmer skin
- Natural tightening, Less puffiness

- Softer, more refreshed rejuvenation

This is where collagen biostimulators have become increasingly popular.

JULÄINE is a newer generation Poly-L-Lactic Acid (PLLA) biostimulator developed in Sweden and designed to stimulate collagen production gradually over time.

Unlike traditional dermal fillers that create immediate volume, JULÄINE works by activating fibroblasts within the skin to encourage the body to produce its own collagen naturally.

The treatment focuses on improving:

- Skin firmness, Elasticity, Facial laxity, Fine lines, Skin texture, Mild volume loss

Rather than dramatically changing facial shape, the aim is to improve the quality and structure of the skin itself.

How JULÄINE Works

JULÄINE contains PLLA microspheres which stimulate collagen production after injection into the tissue.

Over time, the body responds by producing new collagen around the treated areas. This gradual collagen formation can help restore support, improve skin thickness, and create a firmer appearance.

Results are not immediate. Improvements develop progressively over several weeks to months as collagen production increases.

This gradual process is one reason biostimulators often appear more natural than traditional fillers.

LASYNPRO™ Microsphere Technology

One of the major features of JULÄINE is its LASYNPRO™ microsphere technology.

The PLLA particles are designed to be highly uniform in size and shape. This more consistent particle structure is intended to:

- Improve tissue integration, Allow smoother product distribution
- Reduce uneven clustering, Create a more controlled collagen response

JULÄINE is also promoted as stimulating predominantly Type I collagen, which is the strong structural collagen associated with youthful skin firmness and resilience.

Reconstitution and Preparation

Unlike older PLLA technologies that often required lengthy hydration times before use, JULÄINE has been developed for faster and easier preparation.

The product is designed to hydrate more rapidly and form a smoother suspension.

Treatment protocols vary between practitioners, however JULÄINE generally requires less preparation time before injection compared to traditional PLLA products.

There is also less emphasis on aggressive post-treatment massage protocols.

Areas Commonly Treated

JULÄINE may be used for:

- Midface laxity, Lower face ageing
- Jawline softening, Temples, Thin ageing skin
- General facial rejuvenation, Skin quality improvement

It is particularly suited to patients seeking subtle rejuvenation and improved skin quality without looking overfilled.

Difference Between JULÄINE and Sculptra

Although both JULÄINE and Sculptra are PLLA collagen biostimulators, there are several important differences.

JULÄINE	Sculptra
Newer PLLA technology	Original established PLLA biostimulator
Uses LASYNPRO™ uniform microspheres	Uses traditional PLLA particles
Designed for smoother tissue integration	Relies more on dilution and technique
Faster hydration and preparation	Traditionally reconstituted 24–48 hours prior
Lower inflammatory stimulation	Works through controlled inflammatory response
Less emphasis on massage protocols	Historically required massage after treatment
Focuses strongly on Type I collagen stimulation	General collagen stimulation
Designed for subtle regenerative skin improvement	Often used for volume restoration and collagen stimulation

Both products stimulate collagen gradually over time and belong to the regenerative aesthetics category rather than traditional volumising fillers.

Profhilo® Structura: Advanced Facial Rejuvenation

Profhilo® Structura is an innovative injectable treatment developed to address deeper structural changes in the face associated with ageing. Building upon the original Profhilo® formulation, Structura focuses on regenerating and repositioning superficial facial fat layers to enhance facial contours and provide a natural lifting effect.

Composition and Technology

Utilizing the patented NAHYCO® technology, Profhilo® Structura combines 45 mg of high molecular weight hyaluronic acid (H-HA) with 45 mg of low molecular weight hyaluronic acid (L-HA) per 2 mL syringe. This thermal stabilization process creates hybrid cooperative complexes (HCC) without the need for chemical cross-linking agents, resulting in a purer and more biocompatible product.

Mechanism of Action

Injected into the superficial fat compartments of the face, particularly the preauricular area, Profhilo® Structura stimulates the regeneration of adipose tissue. This process counteracts age-related fat loss and tissue descent, effectively restoring facial volume and contour. The treatment promotes collagen production and enhances skin firmness, leading to a rejuvenated and lifted appearance.

Treatment Protocol

The recommended protocol involves two treatment sessions spaced one month apart. Each session consists of injecting 1 mL of Profhilo® Structura into each side of the face using a 25G x 50 mm cannula, targeting the superficial fat compartments. Clinical studies have demonstrated significant improvements in facial volume and wrinkle reduction, with results maintained for at least three months post-treatment.

Distinction from Original Profhilo®

While both Profhilo® and Profhilo® Structura utilize hyaluronic acid-based formulations, they serve different purposes:

Profhilo®: Primarily enhances skin hydration and elasticity by stimulating collagen and elastin production in the dermis, without adding volume.

Profhilo® Structura: Targets deeper layers to restore facial fat compartments, providing structural support and a lifting effect, thereby addressing more pronounced signs of ageing.

In summary, Profhilo® Structura offers a novel approach to facial rejuvenation by focusing on the restoration of subcutaneous fat and structural support, delivering natural-looking results for individuals experiencing age-related facial volume loss and sagging.

Profhilo Structura: for Sinkers & Saggers.

Unlike regular Profhilo, which uses the BAP (Bio Aesthetic Points) technique with needle injections, Profhilo Structura is administered exclusively with a cannula, allowing for better diffusion, reduced trauma, and targeted tissue support.

Profhilo Structura

Sinkers

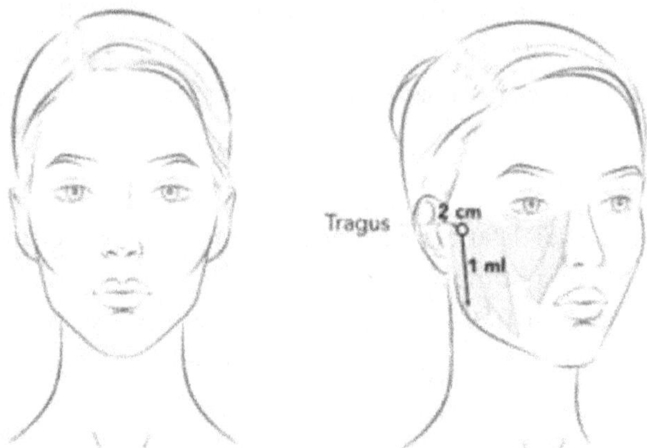

Saggers

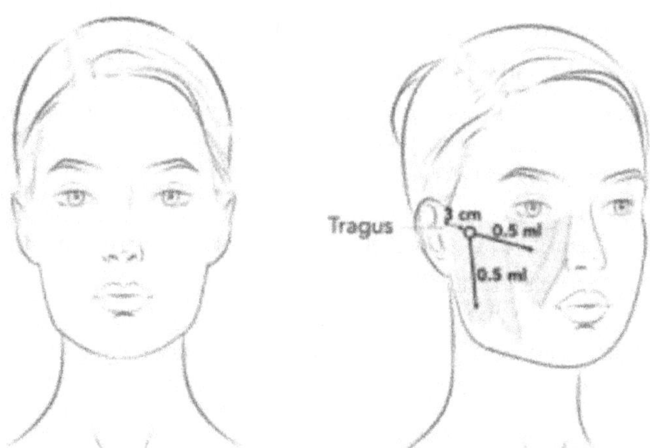

Sinkers vs. Saggers: Understanding the Two Ageing Patterns

1. Sinkers – Individuals who lose volume due to fat pad depletion, bone resorption, and skin thinning.

Common Areas: Midface, temples, preauricular region, jawline

Treatment Goal: Restore support and prevent further structural collapse

2. Saggers – Individuals with skin laxity and tissue descent, causing jowling, deep marionette lines, and lower face drooping.

Common Areas: Jawline, submalar (SUMO) region, neck

Treatment Goal: Tighten and lift skin by enhancing collagen and elastin production

Injection Techniques for Profhilo Structura: Sinkers vs. Saggers
1. Injection Technique for Sinkers (Structural Loss & Volume Depletion)

Cannula: 22G

Entry Point: Preauricular (near the ear)

Injection Plane: Deep subcutaneous layer (above SMAS)

Technique:

Retrograde threading – Injecting product while withdrawing the cannula, ensuring even distribution

Targeting deep fat compartments for improved facial support

Goal:

Reinforce structural integrity of volume-depleted areas, Improve hydration and skin quality, Prevent further sinking of facial tissues

2. Injection Technique for Saggers (Skin Laxity & Drooping)

Cannula: 25G

Entry Points:

SUMO area (submalar fat pad) – To support midface tissue

Preauricular (near the ear) – To tighten jawline and reduce jowling

Injection Plane: Superficial subcutaneous layer

Technique:

Soft fanning technique – Spreading the product evenly across legs zygmatic bone and pre auricular (lateral cheek) .

Emphasis on collagen stimulation rather than volume replacement

Goal:

Strengthen skin support structures, Enhance elasticity and skin density, Reduce sagging and improve skin texture

Why Use a Cannula for Profhilo Structura?

Safer Delivery – Reduces risk of vascular compromise

Less Bruising & Swelling – Fewer entry points compared to multiple needle injections

Better Product Diffusion – Spreads smoothly across treatment zones for natural integration.

GOURI

GOURI is an innovative, fully liquid polycaprolactone (PCL) injectable developed to stimulate natural collagen production, offering comprehensive skin rejuvenation. Unlike traditional fillers that primarily add volume, GOURI enhances the skin's structural integrity by promoting collagen synthesis, leading to improved elasticity and a more youthful appearance.

Key Features of GOURI:

- **Composition**: GOURI utilizes 100% liquid PCL, a biodegradable and biocompatible polymer, ensuring a natural integration into the skin.

- **Mechanism of Action**: Upon injection, GOURI spreads evenly across the treatment area, stimulating fibroblasts to produce collagen. This process gradually restores skin elasticity and firmness, addressing signs of ageing such as fine lines and wrinkles.

- **Treatment Areas**: GOURI is versatile and can be used on various facial regions, including the cheeks, nasolabial folds, and areas with noticeable sagging or loss of elasticity.

- **Procedure**: The treatment involves injecting GOURI into specific points of the face using either a 5-point injection technique or a cannula method. The choice of technique depends on the patient's needs and the practitioner's assessment.

- **Results and Longevity**: Patients may begin to notice improvements within a few weeks post-treatment, with optimal results typically observed after multiple sessions. The effects of GOURI can last between 6 to 12 months, depending on individual factors and the treatment plan.

Benefits of GOURI:

- **Natural Rejuvenation**: By stimulating the body's own collagen production, GOURI provides a natural-looking enhancement without adding excessive volume.

- **Minimal Downtime**: Most patients experience mild swelling or redness post-procedure, which typically resolves within a few days, allowing for a quick return to daily activities.

- **Safety Profile**: As a biocompatible and biodegradable product, GOURI integrates seamlessly with the body's tissues, minimizing the risk of adverse reactions.

GOURI represents a significant advancement in aesthetic medicine, offering a non-surgical option for individuals seeking to rejuvenate their skin by harnessing the body's natural regenerative processes. Consultation with a qualified aesthetic practitioner is essential to determine suitability and develop a personalized treatment plan.

Ellansé

Ellansé is a unique dermal filler that not only provides immediate volume correction but also stimulates the body's natural collagen production, leading to longer-lasting and natural-looking results.

Key Features of Ellansé:

• **Immediate Volume Restoration**: Upon injection, Ellansé provides instant correction of wrinkles and folds, restoring facial volume and contours.

• **Collagen Stimulation**: Beyond immediate effects, Ellansé stimulates the body's own collagen production, enhancing skin elasticity, firmness, and overall quality over time.

• **Long-Lasting Results**: Depending on the specific Ellansé product used, results can last from 18 months up to 3 years, reducing the need for frequent touch-ups.

• **Biocompatible and Biodegradable**: Composed of polycaprolactone (PCL) microspheres suspended in a carboxymethylcellulose (CMC) gel, Ellansé is both biocompatible and biodegradable, ensuring safety and natural integration into the skin.

Treatment Areas:

Ellansé is versatile and can be used to address various facial areas, including:

• Nasolabial folds, Marionette lines, Cheek volume loss, Jawline contouring, Chin augmentation, Temple hollows, Hand rejuvenation

Procedure and Recovery:

The treatment involves injecting Ellansé into the desired areas using fine needles or cannulas. The procedure typically takes about 30 to 45 minutes, depending on the number of areas treated. Most patients experience minimal downtime, with possible mild swelling or redness that usually subsides within a few days.

Safety and Considerations:

Ellansé has a strong safety profile; however, as with any injectable treatment, there are potential side effects, including:

• Redness, Swelling, Bruising, Tenderness at the injection site

These side effects are typically mild and resolve spontaneously within a few days. Rare but serious complications, such as vascular occlusion, have been reported; thus, it is crucial to have the procedure performed by a qualified and experienced medical professional.

Why Choose One Over the Other?

For Full-Face Rejuvenation & Gradual Volume: → Sculptra (Best for global collagen stimulation)

For Instant Lift with Long-Term Collagen Boost: → Radiesse (Gives immediate structure & tightens skin)

For Skin Tightening & Subtle Refinement: → Gouri (Best for mild laxity & fine lines without adding bulk)

For Long-Lasting Structural Support & Contouring: → Ellansé (Acts as a filler with collagen-stimulating benefits)

Juvelook and Lenisna are advanced injectable treatments designed to rejuvenate the skin by stimulating collagen production. Both products combine Poly-D,L-lactic acid (PDLLA) with non-cross-linked hyaluronic acid (HA), offering both immediate hydration and long-term skin improvement.

Juvelook:

- **Composition**: Contains 42.5 mg of PDLLA and 7.5 mg of HA, with particle sizes ranging from 10 to 40 micrometers.
- **Application**: Suitable for addressing fine lines, improving skin texture, treating under-eye concerns, and reducing acne scars.
- **Injection Depth**: Administered into the dermis to superficial subcutaneous layers.
- **Results**: Typically visible around two weeks after treatment and can last between 12 to 16 months.

Lenisna:

- **Composition**: Contains 170 mg of PDLLA and 30 mg of HA, with particle sizes between 50 to 60 micrometers.
- **Application**: Effective for treating deep wrinkles, volume loss in the face or hands, and significant tissue defects.
- **Injection Depth**: Targeted at the superficial subcutaneous layer.
- **Results**: Effects appear after about two weeks and can last approximately 18 to 24 months.

Both treatments work by gradually absorbing into the skin, activating fibroblasts to stimulate the production of collagen and elastin, leading to improved skin elasticity and firmness. The choice between Juvelook and Lenisna depends on individual skin concerns and desired outcomes.

Ariessence™ Pure PDGF+: A Next-Gen Biostimulant

Among the evolving range of biostimulants making waves in aesthetic medicine, Ariessence™ Pure PDGF+ stands out as a groundbreaking innovation. Rooted in advanced regenerative science, this treatment harnesses the power of Platelet-Derived Growth Factor (PDGF)—a potent signaling protein that plays a pivotal role in tissue regeneration, collagen synthesis, and cellular communication.

Unlike traditional autologous treatments such as Platelet-Rich Plasma (PRP), which depend on the variability of the patient's own platelets, Ariessence delivers pharmaceutical-grade, recombinant PDGF in a highly purified and consistent format. This ensures predictability, potency, and safety—key components in achieving reliable clinical outcomes.

What Makes Ariessence Unique?

- **Ultra-Purified Formula**: With only four ingredients, Ariessence's formulation eliminates unnecessary additives and focuses on delivering bioactive growth factors at an unparalleled level of purity.
- **Potency**: According to the manufacturer, Ariessence boasts up to 300,000 times the concentration of growth factors found in typical PRP preparations—an extraordinary leap in therapeutic strength.
- **Consistency**: Because it is lab-engineered rather than patient-derived, it removes variability between individuals, offering more uniform outcomes across diverse skin types and conditions.
- **Clinical Heritage**: PDGF has been extensively studied and utilized in medical-grade wound healing and tissue repair, with a strong safety profile and FDA approval in other therapeutic categories.

Treatment Applications

Ariessence can be used as a standalone injectable treatment or combined with microneedling, RF microneedling, laser resurfacing, or dermal fillers. Its regenerative capabilities make it ideal for addressing:

- Skin laxity, Fine lines and wrinkles, Dull or uneven skin tone, Post-procedural recovery, Acne scarring

Who Is It For?

Ariessence is particularly well-suited to clients seeking visible skin rejuvenation without volumizing, such as those wary of hyaluronic acid fillers but still desiring a refreshed, youthful appearance. It's also excellent for younger patients focused on prevention and mature clients looking for firming and texture improvement.

Comparative Chart Ariessence with Natural Biostimulant PRP, Synthetic Bio stimulant Sculptra.

Feature	Ariessence Pure PDGF+	PRP (Platelet-Rich Plasma)	Sculptra (Poly-L-lactic Acid)
Source	Lab-engineered PDGF (non-autologous)	Autologous (patient's own blood)	Synthetic poly-L-lactic acid (biodegradable polymer)
Key Action	Regenerative signaling for collagen and cell renewal	Moderate collagen stimulation and healing via growth factors	Strong fibroblast stimulation via inflammatory cascade
Onset of Results	Visible results within 2 to 4 weeks	4 to 6 weeks	Gradual, 8 to 12 weeks
Duration	Several months (varies depending on treatment plan)	Typically 3to 6 months	Up to 2 years or longer with full course
Consistency	Highly consistent lab-purified and controlled	Variables depends on patients platelet concentration	Consistent once injected correctly
Texture & Volume	No volume; improves tone, firmness, clarity	Little to no volume; more regenerative	Volumizing effect as collagen builds
Ideal For	Skin quality, texture, early ageing, post-laser or microneedling	Prevention, healing, dullness, hair loss	Volume loss, deep folds, structural rejuvenation
Contraindications	Very fewer non-autologous, no allergy risk	Autoimmune disorders, anemia, low platelet counts	History of keloids, active inflammation
Treatment Comfort	Mild topical or needle-based application	Blood draw + microinjections or microneedling	Deep dermal injections; requires massage post-treatment

Biostimulants Guide

Product	Main Ingredient	Mechanism of Action	Best For	Longevity
Sculptra	Poly-L-Lactic Acid (PLLA)	Stimulates deep collagen production for gradual volume restoration	Global volume loss, hollow cheeks, temples, buttocks augmentation	Up to 2 yrs
Radiesse	Calcium Hydroxylapatite (CaHA)	Provides immediate lift & stimulates collagen production	Jawline contouring, cheek augmentation, hand rejuvenation	12-18 m
Gouri	Liquid polycaprolactone (PCL)	Fully liquid form spreads evenly to stimulate collagen	Skin laxity, fine lines, overall skill tightening	6-12 m
Ellansé	Polycaprolactone (PCL) microspheres in CMC gel	Immediate volume correction + collagen stimulation for long term skin support	Facial contouring, deep folds, chin & Jawline enhancement	1 to 4 yrs
Profhilo Structura	Hybrid Cooperative Complex (HCC) HA	Hydrates deeply while stimulating collagen, elastin & adipose tissue for skin tighten and volume restoration	Skin laxity, fine lines , overall skin firmness & elasticity	6-12 m
Juvelook	Poly-D,L-lactic acid (PDLLA) and non-cross-linked Hyaluronic Acid (HA)	HA provides immediate hydration and plumping; PDLLA stimulates collagen production for long-term skin rejuvenation	Fine lines, wrinkles, acne scars, skin hydration, peri-orbital rejuvenation	24 m
Lenisna	Poly-D,L-lactic acid (PDLLA) and Hyaluronic Acid (HA)	HA offers immediate volume; PDLLA acts as a collagen stimulator, enhancing skin elasticity and firmness over time	Deep wrinkles, facial volume loss, skin laxity, body rejuvenation	2 yrs
Ariessence	Poly D,L-lactic acid (PDLLA) + Hyaluronic Acid (HA)	PDLLA stimulates type I&III Collagen via a controlled inf. response, HA Provides hydration and elasticity	Under eyes, cheeks, temples, jawline	12-18 m

BIOSTIMULANT MECHANISM OF ACTION

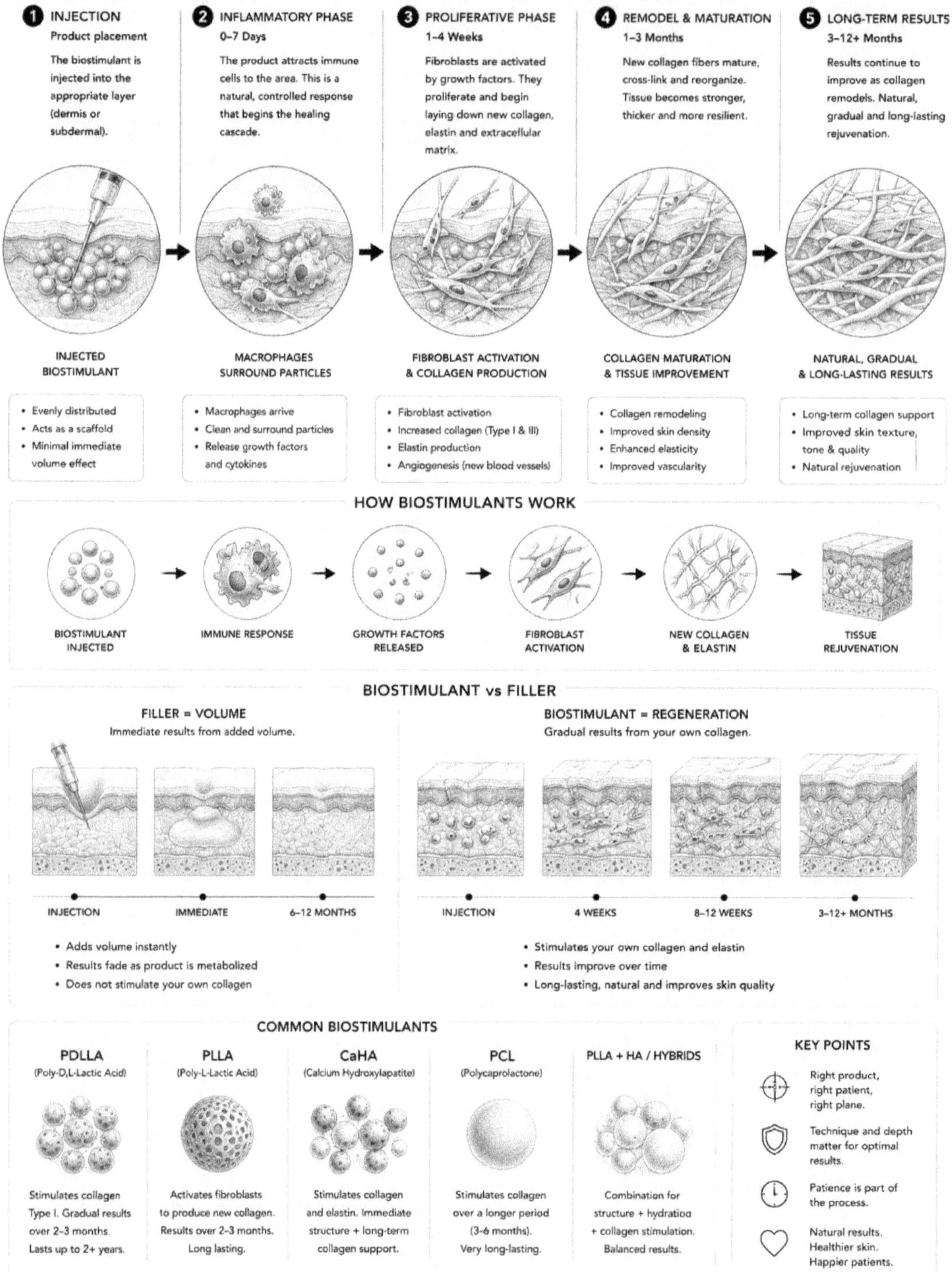

What Is Collagen?

Collagen is the most abundant structural protein in the human body. It provides firmness, strength, and elasticity to the skin, and is also a major component of bones, tendons, ligaments, and connective tissue. From our mid-20s, natural collagen production begins to decline—accelerated by sun exposure, smoking, poor diet, and stress—leading to visible signs of ageing such as skin laxity, fine lines, and volume loss. Cosmetic biostimulant treatments aim to reawaken the body's natural collagen production, resulting in gradual, long-lasting rejuvenation.

Types of Collagen Relevant to Aesthetics

While there are 28 different types of collagen in the body, only a few are relevant when it comes to skin health and aesthetics:

Type I Collagen: The most abundant type, found in skin, tendons, bones, and ligaments. It provides tensile strength and structure.

Type III Collagen: Often found alongside Type I. It plays a key role in the early stages of wound healing and is abundant in youthful skin.

Type IV Collagen: Found in the skin's basement membrane, supporting cell layers and filtration.

Most collagen-inducing injectables used in aesthetics target the stimulation of Type I and Type III collagen.

What Types of Collagen Do Biostimulants Stimulate?

Different biostimulants stimulate collagen at varying depths and rates. Below is a summary of popular collagen-stimulating injectables:

Sculptra (Poly-L-lactic acid): Stimulates Type I collagen. Results begin to appear after 6 to 12 weeks, with full effects developing over several months. Typically requires a series of 2 to 3 treatments, spaced 4 to 6 weeks apart. Longevity: up to 2 to 3 years.

Radiesse (Calcium Hydroxylapatite): Stimulates Type I & III collagen. Offers immediate volume from its carrier gel, with collagen forming over 8 to 12 weeks. Longevity: 12 to 18 months.

Lenisna (Hybrid PLLA + HA): Stimulates Type I and III collagen. Begins working within 6 to 8 weeks and continues to improve skin quality over time. Longevity: 12 to 24 months.

Gouri (Liquid PLLA): A fully solubilised PLLA that spreads evenly. Stimulates Type I and III collagen. Onset around 4 to 6 weeks. Longevity: 6 to 12 months.

Ariessence (Polycaprolactone or PCL): A newer biostimulant that also targets Type I and III collagen. Results typically start after 8 to 10 weeks. Longevity: up to 24 months or more.

How Long Does It Take for Collagen to Form?

Collagen production typically begins around 4 to 8 weeks post-treatment, with visible improvements continuing to build up over 3 to 6 months. This delayed onset is why biostimulants require patience but reward consistency.

Hyperdilution: What Is It and Why Use It?

Hyperdilution involves mixing a biostimulant product with saline and/or lidocaine to reduce its thickness and allow for even spread across a larger treatment area. This technique is ideal when the goal is skin tightening or improving texture, rather than volume restoration.

Products that can be hyperdiluted include:

Radiesse: Commonly hyperdiluted for treating neck, décolletage, arms, buttocks, and thighs to improve skin firmness and crepey texture.

Sculptra: Can be diluted for broader collagen stimulation, such as buttocks or large surface areas like the chest.

Lenisna: May be diluted for superficial collagen induction and skin quality improvement.

Ariessence: Although newer, clinicians are adapting it for dilution-based use in larger treatment zones.

How Do You Choose the Right Biostimulant?

Choosing the appropriate product depends on several factors: skin condition, area treated, desired result, patient tolerance for downtime, and treatment goals.

Here's a simplified guide: For volume and deep collagen induction: Sculptra or undiluted Radiesse , Ellanse.

For skin tightening and texture improvement: Hyperdiluted Radiesse, Ariessence, and Sculptra.

For subtle, natural glow and hydration: Gouri or Lenisna

For long-lasting collagen stimulation: Ariessence or Sculptra

It's essential to match the product not only to the indication but also to the injector's experience and the patient's expectations.

THE COLLAGEN & ELASTIN NETWORK OF FACIAL SKIN

DIFFERENT TYPES. DIFFERENT ROLES. ONE STRUCTURE.

TYPES OF COLLAGEN IN FACIAL SKIN

TYPE I
The most abundant collagen. Provides tensile strength, structure and firmness. Found in dermis and subcutaneous tissue.

TYPE III
Works alongside Type I to provide elasticity and support. More prevalent in younger skin.

TYPE IV
Forms the basement membrane. Supports structure and filtration between epidermis and dermis.

TYPE VII
Anchoring fibrils that secure the epidermis to the dermis. Essential for skin stability.

ELASTIN
Provides elasticity and resilience. Allows skin to stretch and recoil.

OTHER COLLAGENS

Type V & XII: Regulate collagen fibril formation and organization.

Type XIV & XVI: Involved in cell adhesion and skin integrity.

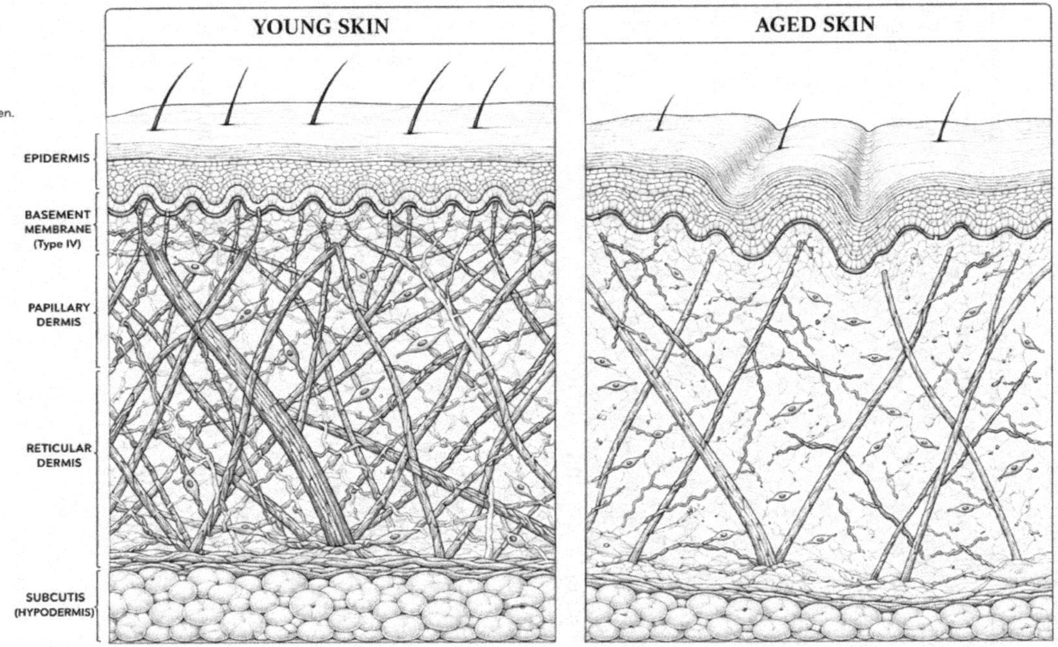

Young skin

- ✓ High density of Type I & III collagen
- ✓ Strong, organized collagen structure
- ✓ Abundant elastin for stretch and recoil
- ✓ Thick dermis and strong skin support
- ✓ Smooth, firm, resilient appearance

Aged skin

- ✗ Reduced Type I & III collagen
- ✗ Disorganized and fragmented fibers
- ✗ Decreased and degraded elastin
- ✗ Thinner dermis, loss of structural support
- ✗ Wrinkles, laxity, thinning, dull appearance

KEY

- Type I Collagen
- Type III Collagen
- Type IV Collagen
- Type VII Collagen
- Elastin
- Fibroblast

WHY IT MATTERS

As we age, we lose not only collagen, but the quality, organization, and communication between these essential proteins.

Healthy, youthful skin depends on a strong, balanced network of collagen and elastin.

PRX-T33 Non-Invasive Biostimulant:

PRX-T33 is a next-generation, non-invasive skin biostimulator designed to rejuvenate and revitalize the skin without causing peeling or significant downtime. Unlike traditional chemical peels that focus on exfoliation and resurfacing, PRX-T33 works at a deeper level to stimulate the skin's natural regenerative processes. It is applied topically in a clinical setting and is often referred to as a "peel without peeling" due to its ability to deliver results without visible flaking or irritation.

What Does PRX-T33 Stimulate?

This treatment stimulates fibroblast activity, which plays a key role in collagen production, skin hydration, and overall tissue repair. The active ingredients penetrate the dermis without disrupting the outer skin barrier, prompting cellular renewal, dermal remodelling, and enhanced hydration. The result is improved skin texture, elasticity, and firmness.

Key benefits include:

- Increased collagen and elastin production for firmer skin
- Enhanced hydration without causing dryness
- Reduction in fine lines, wrinkles, and superficial scarring
- Improvement in pigmentation and skin tone
- Tighter pores and a more radiant complexion

How Is It Different from Skin Peels?

Unlike conventional skin peels that work by exfoliating the epidermis (outer skin layer), PRX-T33 is a biostimulatory treatment that bypasses the epidermis and works within the dermis. It does not cause significant peeling or downtime while still achieving deep rejuvenation.

No visible peeling: Traditional chemical peels cause layers of skin to shed, leading to downtime. PRX-T33 stimulates skin renewal without excessive flaking or irritation.

Non-ablative: It does not damage the epidermis, unlike aggressive peels that require recovery time.

Stronger regenerative action: The formulation activates fibroblast cells, leading to long-term skin improvements beyond surface exfoliation.

Can be used year-round: Many chemical peels require caution in summer due to photosensitivity risks, whereas PRX-T33 is safe even in warmer months.

Mode of Action: How Does PRX-T33 Work?

PRX-T33 is a patented formula that combines trichloroacetic acid (TCA) at 33%, hydrogen peroxide (H2O2), and kojic acid. Each component plays a specific role:

1. Trichloroacetic Acid (TCA, 33%)

• Traditionally used in peels, but in this formulation, it penetrates the dermis without damageing the epidermis.

• Stimulates fibroblasts to increase collagen production and skin renewal.

• Helps with wrinkles, sagging, and scars.

2. Hydrogen Peroxide (H2O2)

• Modulates the action of TCA, preventing excessive peeling.

• Promotes growth factor release and speeds up skin regeneration.

• Has an antiseptic and anti-inflammatory effect.

3. Kojic Acid

• Helps to brighten and even out skin tone, reducing hyperpigmentation.

• Works as a melanin inhibitor, making it beneficial for treating sun spots and post-inflammatory pigmentation.

The treatment is massaged into the skin by a professional using a specific technique to ensure deep penetration. The skin absorbs the product quickly, activating collagen synthesis and tissue remodelling from within.

What to Expect:

PRX-T33 delivers instant and progressive results, meaning the skin looks fresher and more hydrated after just one session, but the full benefits build up over multiple treatments.

Immediate effects (after 1 session):

Firmer, plumper skin, A visible glow and improved hydration, Tighter pores

Long-term effects (after a full course):

Increased collagen and elastin production,

Reduction in fine lines, wrinkles, and mild sagging

Improved skin tone and texture

Reduction in pigmentation, sun spots, and acne scars

Since the treatment does not cause flaking or downtime, clients can return to their normal activities immediately after.

How Many Treatments Are Needed?

For optimal results, a course of 4–6 sessions is typically recommended, spaced one week apart. The exact number of sessions depends on the skin concern being treated.

• For general skin rejuvenation → 4 sessions

• For deeper wrinkles, scars, or hyperpigmentation → 5–6 sessions

• For acne-prone or dull skin → 3–4 sessions

Many clients opt for maintenance treatments every few months to prolong the effects. PRX-T33 is often combined with other treatments like microneedling, RF skin tightening, or PRP to enhance its benefits.

Is PRX-T33 FM (For Men)?

Yes! PRX-T33 is suitable for both men and women who want to improve their skin without undergoing aggressive treatments. Since it doesn't involve needles or visible peeling, it's an excellent choice for men who prefer a non-invasive, low-maintenance approach to skin rejuvenation.

PRX-T33 is a powerful yet gentle alternative to traditional peels, offering deep skin rejuvenation with no peeling, no pain, and no downtime. By stimulating collagen and fibroblast activity without damaging the surface layer, it provides an effective, year-round skin solution for those looking to enhance their complexion naturally.

PRX-T33 vs PRX-PLUS

PRX-T33 and PRX-PLUS are both needle-free skin biorevitalisation treatments developed by WiQo®, however they are formulated for slightly different treatment objectives. PRX-T33 combines 33% trichloroacetic acid (TCA), hydrogen peroxide and kojic acid to stimulate fibroblast activity, encourage collagen production and improve skin firmness, laxity, acne scarring and overall skin quality without visible peeling or significant downtime. PRX-PLUS is the newer generation formulation, designed to provide enhanced rejuvenation for mature, photodamaged and textured skin, with a greater focus on improving pigmentation, skin luminosity, enlarged pores and superficial wrinkles while maintaining collagen-stimulating benefits.

A practical difference for clinicians and patients is the treatment protocol and vial usage. A single vial of **PRX-T33 is generally used for one treatment session**, making it ideal for individual procedures. In contrast, **one vial of PRX-PLUS typically provides approximately four treatment sessions**, offering a more economical option when performing a treatment series.

PRX-T33 is often selected when skin tightening and collagen stimulation are the primary goals, whereas PRX-PLUS may be preferred when treating pigmentation concerns, uneven skin tone, photoageing and surface texture. Both treatments can be performed year-round and are commonly incorporated into combination protocols with microneedling, skin boosters, LED therapy and other regenerative aesthetic treatments.

Chapter 50: Using Your Own Cells to Rejuvenate

PRP, PRF, and PRP Filler (Cellenis)

Regenerative medicine has brought ground breaking advancements in aesthetics, with platelet-derived treatments like PRP (Platelet-Rich Plasma), PRF (Platelet-Rich Fibrin), and PRP Filler (Plasma Biofiller) offering natural ways to restore volume, improve skin quality, and stimulate tissue repair. These treatments use your own blood to harness the power of platelets and growth factors, making them a powerful tool in aesthetic and anti-ageing treatments.

What Are They?

1. PRP (Platelet-Rich Plasma)

PRP is a concentrated plasma solution derived from your blood, rich in growth factors and platelets. It has been widely used in aesthetic medicine, orthopedics, and wound healing to stimulate collagen production, tissue repair, and overall skin rejuvenation.

2. PRF (Platelet-Rich Fibrin)

PRF is a more advanced version of PRP, containing a fibrin matrix that allows for a slower release of growth factors. This means longer-lasting stimulation of healing and collagen production. Unlike PRP, PRF is obtained without anticoagulants, which results in a thicker, gel-like consistency.

3. PRP Filler (Plasma Biofiller) - Cellenis

PRP Filler, also called Plasma Biofiller, is a thickened version of PRP achieved by heating plasma to create a gel-like consistency. This allows it to act as a natural filler, providing temporary volume while also delivering regenerative benefits.

What is the Difference?

Features	PRP	PRF	PRP Filler
Growth Factor Release	Immediate	Sustained (slow release)	Slow release + volume effect
Consistency	Liquid	Gel-like	Thickened gel (filler-like)
Longevity	Short-term (1-2 weeks)	Longer-lasting (2-4 weeks)	Temporary volume (3-6 months)
Anticoagulants	Yes (prevents clotting)	No (allows natural clotting)	No (plasma thickened by heat)

Use Skin rejuvenation, hair restoration Wound healing, collagen production Facial volume, contouring, regenerative benefits

Purpose of All Three Treatments

PRP: Improves skin texture, boosts collagen, accelerates healing, and is commonly used for hair restoration and facial rejuvenation.

PRF: Provides a longer-lasting release of growth factors, making it ideal for skin rejuvenation, under-eye hollows, and wound healing.

PRP Filler (Plasma Biofiller): Acts as a natural dermal filler while delivering regenerative properties, making it suitable for volume loss in areas like cheeks, nasolabial folds, and lips.

How Do You Get PRP?

1. A small amount of blood is drawn from your arm.

2. The blood is spun in a centrifuge to separate the platelets and plasma from red and white blood cells.

3. The platelet-rich plasma is extracted and used for treatment.

How Do You Get PRF?

1. Blood is drawn from the patient.

2. The blood is centrifuged at a lower speed and for a shorter time than PRP to preserve fibrin and white blood cells.

3. Since no anticoagulant is used, the PRF forms a clot-like gel that is then applied to the treatment area.

How Do You Get PRP Filler?

1. PRP is obtained using the same process as standard PRP.

2. The plasma is then heated at a controlled temperature, causing it to thicken into a gel-like consistency.

3. Once cooled, it is ready for injection as a natural volumizer.

What Do They Do in the Body?

PRP: Stimulates collagen production, enhances tissue repair, and promotes healing.

PRF: Releases growth factors slowly over time, leading to prolonged regenerative effects.

PRP Filler: Provides immediate volume and stimulates collagen while gradually being absorbed by the body.

Which One to Choose & Why?

Choose PRP if you want a quick boost in collagen production, skin rejuvenation, or hair restoration without volume enhancement.

Choose PRF if you want a longer-lasting effect with sustained growth factor release, particularly for delicate areas like the under-eyes.

Choose PRP Filler (Plasma Biofiller) if you need both volume replacement and regenerative benefits, making it ideal for areas of volume loss.

Each treatment has its strengths, and the best choice depends on your goals whether it is rejuvenation, repair, or natural volume restoration. By using your own cells, these treatments provide a safe, effective, and natural approach to maintaining youthful, healthy skin.

Treatment	What is it	Indications of Use	How Long Does it Last	How Many Treatments
PRP (Platelet -Rich Plasma)	A concentration of platelets from your own blood, spun at high speed to separate plasma rich in growth factors.	Skin rejuvenation, fine lines, texture, acne scars, hair restoration.	3–6 months (biological stimulation, not volumizing).	Initial series of 3–4 treatments spaced 4–6 weeks apart, then maintenance 1–2 times/year.
PRF (Platelet -Rich Fibrin)	Second-generation PRP, spun at lower speeds, no anticoagulant, forming a fibrin matrix that slowly releases growth factors.	Under-eye hollows, fine lines, crepey skin, early volume loss, slow-healing areas.	Up to 12 months (longer release of growth factors).	2–4 sessions spaced 6–8 weeks apart, then 1–2 annually.
PRP Filler (Bio-filler / Plasma Gel)	Heated PRP converted into a gel consistency and injected like a filler for volume.	Tear troughs, cheeks, nasolabial folds, lips, skin creping, facial hollows.	3–6 months (depends on technique and patient).	1–2 sessions initially; may repeat every 3–6 months for volume

Chapter 51: Genital Rejuvenation with Platelet-Rich Plasma (PRP)

Platelet-Rich Plasma (PRP) therapy has emerged as a promising non-surgical option for genital rejuvenation in both men and women. By utilizing the body's own healing mechanisms, PRP aims to enhance the appearance and function of genital tissues.

PRP for Female Genital Rejuvenation

In women, PRP injections target the vulvar and vaginal areas to address various concerns:

Enhanced Appearance: PRP can improve skin texture and elasticity, leading to a more youthful vulvar appearance.

Improved Function: Benefits may include increased lubrication, heightened sensitivity, and enhanced sexual satisfaction.

Treatment of Conditions: PRP has been explored for manageing symptoms of vaginal atrophy, laxity, and lichen sclerosis a condition causing thin, patchy skin in the genital area.

PRP for Male Genital Rejuvenation

For men, PRP therapy focuses on penile enhancement and addressing erectile dysfunction (ED):

Revascularization: PRP promotes the formation of new blood vessels, potentially improving blood flow to the penis, which is crucial for erectile function.

Enhanced Sensation and Performance: Men may experience increased sensitivity and improved sexual performance following PRP treatments.

The PRP Injection Procedure

The PRP treatment process is straightforward and minimally invasive:

1. **Blood Collection**: A small amount of the patient's blood is drawn.

2. **PRP Preparation**: The blood is processed in a centrifuge to concentrate the platelets, resulting in PRP rich in growth factors.

3. **Application**: The PRP is injected into specific areas of the genitalia, depending on the desired outcomes.

To minimize discomfort during the procedure, a topical anaesthetic cream, such as BLT (Benzocaine, Lidocaine, Tetracaine) cream, is applied to the treatment area prior to injection.

Treatment Frequency and Onset of Effects

Number of Treatments: Protocols vary, but a common approach involves multiple sessions. For instance, in treating female sexual dysfunction, 2 mL of PRP may be injected into the distal anterior vaginal wall once a month for three months.

Time to Notice Effects: Patients may begin to observe improvements within a few weeks after the initial treatment, with optimal results typically developing over several months.

Safety and Considerations

PRP therapy utilizes the patient's own blood components, reducing the risk of allergic reactions or rejection. However, as with any medical procedure, it's essential to consult with a qualified healthcare provider to determine if PRP is appropriate for your specific needs and to understand the potential risks and benefits involved.

By harnessing the body's natural healing processes, PRP offers a promising avenue for those seeking genital rejuvenation, aiming to enhance both aesthetic and functional aspects of the genitalia.

The O-Shot® and P-Shot® procedures were developed by Dr. Charles Runels, a physician from Alabama, USA, who pioneered the use of Platelet-Rich Plasma (PRP) in sexual wellness and regenerative medicine. Both treatments utilise a patient's own blood, which is processed to concentrate platelets and growth factors before being reinjected into targeted tissues. The O-Shot® (Orgasm Shot) is designed to enhance female sexual function, improve vaginal lubrication, increase sensitivity, and may assist with mild urinary incontinence. The P-Shot® (Priapus Shot) is used in men to support erectile function, improve penile blood flow, enhance sensation, and promote tissue regeneration. These procedures are based on the regenerative properties of PRP, which contains growth factors that stimulate collagen production, angiogenesis (new blood vessel formation), and tissue repair. While many patients report positive outcomes, results can vary, and ongoing research continues to evaluate long-term efficacy .

Chapter 52: Bio-Filler

In the evolving landscape of aesthetic medicine, the quest for natural and effective rejuvenation techniques has led to the development of autologous treatments those utilizing the patient's own biological materials. One such innovation is the Platelet-Rich Plasma (PRP) Bio-Filler, a treatment that serves both as a dermal filler and a biostimulant, offering a holistic approach to facial rejuvenation.

Understanding PRP Bio-Filler

PRP Bio-Filler is an advanced aesthetic procedure that harnesses the regenerative properties of a patient's blood to restore facial volume and enhance skin quality. Unlike traditional synthetic fillers, this method reduces the risk of allergic reactions and ensures better biocompatibility.

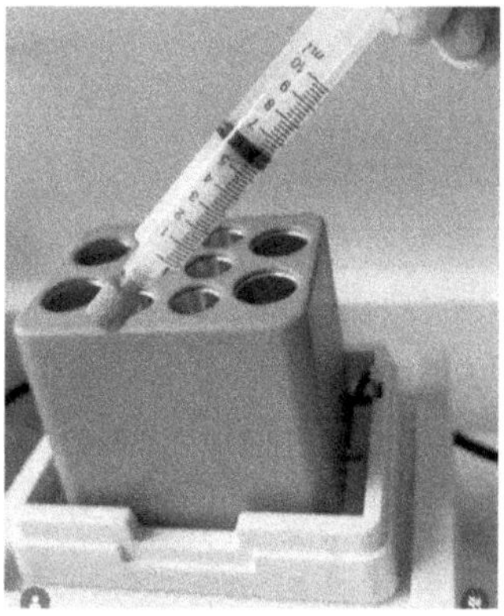

Platelet poor plasma is heated and the albumin thickens. Once it cools Platelet Rich Plasma is mixed with the Platelet Poor plasma and forms a bio stimulating filler.

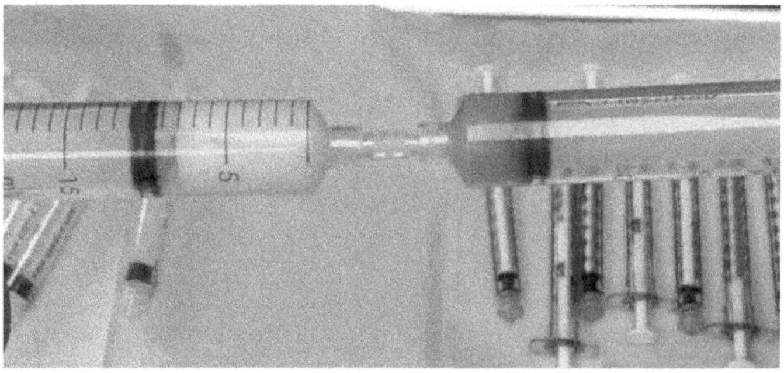

Thickened PPP mixed with PRP to make biofiller.

Application and Benefits

PRP Bio-Filler is versatile and can be used in various facial regions, with notable efficacy in treating tear trough deformities:

Tear Trough Rejuvenation: The under-eye area often exhibits signs of ageing, such as hollowness and dark circles. Injecting PRP Bio-Filler into this region not only restores volume but also stimulates collagen production, leading to improved skin texture and elasticity. This dual action addresses both the superficial and underlying causes of under-eye concerns.

Duration and Longevity

The effects of PRP Bio-Filler are both immediate and progressive:

Immediate Results: Post-injection, patients may notice an instant improvement in volume and skin tightness.

Long-Term Benefits: The biostimulatory properties of the filler promote ongoing collagen synthesis and tissue regeneration. Typically, the results can last between 3 to 6 months, with some variations based on individual factors such as age, skin condition, and lifestyle.

Advantages over Traditional Fillers

PRP Bio-Filler offers several benefits compared to conventional dermal fillers:

Natural Composition: Utilizing the patient's own blood eliminates the risk of allergic reactions and ensures high biocompatibility.

Dual Functionality: It acts as a filler to restore volume and as a biostimulant to enhance skin quality intrinsically.

Safety Profile: The autologous nature of the treatment minimizes potential complications associated with synthetic fillers.

PRF vs Cellenis® Derma Filler: Natural Healing vs Structural Support

Platelet-Rich Fibrin (PRF) and Cellenis® DermaFiller both harness the regenerative power of the patient's own blood, but they serve different purposes in aesthetic medicine.

- **PRF** forms a natural fibrin clot after injection. This clot acts as a short-lived scaffold that supports wound healing, collagen production, and tissue repair. It is fully metabolised within 5–10 days, making it ideal for stimulating the skin's natural rejuvenation processes without adding volume.

- **Cellenis® DermaFiller** on the other hand, forms a proteinic scaffold—a more durable structure designed to mimic the body's extracellular matrix. This scaffold supports cell regeneration while also providing immediate volume and structural lift, especially useful in delicate areas like the tear troughs. It remains active in the tissue for 3 to 6 months, offering both regenerative and volumising effects.

In summary:

- **PRF** = Temporary fibrin matrix for healing and collagen boost
- **Cellenis DermaFiller** = Longer-lasting protein scaffold for regeneration + volume

PRF vs Cellenis® DermaFiller Comparison

Feature	PRF (Platelet-Rich Fibrin)	Cellenis® DermaFiller
Type of Structure	Fibrin Clot	Proteinic Scaffold
Primary Function	Stimulate healing & collagen production	Regeneration + structural support
Composition	Natural fibrin from blood	Engineered protein matrix
Duration in Tissue	5-10 days	3-6 Months
Mechanism of Action	Forms clot post-injection; supports natural repair	Scaffold integrates with tissue, supports regeneration
Best Used For	Skin texture, fine lines, crepey skin	Tear troughs, volume restoration, support
Volume Effect	No immediate volume	Immediate volume + lift

Why Cellenis® DermaFiller

- Induce new collagen to form and enhance skin radiance and revitalization
- Effective for face and body rejuvenation
- Derived from completely autologous materials
- Decelerate ageing by immediately replacing missing volume while bio-stimulating to prevent further tissue lost
- One kit provides 13ml of regenerative material for a comprehensive treatment.

How Cellenis Dermal Filler is Created – In Simple Terms

Cellenis Dermal Filler is made from your own blood, so it's completely natural and unique to you. Here's how it works:

1. A small blood sample is taken – just like having a routine blood test.

2. The blood goes into a special tube designed to separate its components.

3. We spin the tube in a centrifuge – this rapid spinning separates the blood into layers:

• Platelet Poor Plasma (PPP) – the clearer top layer, which we can transform into a gel.

• Platelet Rich Plasma (PRP) – the golden layer rich in growth factors and healing platelets.

4. The PPP is gently heated – this changes its texture from a liquid into a smooth, gel-like consistency (about 8 mls).

5. The PRP is collected – usually around 3 mls of this powerful, rejuvenating liquid.

6. The two are combined – the PRP is mixed back into the PPP gel. This creates a natural filler that is rich in your own platelets.

The end result is a bio-filler that not only restores volume but also stimulates your skin's natural rejuvenation process — improving texture, tone, and overall vitality over time. Because it's made from your own blood, the risk of allergic reaction is extremely low, and you're giving your skin a boost from the inside out.

Conclusion

PRP Bio-Filler represents a significant advancement in aesthetic treatments, merging the benefits of dermal fillers with the regenerative potential of biostimulants. Its natural composition, combined with its efficacy in areas like the tear troughs, makes it a compelling option for individuals seeking holistic facial rejuvenation. As with any medical procedure, it is essential to consult with qualified healthcare professionals to determine suitability and ensure optimal outcomes.

Regenerative Volume: From Biofiller to Adipose Matrix

For many years in aesthetic medicine, restoring volume meant one thing — filling.

We placed hyaluronic acid into the face to replace what had been lost. And while this has its place, it is still, at its core, an implant. A product sitting within the tissue to mimic volume.

But over time, both practitioners and patients have begun to ask for something different.

Something softer. More natural. More aligned with the body.

And this is where regenerative aesthetics begins.

Not replacing. But restoring.

Understanding What We Lose

As we age, we don't just develop lines.

We lose: Bone support, Ligament strength, Fat volume, Skin integrity

It is the loss of fat — particularly deep structural fat — that creates hollowing, heaviness, and imbalance.

So the question becomes:

Can we restore that fat... rather than simply filling around it?

Biofiller — Using Your Own Biology

Biofiller was one of the first steps in this direction.

It is created using the patient's own blood.

Through a process of: Centrifugation, Heating, Transformation of plasma proteins

We convert plasma into a gel-like substance that can be injected.

This creates: Soft, natural volume, Improved skin quality, Mild collagen stimulation

What I like about biofiller is its simplicity.

It is: Autologous, Natural, Biocompatible

And it gives an immediate, subtle result.

But it is still temporary.

It behaves like a soft filler — one that integrates beautifully — but ultimately gets reabsorbed over time.

Adipose Matrix — A Different Concept Entirely

Adipose matrix treatments, such as Renuva, take regenerative aesthetics to another level.

They are not created from blood. They are derived from human fat tissue, but in a very specific way.

Not living fat. Not transplanted fat. But the structure of fat, without the cells.

Where Does It Come From?

The source is donated human fat, obtained through regulated tissue banks.

Donors are: Carefully screened, Medically assessed, Tested for infectious diseases

The fat is then processed using specialised techniques.

How Are the Cells Removed?

This is the critical step.

The tissue undergoes a process designed to:

Remove all living fat cells, Remove lipids and cellular material, Eliminate anything that could trigger an immune response

What remains is something called a decellularised extracellular matrix.

In simple terms: The living component is removed, leaving behind the structural blueprint of fat.

This matrix is: Sterile, Biocompatible, Non-immunogenic

How Does It Work?

Once injected, it behaves very differently from a filler.

It doesn't simply sit there and create volume.

Instead, it acts as a scaffold.

A framework that invites the body to respond.

The process looks like this:

The matrix is placed into the tissue

The body recognises it as a natural structure

It sends in: Stem cells, Blood vessels, Support cells

The area becomes revascularised

Over time, the scaffold is replaced with: New fat cells, New connective tissue

What you are left with is not product — but your own tissue.

How Does It Stimulate Fat Formation?

The extracellular matrix contains: Structural proteins like collagen, Signalling molecules

Binding sites that guide cell behaviour, These elements act as instructions.

They tell incoming stem cells: *This is fat. This is where you belong.*

The cells then differentiate into adipocytes, and new fat tissue forms.

This is not forced. It is guided regeneration.

Biofiller vs Adipose Matrix — Understanding the Difference

Although both sit under the umbrella of regenerative treatments, they are not the same.

Biofiller comes from: Your own blood

Adipose matrix comes from: Donated fat tissue (processed and purified)

How They Work

Biofiller: Acts as a soft, temporary volumiser, Provides immediate improvement, Stimulates collagen modestly

Adipose matrix: Acts as a scaffold, Does not rely on immediate volume, Stimulates actual fat regeneration

Timing

Biofiller: Immediate result, Gradually fades

Adipose matrix: Minimal immediate change, Builds slowly over time

Longevity

Biofiller: Short to medium duration

Adipose matrix: Longer-lasting, as it becomes living tissue

Feel and Integration

Biofiller: Soft and natural, But still a temporary gel

Adipose matrix: Integrates into the tissue, Feels like natural fat

When Would I Choose One Over the Other?

This is where experience matters.

Biofiller is beautiful for: Skin quality, Fine lines, Subtle, immediate refresh

Patients wanting something completely autologous

Adipose matrix is more suited to: Volume loss, Contour irregularities, Early hollowing

Patients willing to wait for a regenerative outcome

And in some cases, they can complement each other.

Biofiller for the surface.

Adipose matrix for the structure.

The Bigger Picture

What both of these treatments represent is a shift in thinking.

We are moving away from: Overfilling, Chasing lines, Artificial volume

And towards: Supporting the skin, Stimulating collagen, Restoring fat

Respecting anatomy, Not one treatment. But a layered approach.

Final Thoughts

In the past, we asked: *What can I inject to fix this?*

Now, the question is changing. *How can I help the body restore what it has lost?*

Biofiller was one of the first steps.

Adipose matrix is the next.

And this is only the beginning.

Because the future of aesthetic medicine is not about adding more.

It is about working with the biology that is already there.

Chapter 53: Mesoderm & Mesotherapy Injections

The word mesotherapy comes from the term mesoderm, which is another name for the middle layer of tissue in the body during embryological development. In aesthetics, the mesoderm relates closely to the dermis — the middle layer of the skin where collagen, elastin, blood vessels, and connective tissue exist.

Mesotherapy involves placing tiny injections into this middle layer of the skin to deliver active ingredients directly where they are needed. Rather than creating large amounts of volume like traditional dermal fillers, mesotherapy focuses on improving skin quality, hydration, circulation, and cellular activity.

The technique was first developed in France and has evolved into a popular treatment for skin rejuvenation, hair restoration, pigmentation, and even fat reduction.

Mesotherapy injections may contain customised combinations of:

Vitamins, Amino acids, Hyaluronic acid, Antioxidants, Peptides, Minerals, Growth factors

These ingredients are placed superficially into the skin using very small needles over multiple injection points.

Unlike structural fillers, mesotherapy works more like "feeding the skin." The goal is to stimulate and nourish the dermis to improve hydration, glow, elasticity, and overall skin health.

Mesotherapy can be used for:

Skin Rejuvenation

Treatments often include hyaluronic acid, vitamins, antioxidants, and amino acids to improve hydration, texture, fine lines, and radiance.

Hair Restoration

Cocktails containing biotin, amino acids, minerals, and growth factors may be injected into the scalp to support circulation and nourish hair follicles.

Pigmentation & Ageing Skin

Brightening ingredients and antioxidants may help improve uneven skin tone and sun damage.

Fat Dissolving Treatments

Some mesotherapy solutions contain ingredients such as phosphatidylcholine and deoxycholate, which are used to target small localized fat deposits.

Mesotherapy is often referred to as “skin boosting” because it focuses on improving skin function rather than dramatically changing facial shape.

Today, many modern injectable treatments have evolved from mesotherapy principles, including skin boosters, bioremodelling products, PRP, PRF, and regenerative injectable therapies.

While mesotherapy is generally considered minimally invasive, patients can still experience temporary swelling, bruising, redness, or tenderness after treatment. As with all cosmetic procedures, treatments should only be performed by qualified and experienced practitioners.

Mesotherapy originated in France and involves the superficial injection of vitamins, amino acids, minerals, antioxidants, hyaluronic acid and regenerative ingredients into the dermis to improve skin quality and hydration.

Modern mesotherapy products vary significantly in composition. Some focus on hydration, others stimulate collagen, while some target pigmentation, hair loss or ageing skin.

1. Classic French Mesotherapy Cocktail

Ingredients

- Hyaluronic Acid (non-crosslinked)
- Vitamin C, Vitamin A, Vitamin E
- B Vitamins (B1, B2, B3, B5, B6, B12)
- Amino acids, Minerals, Coenzymes

Purpose

- Hydration, Dull skin, Prevention of ageing, Fine lines

Injection Depth

1–2 mm superficial dermis

Areas

- Face, Neck, Décolletage, Hands

2. NCTF® 135 HA (Filorga)

Composition

- 5 mg/ml Hyaluronic Acid
- 12 Vitamins, 24 Amino Acids, 6 Minerals
- 6 Coenzymes, 5 Nucleic Acids, Antioxidants

What It Does

- Improves hydration, Brightens skin, Improves elasticity, Stimulates fibroblasts

Best For

- Ageing skin, Smokers, Dull skin, Fine lines

3. Redensity I (Teoxane)

Composition

- 15 mg/ml Hyaluronic Acid, Amino Acids
- Antioxidants, Minerals, Vitamin B6

What It Does

- Deep hydration, Improves skin density, Improves radiance

Best Areas

- Face, Neck, Periorbital area

4. Sunekos 200

Composition

- Low Molecular Weight HA
- Patented Amino Acid Complex

Includes:

- Glycine, Proline, Hydroxyproline, Lysine, Valine, Alanine

What It Does

- Stimulates collagen
- Stimulates elastin, Improves crepey skin

Best Areas

- Under eyes, Neck, Arms, Décolletage

5. Sunekos 1200

Composition

- Higher concentration HA, Amino acid complex

What It Does

- Structural support, Tissue regeneration, Volume restoration

Best Areas

- Midface, Temples, Jawline

6. Jalupro Classic

Composition

- Hyaluronic Acid, Glycine, L-Proline, L-Leucine, L-Lysine

Benefits

- Fibroblast stimulation, Collagen production, Skin rejuvenation

Areas

- Face, Neck, Hands

7. Jalupro HMW

Composition

- Higher Molecular Weight HA, Amino Acid Complex

Benefits

- More hydration, More collagen stimulation, Greater support

8. RRS® HA Long Lasting

Composition

- Hyaluronic Acid, Antioxidants, Vitamins, Trace Elements

Benefits

- Skin rejuvenation, Brightening, Hydration

9. BCN Cocktails

Common Formulas

BCN Revita HA

- Hyaluronic Acid, Vitamins, Amino Acids

BCN Melano

- Tranexamic Acid, Vitamin C, Glutathione

BCN Hair

- Biotin, Vitamins, Growth Factors

10. Hair Mesotherapy Formula

Common Ingredients

- Biotin, Panthenol, Amino Acids
- Zinc, Copper, Growth Factors, Hyaluronic Acid

Uses

- Female pattern hair loss, Male pattern hair loss
- Hair thinning

11. Polynucleotide Mesotherapy

Ingredients

- Purified Polynucleotides

Products

- Plinest, Newest, Rejuran

Benefits

- DNA repair, Improved elasticity
- Tissue regeneration

12. Exosome / Secretome Mesotherapy

Ingredients

- Growth Factors, Cytokines, Peptides, Exosomes or Secretomes

Benefits

- Cellular communication, Collagen stimulation, Improved healing

Mesotherapy Treatment Categories

Goal	Best Product
Hydration	Profhilo, Redensity I
Skin Glow	NCTF 135
Fine Lines	Redensity I
Collagen Stimulation	Sunekos
Crepey Skin	Sunekos
Hair Loss	Hair Mesotherapy
Pigmentation	BCN Melano
Regeneration	Polynucleotides
Tissue Repair	Exosomes / Secretomes

Author's Tip

"Mesotherapy is often described as feeding the skin from within. While moisturisers work from the surface, mesotherapy delivers active ingredients directly into the dermis where fibroblasts, collagen and elastin are produced. The choice of formula depends on whether your goal is hydration, collagen stimulation, regeneration, pigmentation correction or hair restoration."

INJECTION DEPTH IN THE SKIN – A GUIDE TO COMMON TREATMENTS

Different products work at different depths for optimal results.

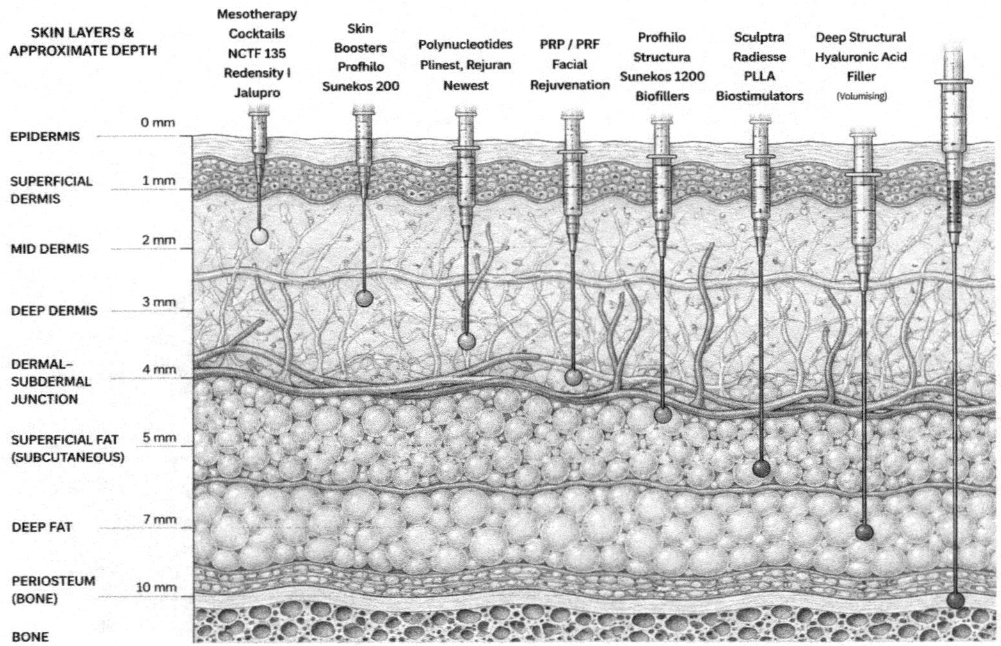

TREATMENT / PRODUCT	TYPICAL DEPTH	MAIN PURPOSE
Mesotherapy Cocktails (NCTF 135, Redensity I, Jalupro, Vitamins, Amino Acids)	1 – 2 mm (superficial dermis)	Hydration, glow, fine lines, prevention, nourishment
Skin Boosters (Profhilo, Sunekos 200, Redensity I)	2 – 4 mm (mid to deep dermis)	Hydration, elasticity, skin quality, radiance
Polynucleotides (Plinest, Rejuran, Newest)	2 – 4 mm (deep dermis)	DNA repair, regeneration, improves elasticity and texture
PRP / PRF (Facial Rejuvenation)	3 – 5 mm (dermis to subcutaneous)	Cell regeneration, collagen stimulation, improved skin quality
Profhilo Structura Sunekos 1200 (Biofillers)	4 – 6 mm (subcutaneous)	Support, remodelling, volume improvement, tissue quality
Sculptra / Radiesse / PLLA (Biostimulators)	5 – 10 mm (deep fat)	Collagen stimulation, volume restoration, structure
Deep Structural HA Filler (Volumising Fillers)	On periosteum (> 8 – 10 mm)	Structural support, contour, lift

- Superficial Dermis (1–2 mm): Fine lines, dullness, dehydration – Mesotherapy cocktails work here.
- Deep Dermis (2–4 mm): Skin boosters and polynucleotides hydrate, improve elasticity and stimulate fibroblasts.
- Dermis–Subdermis (3–5 mm): PRP/PRF works across the junction to enhance healing and collagen.
- Subcutaneous (4–6 mm): Biofillers and structural boosters improve support and tissue quality.
- Deep Fat / Periosteal (5–10+ mm): Biostimulators and volumising fillers restore lost volume and provide structural lift.

AUTHOR'S NOTE

The depth of injection is as important as the product used. Correct plane placement ensures safety, optimal results and reduces the risk of complications.

Chapter 54: Thread Lifting, Collagen Stimulation, and Considerations for Long-Term Rejuvenation

Thread lifts have gained popularity as a minimally invasive alternative to facelifts, offering skin tightening and collagen stimulation with minimal downtime. With advancements in technology, thread procedures have evolved from simple skin repositioning to bio-stimulating treatments that improve overall skin quality.

This chapter explores the different types of threads, their longevity, best patient selection, combination treatments, complications, and long-term considerations especially for those considering a future surgical facelift.

Types of Threads Available on the Market

Thread lifts are categorized based on their composition and function:

1. Mini (Mono) Threads For Collagen Stimulation

Thin, smooth threads placed in a mesh pattern under the skin.

Do not lift but stimulate collagen production over time.

Best for improving skin texture, fine lines, and mild laxity.

Common areas: Cheeks, neck, under-eye, jawline, and decolletage.

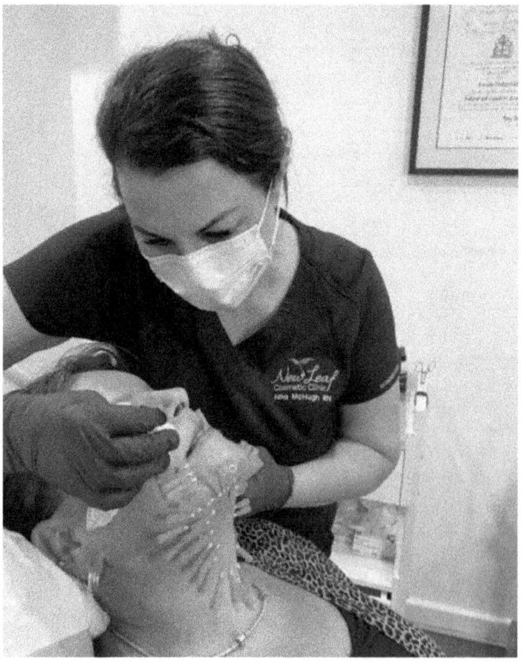

2. Cogged (Barbed) Thread: For Lifting & Contouring

Have tiny barbs/hooks that anchor into tissue, allowing mechanical lifting of sagging skin.

Best for jawline definition, mid-face lifting, and reducing jowls. Stimulate collagen as they dissolve, improving firmness and elasticity.

3. Screw & Tornado Threads For Volume Enhancement

Twisted threads that create mild volumization in areas of hollowing.

Best for nasolabial folds, cheeks, and temples.

4. PLLA & PCL Threads Longer-Lasting Bio-Stimulatory Threads

Made from poly-L-lactic acid (PLLA) or polycaprolactone (PCL), which stimulate collagen for a longer period than traditional PDO threads.

Best for long-term skin rejuvenation rather than lifting.

How Do Threads Work?

Mechanical Lift (for cogged threads) Immediate lifting effect as the barbs hook into tissue.

Collagen Stimulation (for all threads) The body responds to the threads as a foreign material, triggering fibroblast activity and new collagen synthesis.

Gradual Dissolution :Threads break down over time while leaving new collagen in place for longer-lasting effects.

Best Patient Selection for Thread Lifts

Ideal Candidates:

Mild to moderate skin laxity (not excessive sagging).

Good skin quality with some elasticity (threads work best if the skin still has some natural firmness). Patients who want a non-surgical option for lifting or rejuvenation. Those who are open to combined treatments (threads alone may not be enough for full correction).

Not Suitable For:

Severe skin laxity or heavy sagging these patients would benefit more from a facelift. Very thin, atrophic skin (threads may not hold well). Patients with active infections or autoimmune conditions affecting healing.

Threads Work Best in Combination with Fillers & Bio-Stimulants While threads provide lift and collagen stimulation, they do not restore lost volume. The best results are seen when threads are combined with dermal fillers, PRP, or bio-stimulants like Sculptra or Radiesse.

Threads + Fillers: Restores both structure and volume, preventing a flat or tightened but hollow look.

Threads + PRP/Exosomes: Enhances healing and collagen production.

Threads + Skin Boosters: Improves skin hydration and elasticity.

How Long Do Threads Last?

Immediate lifting effect : Visible right after the procedure, but best results are seen 3-6 months later due to collagen remodeling.

Longevity depends on the type of thread used:

Thread Type	Dissolution Time	Collagen Stimulation Duration
PDO (Polydioxanone)	4-6 months	Up to 12 months
PLLA (Poly-L-Lactic Acid)	12-18 months	Up to 2 years
PCL (Polycaprolactone)	18-24 months	Up to 3 years

Maintenance treatments every 12-18 months help maintain results over time.

What Happens to Threads in the Body?

Threads are absorbable .They break down naturally through hydrolysis (a process where water molecules dissolve the material). As they dissolve, the body replaces them with collagen, prolonging the skin-tightening effects. No permanent foreign material remains after full absorption.

Potential Complications of Thread Lifts

While thread lifts are generally safe, complications can occur, particularly if the procedure is performed by an inexperienced injector.

Mild Side Effects (Expected & Temporary): Swelling and bruising (common for 1-2 weeks). Mild discomfort or tightness.

Possible Risks:

Thread migration (if placed incorrectly, threads can move). Visible or palpable threads (especially in thin skin). Asymmetry if one side tightens more than the other. Dimples or puckering (usually resolves as swelling subsides).

Chapter 55: Combination and Stacked Treatments

The Secret to Natural, Long-Lasting Results

One of the biggest misconceptions in aesthetic medicine is that one treatment can fix everything.

Many patients come in asking for:

- "Just a bit of Botox"
- "One syringe of filler"
- "Something for these lines"

But the face is not made of one layer, and it does not age in one way.

Ageing affects:

- Bone, Fat pads, Ligaments, Skin, Muscle movement, Collagen quality

That's why the most natural, long-lasting results come from combination treatments—also known as stacking or layering treatments.

What Are Combination or Stacked Treatments?

Combination treatments involve using more than one type of procedure, either:

- In the same session, or Over a series of treatments

Each treatment targets a different layer or function of the face.

Instead of trying to fix everything with filler, we treat:

- Muscle movement, Volume loss, Skin quality, Collagen stimulation, Structural support

This creates results that are:

- More natural, Longer lasting
- More balanced, Harder to detect

People won't say:

"You've had filler."

They'll say:

"You look amazing. What's your secret?"

Understanding the Layers of the Face

Think of the face like a house with several levels:

The Foundation: Bone

As we age: Bone density decreases, The eye sockets widen, The jawline recedes

This causes: Sagging, Hollowing, Loss of structure

Treatment: Structural fillers, Biostimulants

The Support Layer: Fat Pads and Ligaments

With time: Fat pads shrink or descend, Ligaments loosen

This leads to: Drooping cheeks, Nasolabial folds, Jowls

Treatment: Strategic filler placement, Biostimulators

The Movement Layer: Muscles

Repeated expressions cause: Frown lines, Crow's feet, Forehead lines

Treatment: Botulinum toxin

The Surface Layer: Skin

Skin changes include: Loss of collagen, Dehydration, Fine lines, Pigmentation, Dullness

Treatment: Skin boosters, PRP, Biostimulants, Medical-grade skincare

Why One Treatment Alone Isn't Enough

For example:

Treating only lines with filler

This may: Overfill the face, Create heaviness, Look unnatural

Treating only with toxin

This may: Soften lines, But not address volume loss or skin quality

The result may still look: Tired, Flat, Hollow

True rejuvenation requires addressing multiple layers.

The Main Treatment Categories

1. Botulinum Toxin

Targets: Muscle movement, Expression lines

Benefits: Softens frown lines, Reduces crow's feet, Prevents deeper wrinkles

2. Dermal Fillers

Targets: Volume loss, Structural support, Facial contours

Benefits: Restores cheek volume, Defines jawline, Softens folds

3. Biostimulants

Examples: Sculptra, Radiesse, PRP/PRF

Targets: Collagen production, Skin thickness, Structural support over time

Benefits: Gradual, natural improvement, Long-lasting results

4. Skin Boosters

Targets: Hydration, Skin texture, Fine lines

Benefits: Smoother skin, Improved glow, Better elasticity

The Stacking Approach: How It Works

Instead of doing everything in one session, treatments are often layered over time.

Step 1: Relax the muscles

Botulinum toxin: Softens harsh expressions, Prevents deeper lines

Step 2: Restore structure

Filler or biostimulants: Replace lost volume, Support the face

Step 3: Improve skin quality

Skin boosters or PRP: Improve texture, Stimulate collagen, Add hydration

This approach creates: Softer expressions, Better structure, Healthier skin

The result is a naturally refreshed face, not an overfilled one.

Example of a Stacked Treatment Plan

Patient in her mid-40s

Concerns: Tired eyes, Drooping cheeks, Fine lines

Month 1

- Botulinum toxin: frown, forehead, crow's feet

Month 2

- Cheek filler or biostimulant for structure

Month 3

- Skin booster or PRP for skin quality

Maintenance

- Toxin every 3–4 months
- Skin boosters twice a year
- Structural treatment every 12–24 months

This creates: Natural, progressive improvement. No sudden, obvious changes

The Advantages of Combination Treatments

More Natural Results

No single area is overtreated.

Longer-Lasting Outcomes

Biostimulants and skin treatments improve collagen over time.

Better Value

Balanced treatments reduce the need for constant touch-ups.

Healthier Skin

The face looks not just fuller—but brighter and more youthful.

The Biggest Mistake: Overfilling

One of the most common problems in modern aesthetics is overuse of filler.

When filler is used to: Lift the face, Improve skin quality, Replace collagen, Correct every line

…the result can be:

- Puffy cheeks, Heavy faces, Distorted proportions

This is often called:

- Pillow face, Overfilled face, Filler fatigue

Combination treatments reduce the need for excessive filler.

Chapter 56: Emerging Trends in Aesthetic Medicine

The field of aesthetic medicine is rapidly evolving, with continuous advancements in injectables, regenerative treatments, and technology-driven solutions. While Korea remains at the forefront of skin innovation, Australia and the USA have strict regulatory frameworks, meaning that many of these cutting-edge treatments are not yet widely available. However, Europe and Korea are leading the way in pioneering new therapies that will likely shape the future of aesthetic medicine.

This chapter explores some of the latest developments, including exosomes, stem cell therapies, AI-driven treatments, non-invasive skin tightening, and the trend toward natural-looking enhancements.

Exosome Therapy : A New Frontier in Skin Rejuvenation

Exosomes are extracellular vesicles that carry proteins, lipids, and genetic material between cells, promoting cell regeneration, repair, and communication. In aesthetic medicine, exosome-based treatments are gaining attention for their potential to improve skin texture, boost collagen, and accelerate wound healing.

Notable Exosome-Based Products & Treatments

Skin Booster Exosome Therapy (Korea) Enhances collagen synthesis, improving elasticity, hydration, and skin tone. Popular in high-end Korean aesthetic clinics.

Platelet Skin Sciences Renewosome Serums (Europe) Uses platelet-derived exosomes to reduce fine lines, wrinkles, and improve hair density.

Rose Stem Cell-Derived Exosomes Under research for their anti-ageing effects and ability to promote youthful skin renewal.

Regulatory Considerations: Exosome therapy is still undergoing clinical validation, with varying levels of approval across different countries.

Stem Cell Therapies : The Next Generation of Regenerative Aesthetics. Stem cell treatments harness the body's natural healing abilities for skin rejuvenation, tissue repair, and volume restoration.

Innovations in Stem Cell Aesthetics

Stem Cell Fat Grafting : Uses adipose-derived stem cells (ADSCs) extracted from fat deposits to restore volume in the face, breasts, and hips.

Exosome-Infused Stem Cell Serums Combining exosomes and stem cells to accelerate skin regeneration. While promising, stem cell therapies face regulatory hurdles in many countries due to concerns over safety, consistency, and ethical sourcing.

Artificial Intelligence (AI) in Aesthetics

AI is revolutionizing the diagnosis, treatment planning, and outcome prediction in aesthetic medicine.

AI-Powered Facial Analysis : Software that scans a patients' face to recommend customized treatment plans.

AI-Assisted Injectables Algorithms that help determine the optimal placement of fillers and botulinum toxin for symmetry and balance.

Virtual Try-On Technology : Allows patients to preview their post-treatment results before undergoing procedures. AI-driven tools will enhance precision and personalize treatments for superior patient outcomes.

Non-Invasive Skin Tightening & Lifting

Patients are increasingly seeking non-surgical alternatives to facelifts, leading to advancements in energy-based treatments:

High-Intensity Focused Ultrasound (HIFU) Stimulates collagen production deep within the skin to provide a lifting effect.

Radiofrequency Microneedling (Morpheus8, Profound RF) Combines microneedling with RF energy to tighten loose skin and improve texture.

Plasma Energy Devices (Jett Plasma, Plexr) Use plasma energy to tighten excess skin, particularly for non-surgical eyelid lifts. These treatments offer minimal downtime while still delivering visible improvements in skin laxity.

Combination Treatments & Treatments Stacking

The trend of stacking multiple treatments in a single session is gaining popularity. Combining injectables, lasers, and regenerative therapies can address multiple concerns at once for more comprehensive results.

Example of Treatment Stacking:

PRP (Platelet-Rich Plasma) + RF Microneedling = Boosts collagen remodelling & skin tightening.

Exosome Therapy + Skin Boosters = Enhances hydration & cellular repair.

Botox + HA Fillers + Bio-Stimulants = Creates a balanced, natural facial rejuvenation.

Why It Works: By combining synergistic treatments, patients achieve better, longer-lasting results with less downtime.

Natural-Looking Enhancements : The Shift Toward Subtlety Modern aesthetic trends emphasize natural beauty over excessive augmentation. Patients are moving away from overfilled, frozen looks and opting for treatments that enhance their unique facial features.

Bio-Stimulants (Sculptra & Radiesse) Stimulate collagen production for gradual, subtle volume restoration.

Microdosing Botox (Baby Botox) Uses smaller amounts of botulinum toxin for a more natural, expressive appearance.

Skin Boosters & Light Fillers Improve skin hydration and elasticity rather than adding bulk. The future of aesthetics is about refinement, not transformation.

Regenerative Aesthetics : The Future of Beauty & Longevity

The next generation of treatments will move beyond aesthetics to enhancing overall skin health and slowing the ageing process at a cellular level.

Exosome Therapy & Stem Cell Infusions Repair and rejuvenate skin from within.

Peptide & Growth Factor Serums Target cell regeneration and skin longevity.

NAD+ & Anti-Ageing Supplements Support mitochondrial function and collagen synthesis.

The focus is shifting toward preventative and regenerative solutions rather than simply reversing ageing.

Conclusion: The Future of Aesthetic Medicine

Exosomes, stem cell therapies, and AI-driven treatments are shaping the future of aesthetics. Energy-based devices like RF microneedling and HIFU are replacing more invasive procedures. Combination treatments (treatment stacking) enhance results while minimizing downtime. The demand for natural, subtle enhancements is driving innovation in skin boosters, bio-stimulants, and microdosing techniques. Regenerative aesthetics is emerging as the ultimate goal, focusing on long-term skin health and ageing prevention.

Chapter 57: Energy based Rejuvenation Treatments

Light, LED and Lasers

In aesthetics today, we are no longer just treating lines — we are treating the skin itself.

Tone, texture, clarity, redness, pigmentation… these are all driven by what is happening beneath the surface. That is where light-based treatments come in. But to use them well, you need to understand the difference between LED and lasers, because they are often confused — and they should not be.

What is LED and How Does It Work?

LED (light-emitting diode) is a low-level light therapy. It does not burn, cut, or remove skin. It works by delivering light energy into the skin to stimulate cellular activity — a process known as photobiomodulation.

In simple terms, LED encourages your skin cells to function better.

Different wavelengths (colours) of LED penetrate to different depths:

Blue light works at the surface (epidermis), targeting acne bacteria

Red light penetrates into the mid dermis, stimulating collagen and healing

Yellow light works on superficial vessels, calming redness and inflammation

Green light targets pigment at the epidermal level

Near-infrared reaches deeper layers, supporting repair and reducing inflammation

LED can also be delivered as a steady light or in a pulsed (flashing) mode. Pulsed light allows higher energy delivery without overheating the skin, giving a slightly stronger cellular response.

The important thing to understand is this: LED does not create injury. It supports, calms, and enhances the skin. It is not a corrective treatment on its own, but it plays a powerful role in: reducing inflammation, calming sensitive skin, supporting acne treatment, accelerating healing after procedures and improving overall skin function.

In my practice, LED is often the quiet achiever — the treatment that makes everything else work better.

What Are Lasers and How Are They Different?

Lasers are completely different.

Where LED supports the skin, lasers are designed to change it.

A laser is a focused beam of high-energy light that targets specific structures in the skin.

Depending on the wavelength, lasers can target: pigment (melanin), blood vessels (haemoglobin) and water in the skin (used in resurfacing)

Some lasers remove layers of skin. Others heat deeper tissues without breaking the surface. Most stimulate collagen by creating a controlled response in the skin.

This is why lasers can: Resurface, tighten, remove pigmentation, reduce redness, improve scars But it is also why they require:

more precision, more careful selection and sometimes downtime

The Key Difference

This is the simplest way I explain it: LED supports the skin without injury

Lasers correct the skin by creating change

Both are valuable. They just serve different roles.

Understanding Laser Types

Lasers vary in strength and depth.

CO2 laser is the most aggressive resurfacing treatment. It removes layers of skin and stimulates strong collagen production. It is used for deep wrinkles and acne scarring, but requires significant downtime — usually one to two weeks, with redness lasting longer.

Erbium YAG is a lighter resurfacing option. It treats more superficial concerns like fine lines with less downtime, usually a few days.

Fractional lasers, often referred to as Fraxel-type treatments, create microscopic columns of injury while leaving surrounding skin intact. This allows faster healing and makes them ideal for texture, early ageing, and moderate scarring.

Moxi is a newer, gentler fractional laser. It is designed more for prevention and maintenance — improving tone, early pigmentation, and overall skin quality with minimal downtime. It represents a shift in aesthetics toward treating early rather than correcting later.

BBL and IPL are not technically lasers but are used in the same category. They use broad-spectrum light to target pigment and redness. They are excellent for sun damage, freckles, and uneven skin tone, with very little downtime.

Nd:YAG lasers penetrate deeper into the skin and are used for vascular concerns, inflammation, and even acne. They are also safer for darker skin types because they bypass the surface.

Pulsed dye lasers are highly specific for blood vessels and are considered the gold standard for rosacea and redness.

Pico lasers are designed for pigmentation. They deliver ultra-fast pulses that break up pigment without generating excessive heat, making them ideal for melasma and stubborn pigmentation.

Other lasers such as diode and Alexandrite are primarily used for hair removal, while KTP lasers target superficial vessels and pigment.

There are also variations within IPL systems — such as BBL HERO, Lumecca, and Limelight — which differ in how energy is delivered, but fundamentally work on the same principle of targeting pigment and vascular changes.

Indications — Matching the Treatment to the Problem

This is where real clinical understanding matters.

Under-Eye Wrinkling

Fractional lasers and light resurfacing (such as Er:YAG) are commonly used to stimulate collagen without damageing delicate tissue. More advanced ageing may be treated with very controlled CO2 in experienced hands.

Full Face Rejuvenation

This is never one issue — it's a combination of tone, texture, and collagen loss.

BBL or IPL improves overall skin clarity, while fractional lasers and Moxi refine texture and stimulate collagen. The best results come from combining treatments rather than relying on one.

Freckles and Sun Spots

These are pigment-based concerns.

BBL, IPL, Pico, and KTP lasers are highly effective. Pigment typically darkens before it clears, which patients should be prepared for.

Rosacea and Redness

This is a vascular condition.

Pulsed dye lasers are the most effective, with BBL and IPL helping diffuse redness. Nd:YAG can treat deeper vessels. LED can calm the skin but does not replace vascular lasers.

Melasma

One of the most difficult conditions to treat.

Heat can worsen it, so aggressive lasers are often not appropriate. Pico lasers, gentle light-based treatments, and supportive LED are preferred. This is a condition that requires careful, conservative management.

Sun Damage — Especially Décolletage

The chest is more fragile than the face and heals more slowly. BBL and IPL are commonly used for pigmentation and redness, with fractional treatments used cautiously for texture. Moxi is excellent for maintenance in this area.

Chemical Pigmentation (Perfume-Related)

Often seen on the neck or chest.

This type of pigmentation can be stubborn and reactive. Pico lasers and gentle light-based treatments are preferred, with gradual improvement over time rather than aggressive correction.

Acne and Acne Scarring

These must be treated as separate conditions.

Active acne is driven by inflammation, oil, and bacteria. Nd:YAG and acne-specific lasers help calm the skin, while blue LED supports bacterial control.

Acne scarring is a structural issue. CO2 is most effective for deep scars, while fractional lasers treat moderate scarring. Moxi or gentler treatments can help with early texture changes.

Treat the acne first — then the scars.

Bringing It All Together

There is no single "best" treatment.

The outcome depends on: understanding what is driving the problem, choosing the correct depth, using the right technology and timing the treatment appropriately

In my experience, the best results don't come from aggressive, one-off procedures.

They come from: supporting the skin, treating the cause and layering treatments over time

LED to calm and heal. Light-based treatments to improve tone. Lasers to correct when needed. Injectables to restore structure.

That is how natural, balanced, long-term results are achieved.

Not by chasing one treatment — but by understanding the skin and working with it.

HIFU and Ultherapy

Lifting, Tightening — and Knowing When Not To

As aesthetics has evolved, there has been a strong move toward treatments that **lift and tighten without surgery**. This is where HIFU and Ultherapy sit.

They are often marketed as "non-surgical facelifts," and while that sounds appealing, it needs to be understood properly — because these treatments are powerful, and when used incorrectly, they can give results you don't want.

What is HIFU?

HIFU stands for **High-Intensity Focused Ultrasound**.

It uses focused ultrasound energy to deliver heat at specific depths beneath the skin — without damageing the surface.

What makes HIFU different from lasers is this:

- it bypasses the surface entirely, it targets deeper structural layers

The energy creates small thermal ن قاط (heat points) in the tissue, which triggers:

- collagen contraction, collagen production over time

The result is gradual tightening and lifting.

What is Ultherapy?

Ultherapy is a **medical-grade, branded form of HIFU**.

The key difference is:

- it uses **real-time ultrasound imageing**
- allowing the practitioner to actually *see* the tissue layers being treated

This adds a level of precision that standard HIFU devices do not always have.

In experienced hands, this can make a significant difference in safety and outcomes.

What Layer Does It Target?

This is the most important concept to understand.

HIFU and Ultherapy target the **SMAS layer** — the same structural layer tightened during a surgical facelift.

The depths typically treated are:

- 1.5 mm (superficial dermis)
- 3.0 mm (deep dermis)
- 4.5 mm (SMAS layer)

At the deeper level, the energy causes contraction of this fibromuscular layer, leading to lifting.

It does not "fill" the face.

It works by tightening what is already there.

What Does It Treat?

HIFU and Ultherapy are best suited for:

- mild to moderate skin laxity, early jowling
- soft jawline definition, brow lifting, neck tightening

It is not a replacement for volume loss.

If the face has lost fat and structure, tightening alone can sometimes make this more obvious.

The Fat Factor — This Is Where It Matters

This is where I see the biggest mistakes being made.

Ultrasound energy, particularly at deeper levels, can affect **fat** as well as tissue.

This can be beneficial in the right patient.

For example:

- a heavier face, thicker lower face, early jowling with fullness

In these cases, a small degree of fat reduction can improve contour and definition.

But in a Thinner Face…

This is where caution is critical.

If you treat too deeply or too aggressively in someone who:

- already has low facial fat, is naturally thin, or is showing volume loss with age

You can:

- reduce fat further, create hollowing, exaggerate sagging rather than improve it

Because once fat is reduced, the skin has less support.

And tightening without volume can sometimes make the face look:

- older, more drawn, less balanced

Technique Matters

The outcome of HIFU is not just about the machine — it is about:

- depth selection, energy level, placement, patient selection

If a practitioner goes too deep in the wrong area, they may:

- affect fat unnecessarily, miss the structural layer, create uneven results

This is why experience matters.

It is not a "one setting fits all" treatment.

What Does It Feel Like?

Patients often describe HIFU as:

- a deep, zapping or tingling sensation
- sometimes uncomfortable depending on the area

Unlike LED or many laser treatments, it is not relaxing — it is working at a deeper structural level.

Results and Timeline

Results are not immediate.

You may see some early tightening, but the real change happens over:

- 8 to 12 weeks
- sometimes up to 6 months

This is due to collagen remodelling.

Results are subtle and natural — not dramatic like surgery.

Downtime

One of the appealing aspects of HIFU is minimal downtime.

You may experience:

- slight swelling, tenderness, occasional tingling

But most patients return to normal activities immediately.

Where It Fits in Aesthetic Treatment

HIFU is not a standalone solution.

It works best when combined with:

- skin quality treatments, collagen stimulation and, where needed, volume restoration

Because tightening alone does not address: volume loss, skin texture, pigmentation

My Clinical Perspective

I am selective with HIFU.

In the right patient, it can be a beautiful treatment — subtle lifting, improved firmness, and a refreshed look.

But it is not for everyone.

In thinner faces, or in those already showing volume depletion, I approach it with caution — or avoid it altogether.

Because in aesthetics, more is not always better.

Sometimes preserving what is there is far more important than trying to tighten everything.

The Takeaway

HIFU and Ultherapy are powerful tools for lifting and tightening.

But they require:

- the right patient, the right depth
- and the right practitioner

Used well, they can enhance and support the ageing face.

Used incorrectly, they can accelerate the very changes we are trying to prevent.

And that is where knowledge — and experience — makes all the difference.

Radiofrequency Treatments

Heating, Tightening, and Collagen — Without Removing the Skin

If lasers are about light, and HIFU is about ultrasound, then radiofrequency sits in its own category.

It doesn't rely on colour or pigment.

It doesn't depend on light absorption.

Radiofrequency works by delivering **electrical energy** into the skin, which is converted into **heat**.

And that heat is what creates change.

How Radiofrequency Works

RF energy penetrates the skin and heats the deeper layers — particularly the dermis.

At the right temperature, this heat:

- causes **immediate collagen contraction**
- stimulates **new collagen production over time**
- improves skin thickness and elasticity

Unlike lasers, RF is:

- **colour-blind** (it doesn't target pigment)
- generally **safer across different skin types**
- more focused on **tightening and texture** rather than pigment removal

The goal is controlled heating — not burning, not removing — but stimulating the skin to rebuild itself.

Different Types of RF

There isn't just one type of radiofrequency. The delivery method changes how deep it goes and what it treats.

Surface RF (Non-invasive)

These treatments heat the skin from the outside.

They are used for:

- mild skin laxity, early ageing, maintenance

They feel warm, sometimes like a hot stone massage.

Examples include:

- Thermage, Exilis, Venus Legacy

Downtime is minimal, but results are gradual and often require multiple sessions.

RF Microneedling

This is where RF becomes much more powerful

This combines:

- microneedles that penetrate the skin
- with radiofrequency energy delivered directly into the dermis

Instead of heating from the surface, the energy is delivered **inside the skin**, making it far more effective.

Key RF Microneedling Devices

Morpheus8

One of the most well-known systems.

It can treat at multiple depths, including deeper layers where fat sits.

Used for:

- skin tightening, acne scarring
- texture, lower face contouring

Downtime: 2–5 days redness and mild swelling

Important point: At deeper settings, it can affect fat — which can be beneficial in a heavier face, but not in a thin one.

Secret RF

More controlled and often considered gentler.

Used for:

- Texture, fine lines, mild tightening

Downtime: 1–3 days

Sylfirm X

A newer generation device with pulsed wave technology.

Used for:

- Rosacea, pigmentation (including melasma)
- vascular concerns, skin tightening

This is one of the few RF devices used cautiously for melasma due to controlled delivery.

Potenza

Highly versatile with multiple modes and depths.

Used for:

- tightening, acne scars, skin rejuvenation

Downtime: 2–4 days

What RF is Best For

Radiofrequency sits in a very specific space.

It is excellent for:

- skin laxity, mild to moderate sagging
- acne scarring, enlarged pores, skin texture, early ageing

It is not designed for:

- heavy pigmentation (lasers do this better)
- significant volume loss (requires injectables)

RF vs HIFU vs Lasers

This is where people get confused.

- **RF** → heats the dermis → collagen tightening and texture
- **HIFU** → targets deeper structural layers (SMAS) → lifting
- **Lasers** → target pigment, vessels, or resurface skin

They are not competing treatments — they are **different tools for different layers**.

The Fat Discussion (Important)

Just like HIFU, RF — particularly microneedling RF — can affect fat if used deeply.

In the right patient:

- fuller face, heavy lower face

This can help contour and slim.

But in a thinner face:

- too much depth, too much energy

Can lead to:

- hollowing, loss of support, a more aged appearance

This is not talked about enough — but it matters.

What Does It Feel Like?

Surface RF feels warm and comfortable.

RF microneedling is more intense:

- topical numbing is used
- you may feel heat and pressure

It is not painful in most cases, but it is not a relaxing facial.

Downtime

Varies depending on the device and depth.

Surface RF:

- no downtime

RF microneedling:

- redness for 1–3 days, mild swelling
- occasional pinpoint marks

Skin usually feels tighter within a few weeks, with continued improvement over months.

My Clinical Perspective

Radiofrequency is one of the most versatile tools we have.

But like everything in aesthetics, it comes down to:

- patient selection, depth, restraint

I don't use it the same way on every face.

In someone with:

- thicker skin, early laxity, acne scarring

It can be transformative.

In someone who is:

- thin, volume depleted

I am far more conservative.

Because tightening without support can sometimes age the face.

The Takeaway

Radiofrequency is about **controlled heat and collagen stimulation**.

It doesn't replace:

- lasers, HIFU or injectables

But when used correctly, it sits beautifully between them — improving skin quality, tightening gently, and enhancing overall results.

It's another tool.

And like all good tools, it's only as good as the hands using it.

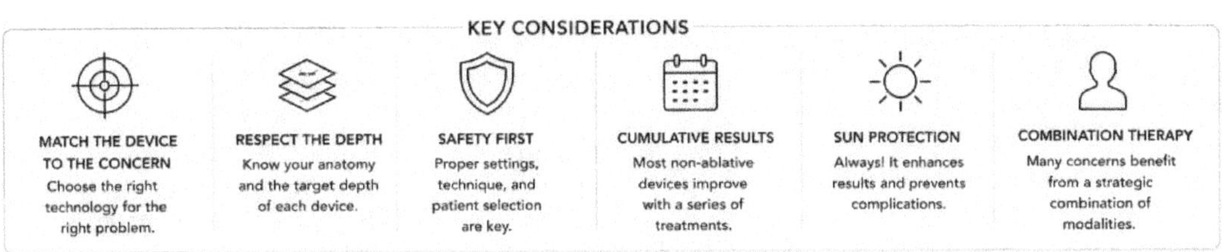

LASER & LIGHT DEVICE COMPARISON CHART

Know your device. Understand the depth. Treat with purpose.

Different wavelengths and technologies target different skin layers and concerns.
Choosing the right device = safer treatments + better results.

DEVICE	IPL *(Intense Pulsed Light)*	BBL HERO™ *(BroadBand Light)*	MOXI® *(Non-Ablative Fractional)*	CLEAR + BRILLIANT® *(Gentle Non-Ablative Fractional)*	FRACTIONAL CO_2 LASER *(Ablative)*	ERBIUM:YAG LASER *(Ablative)*	RF MICRONEEDLING (e.g., MORPHEUS8)	HIFU *(High Intensity Focused Ultrasound)*
	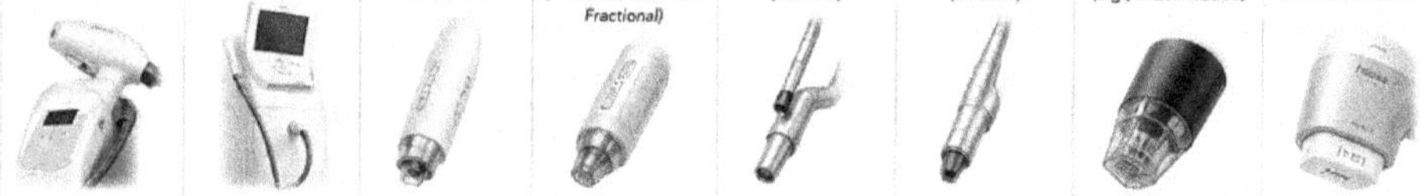							
TECHNOLOGY	Broad spectrum pulsed light	Broad spectrum pulsed light (optimized filters)	Non-ablative fractional laser	Non-ablative fractional laser	Ablative fractional laser	Ablative (thermal)	Radiofrequency energy through microneedles	Focused ultrasound energy
WAVELENGTH / ENERGY	Multiple wavelengths (500–1200 nm)	BroadBand (400–1400 nm) with filters	1927 nm (Thulium)	1440 nm (Diode)	10,600 nm (CO_2)	2940 nm (Er:YAG)	RF Energy (Needle tips)	Ultrasound 4.5mm / 3.0mm / 1.5mm
PENETRATION DEPTH*	Epidermis to superficial dermis (1–2 mm)	Epidermis to superficial dermis (1–2 mm)	Epidermis to dermis (0.3–0.8 mm)	Epidermis to upper dermis (0.2–0.6 mm)	Mid to deep dermis (1–4 mm+)	Epidermis to superficial dermis (0.5–2 mm)	Dermis to subdermal fat (1–4 mm+)	Deep tissue / SMAS (1.5 mm, 3.0 mm, 4.5 mm)
PRIMARY TARGET	Melanin, hemoglobin	Melanin, hemoglobin, acne bacteria	Water in skin cells (thermal coagulation)	Water in skin cells (mild thermal zones)	Water (strong thermal ablation)	Water (surface ablation with minimal heat)	Tissue heating & collagen remodeling	Deep structural support (collagen & SMAS tigthening)
BEST FOR	Pigmentation, redness, sun damage, rosacea, vascular lesions	Pigmentation, redness, rosacea, acne, sun damage, overall tone	Early signs of aging, tone, texture, mild pigmentation	Preventative aging, fine lines, radiance, pore refinement	Wrinkles, acne scars, deep lines, sun damage, skin laxity	Fine lines, texture, scars, surface resurfacing	Skin laxity, acne scars, texture, pores, stretch marks	Skin tightening, jawline lift, neck laxity, brow lift
DOWNTIME	None to minimal	None to minimal	1–2 days (mild redness)	Few hours to 1 day	5–10 days (Depends on depth)	3–5 days (mild peeling)	1–3 days (microneedle marks, redness)	None to minimal
NUMBER OF SESSIONS	3–6 sessions	3–6 sessions	3–4 sessions	3–6 sessions	1–3 sessions	2–4 sessions	1–3 sessions	1–2 sessions
COMFORT LEVEL	Comfortable (Cold gel)	Comfortable (Cold gel)	Mild (Topical anesthetic)	Very Comfortable (Topical only)	Moderate to Low (Numbing required)	Moderate (Numbing recommended)	Moderate (Numbing recommended)	Moderate (Warmth, pressure)

*Penetration depth is approximate and can vary based on settings, handpiece, and individual skin.

SKIN LAYERS & DEPTH VISUAL COMPARISON

IPL | BBL HERO™ | MOXI® | CLEAR + BRILLIANT® | FRACTIONAL CO_2 LASER | ERBIUM:YAG LASER | RF MICRONEEDLING (MORPHEUS8) | HIFU

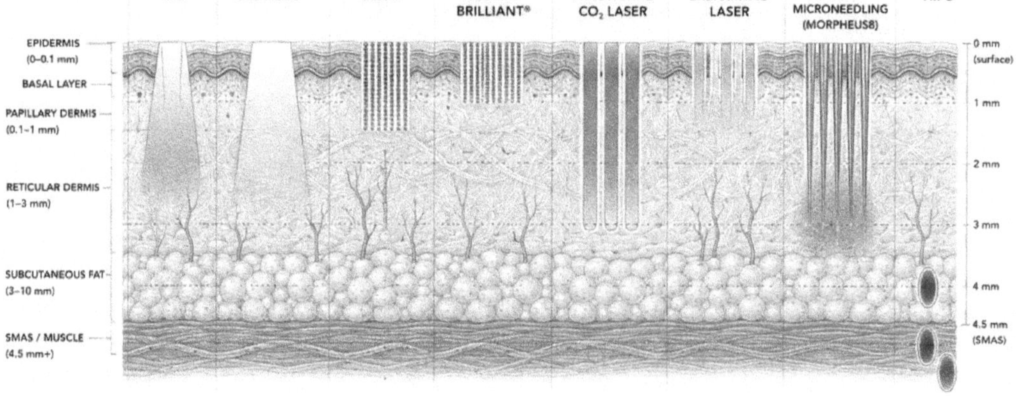

Chapter 58: Peptides- The Next Frontier in Aesthetic, Metabolism and Longevity

There is a quiet shift happening in our industry.

We have moved from creams… to injectables… to regenerative medicine…

…and now we are stepping into the world of peptides.

Peptides are being spoken about everywhere — in clinics, in longevity medicine, in wellness circles — yet there is still a lot of confusion around what they actually do, and where they truly belong.

So let's bring this back to basics, in a way that makes sense clinically.

What Are Peptides?

Peptides are short chains of amino acids — essentially **messenger molecules** in the body.

They tell cells what to do.

Repair. Regenerate. Produce collagen. Reduce inflammation. Improve energy. Support hormones.

Think of peptides as instructions your body already understands. They don't override the body — they communicate with it.

Why Peptides Matter in Ageing

As we age, the body doesn't just "wear out" — it becomes less efficient at communicating.

- Cellular repair slows, Collagen production declines, Inflammation increases, Hormonal signalling changes

Peptides help restore that communication.

They don't force change like some treatments. They support the body to function more effectively.

This is why they sit beautifully alongside:

- PRP
- Biostimulants
- Skin rejuvenation treatments

Skin and Collagen Peptides

These are the most familiar in aesthetics and often used in topical or supportive treatments.

GHK-Cu (Copper Peptide)

One of the most researched peptides in skin. It stimulates collagen and elastin, improves skin thickness, enhances healing, and reduces inflammation.

Matrixyl (Palmitoyl Pentapeptide)

Supports collagen production and improves skin texture and fine lines.

Argireline
Often referred to as a "Botox-like" topical peptide. It softens expression lines but does not replace neuromodulators. In practice, these peptides don't replace injectables — they support and enhance results.

Healing and Regenerative Peptides

These are widely used in recovery and repair.

BPC-157: Known for its ability to support healing of tendons, ligaments, and the gut. It is anti-inflammatory and often used in injury recovery.

TB-500 (Thymosin Beta-4): Supports tissue repair, cell migration, and healing. Often used alongside BPC-157.

These peptides are not aesthetic in the traditional sense, but they support the body's ability to recover — which underpins everything we do.

Growth Hormone and Anti-Ageing Peptides

These influence the body's natural growth hormone pathways.

CJC-1295: Stimulates growth hormone release over a longer duration.

Ipamorelin: Works synergistically with CJC-1295 to promote natural growth hormone pulses.

Sermorelin: A milder option that supports growth hormone release with a more conservative approach.

These peptides can improve:

- Sleep quality, Recovery, Body composition, Skin quality indirectly

This is where aesthetics begins to overlap with longevity medicine.

Fat Loss and Metabolic Peptides

This is one of the fastest-growing areas.

AOD-9604: Supports fat metabolism and fat breakdown.

Tesamorelin: Targets visceral fat and improves body composition.

Semaglutide and Tirzepatide: Well-known metabolic peptides that regulate appetite, insulin, and weight.

Retatrutide: One of the most exciting newer peptides. It acts on multiple metabolic pathways and has shown significant effects on fat loss and metabolic regulation in early studies.

These peptides are changing how we think about weight, insulin resistance, and metabolic health — but they must be approached responsibly.

They are not shortcuts. They are tools.

Mitochondrial and Longevity Peptides

This is where the science becomes very interesting.

MOTS-c: A mitochondrial-derived peptide that supports cellular energy, metabolic function, and insulin sensitivity. It is being explored in longevity and metabolic health.

Epitalon (Epithalon): Linked to cellular ageing and telomere research. Early data suggests potential anti-ageing effects, but more research is needed.

This is still an evolving space, but it represents the future direction of medicine.

Brain and Mood Peptides

These peptides influence the nervous system and cognitive function.

Semax: Supports focus, mental clarity, and neuroprotection. Originally used in neurological settings.

Selank: Has anti-anxiety effects and supports emotional balance.

Dihexa: An emerging peptide linked to memory and neurogenesis, still largely in research phases.

These peptides are interesting, but many are not approved in Australia and should be approached cautiously.

Immune and Systemic Peptides

Thymosin Alpha-1: Supports immune function and reduces inflammation.

LL-37: Has antimicrobial properties and plays a role in immune defence.

These peptides are more medical than aesthetic but support overall health.

Sexual Health and Connection

PT-141 (Bremelanotide): Works centrally to enhance libido in both men and women.

Oxytocin: Often referred to as the "bonding hormone," influencing connection, trust, and emotional wellbeing.

Safety, Regulation and Reality

This is the most important part of this conversation.

Many peptides:

- Are not TGA approved in Australia
- Are sold as "research peptides"
- Have variable quality and purity
- Lack long-term human safety data

This means we must stay grounded and responsible.

Just because something is available does not mean it is appropriate.

Where Peptides Fit in Aesthetics

Peptides are not a replacement for: Neuromodulators, Dermal fillers, Biostimulants

They are supportive.

They improve: Skin quality, Healing, Internal balance, Longevity pathways

They work in the background — quietly enhancing outcomes.

My Perspective

Over the years, I've seen trends come and go.

Peptides are different.

They represent a move away from simply "treating the face" towards **supporting the whole person**.

Less about chasing lines… more about restoring function.

They are subtle. They are intelligent.

And when used appropriately, they can be powerful.

Chapter 59: IV Therapies – Beauty from Within

In aesthetics, we often focus on what we can see—lines, volume loss, pigmentation, and texture. But over the years, I've come to understand that true rejuvenation doesn't just sit on the surface. It begins much deeper, at a cellular level.

This is where IV (intravenous) therapy has found its place in modern aesthetic medicine.

I was first certified in IV nutritional therapy through Australasian College of Nutritional and Environmental Medicine in 2006. At the time, it was considered progressive. Today, it has become a valuable adjunct to aesthetic treatments—supporting skin health, immunity, and overall vitality.

IV therapy is not about quick fixes or miracle cures. It is about replenishing what the body is lacking, supporting cellular function, and enhancing the results of the treatments we already perform.

Why IV Therapy?

When nutrients are taken orally, they must pass through the digestive system, where absorption can be inconsistent. With IV therapy, nutrients are delivered directly into the bloodstream, allowing for higher bioavailability and immediate use by the body.

Think of it as feeding the skin—and the body—from within.

The Role of IV Therapy in Aesthetics

IV therapy complements:

- Skin needling, PRP and regenerative treatments
- Laser procedures, Biostimulants and injectables

It supports: Collagen production, Cellular repair, Hydration, Immune resilience, Recovery

But it must always be approached with the same respect as any medical treatment.

Core IV Therapies

Myers' Cocktail – The Foundation

A blend of: Vitamin C, B-complex, Magnesium, Calcium

Benefits: Energy support, Stress reduction, General skin vitality

Contraindications / cautions: Renal impairment (magnesium clearance), Cardiac conditions (electrolyte sensitivity), Hypotension (magnesium can lower blood pressure)

High-Dose Vitamin C

Benefits: Collagen stimulation, Antioxidant protection, Immune support

Contraindications / cautions: G6PD deficiency (risk of haemolysis), Kidney impairment or history of kidney stones, Iron overload disorders (can increase iron absorption)

Understanding G6PD – A Small Detail That Matters

G6PD (Glucose-6-Phosphate Dehydrogenase) protects red blood cells from oxidative stress.

In deficiency, high-dose Vitamin C can trigger **haemolysis** (breakdown of red blood cells).

This is why: Screening is essential, Treatment must be individualised

Kidney Function – Often Overlooked

The kidneys regulate and excrete excess nutrients.

With IV therapy:

- High doses bypass normal regulation, Poor kidney function can lead to accumulation, Risk of electrolyte imbalance increases

Clinical red flags: Reduced eGFR, History of kidney stones, Dehydration

This is particularly relevant for Vitamin C, magnesium, and electrolyte infusions.

Glutathione – The Master Antioxidant

Benefits: Detoxification, Skin brightening, Anti-inflammatory effects

Contraindications / cautions: Asthma (rare bronchospasm risk), Sulphur sensitivity (rare but relevant), Pregnancy (limited data—use caution)

NAD+ – Cellular Longevity Therapy

NAD+ works at a deep cellular level: Mitochondrial support, DNA repair, Energy production

However, this is also one of the most misunderstood drips.

A clinical observation:

Many patients feel **nauseous, flushed, or unwell during NAD+ infusions**—particularly if infused too quickly.

In my experience, this is often due to:

- Rapid cellular activity, Increased metabolic demand
- The body processing accumulated metabolic waste

Some refer to this loosely as a "detox response," but clinically it is more about **metabolic overwhelm** than toxins alone.

What helps: Slower infusion rates, Lower starting doses, Adequate hydration, Careful patient selection

Contraindications / cautions: Severe liver or kidney impairment, Pregnancy, Patients with low tolerance to infusions or chronic fatigue states (start low)

Biotin (Vitamin B7)

Benefits: Hair growth, Nail strength, Skin hydration

Contraindications / cautions: Can interfere with blood test results (thyroid, troponin), Use cautiously in patients undergoing diagnostic testing

Zinc

Benefits: Immune support, Acne reduction, Wound healing

Contraindications / cautions: High doses may cause nausea, Long-term excess can disrupt copper balance

Magnesium

Benefits: Nervous system calming, Muscle relaxation, Sleep support

Contraindications / cautions: Renal impairment (risk of accumulation), Hypotension, Bradycardia in sensitive patients

Amino Acids – Collagen Support

Benefits: Tissue repair, Skin regeneration, Post-procedure healing

Contraindications / cautions: Severe liver or kidney disease, Rare metabolic disorders

Alpha-Lipoic Acid (ALA)

Benefits: Regenerates antioxidants, Reduces glycation, Supports metabolism

Contraindications / cautions: May lower blood sugar (caution in diabetics), Can cause reflux or nausea in some patients

Hydration and Electrolyte Therapy

Benefits: Rehydration, Improved circulation, Skin plumping

Contraindications / cautions: Heart failure, Kidney disease, Fluid overload risk

Iron Infusions – A Medical Treatment

Iron is essential for: Oxygen transport, Energy, Hair and skin health

When deficient, patients may experience: Fatigue, Hair loss, Pale, dull skin

Important distinction:

Iron infusions are **not cosmetic—they are medical**.

Contraindications / cautions: Iron overload conditions (e.g. haemochromatosis), Active infection, Known hypersensitivity

Must always be: Blood test confirmed, Medically supervised

Combination Drips

Clinics often tailor blends:

Beauty Drip Vitamin C + Glutathione + Biotin. **Immunity Drip** Vitamin C + Zinc + B complex. **Anti-Ageing Drip** NAD+ + ALA + Vitamin C. **Recovery Drip** Magnesium + Amino acids + Electrolytes

Each should still be customised—not one-size-fits-all.

Clinical Considerations

Before any IV therapy: Full medical history, Kidney function assessment, Relevant blood tests, Individualised dosing

This is where experience matters.

A Balanced Perspective

IV therapy is not about chasing youth in a drip. It is about restoring balance.

When used correctly, it enhances: Skin treatments, Energy, Recovery, Overall wellbeing

But when used casually, without assessment, it can do more harm than good.

PART 5- RISKS , SAFETY AND COMPLICATIONS

Chapter 60: How Painful Are Injectable Treatments?

Pain tolerance varies from person to person, but most injectable treatments are well tolerated when performed by a skilled injector. The level of discomfort depends on the type of procedure, technique used, injection depth, and area treated. Fortunately, various pain management strategies, including numbing creams, vibration devices, ice, and anaesthetics can help minimize discomfort. This chapter breaks down the pain levels associated with different injectables and thread lifts, as well as the best methods for pain relief during treatments.

Pain Levels by Treatment Type

1. Dermal Fillers : Minimal Pain with Proper Technique

Skilled injectors can inject gently and precisely, minimizing discomfort.

Numbing cream (topical anaesthetic) is applied before treatment.

Most HA fillers contain lidocaine, which numbs the area as the injection progresses.

Pain Factors:

Needle injections can sting, especially if a blood vessel is accidentally pierced, leading to bruising and swelling.

Swelling and bruising last 1-2 weeks but are temporary.

Cannula technique is often less painful than needles but can feel uncomfortable when breaking through septa (connective tissue compartments), sometimes producing a crunchy sensation.

Pain Relief Options:

1. Topical numbing cream (BLT: Benzocaine, Lidocaine, Tetracaine) Applied 20-30 minutes before treatment.

Dental block (for lips) :Numbs the entire lip area but may cause temporary facial numbness.

Cold compress/ice : Reduces pain and swelling.

Distraction devices (e.g., squeeze balls, vibration pens) Help divert attention from discomfort.

Lips are one of the most sensitive areas, so stronger numbing options like a dental block or BLT cream are often recommended.

2. Cannula vs. Needle : Which Is More Comfortable?

Cannulas require only one or two entry points per treatment area.

Less trauma to blood vessels = fewer bruises and less swelling.

Cannula injections feel more like pressure rather than a sharp sting.

However, the cannula must break through the septa (fibrous tissue), which can feel crunchy and slightly uncomfortable.

A small amount of local anaesthetic is injected at the cannula entry point to reduce pain.

3. Botulinum Toxin (Botox, Dysport, Xeomin, etc.) Stings Slightly Botulinum toxin is mixed with saline, which can cause a mild stinging sensation.

The injections use very fine needles, but they can feel sharper as the needle blunts over multiple injections.

Pain Management:

Ice before and after can reduce discomfort.

Fast injections with minimal passes reduce needle fatigue and pain.

4. Thread Lifts Discomfort During and After

Threads are infused with lidocaine to numb the treatment area during insertion.

However, discomfort and soreness are common after the anaesthetic wears off, lasting up to a week.

Pain Management for Threads:

Oral painkillers (paracetamol, ibuprofen) can help with post-treatment soreness.

Avoid excessive movement or stretching for the first few days to minimize discomfort.

Full-face thread lifts involve multiple entry points, so post-procedure soreness is expected.

5. Nitrous Oxide (Laughing Gas) Available in Some Clinics

Nitrous oxide (laughing gas) is available in some clinics to reduce anxiety and pain.

Provides a relaxing, euphoric effect while keeping the patient conscious.

Wears off quickly, allowing patients to resume normal activities immediately.

Best for patients with low pain tolerance or anxiety about injections.

Pain Reduction Strategies for Injectables

Numbing cream (BLT) Applied before treatment to reduce surface pain.

Cold compress/Ice Numbs the area and reduces swelling.

Vibration anaesthesia devices . Divert the brain's attention from the injection pain.

Squeeze balls or stress-relief tools Provide a distraction.

Shorter, faster injection sessions :Reduce overall discomfort.

Oral pain relievers (paracetamol, ibuprofen) Taken before or after treatment for pain relief.

For patients with very low pain tolerance, discussing stronger numbing options with the injector is recommended.

Conclusion: Is It Painful?

Most injectables are well tolerated, with pain levels ranging from mild to moderate.

Proper numbing and injection techniques make the experience manageable.

Cannulas reduce bruising and pain but can feel uncomfortable when breaking through tissue.

Thread lifts involve more discomfort post-procedure, but pain can be controlled with oral painkillers.

Nitrous oxide, distraction tools, and ice help reduce anxiety and pain during procedures.

A skilled injector ensures a gentle, efficient experience, making aesthetic treatments more comfortable and accessible for all patients.

Chapter 61: Understanding Anaesthetics in Aesthetic Medicine

Aesthetic procedures often involve some level of discomfort, and the right choice of anaesthetic can significantly improve the patient experience. This chapter covers the different types of anaesthetics used in cosmetic injectables, including topical, injectable, and inhalation options, along with nerve blocks and their applications.

1. Topical Anaesthetics:

Topical anaesthetics are commonly used to numb the skin before injectable treatments, reducing pain and discomfort.

Commercially Available Topical Anaesthetics:

Lidocaine 5% (LMX, Emla, Xylocaine gel) ~Used for numbing the skin before procedures such as lip injections, laser treatments, and microneedling.

Tetracaine ~ A more potent topical anaesthetic, often combined with lidocaine for enhanced numbing.

Benzocaine ~ Found in some over-the-counter numbing gels but less commonly used in aesthetic medicine.

Compounded Topical Anaesthetics:

Custom-blended anaesthetics are formulated by compounding pharmacies for stronger and longer-lasting numbing effects.

Lidocaine + Tetracaine (23%/7%) A powerful combination used for high-pain areas like lips and tattoo removal.

BLT Cream (Benzocaine, Lidocaine, Tetracaine) A strong numbing option often used in cosmetic clinics.

Application:

Apply 20~45 minutes before the procedure, depending on formulation.

Occlusion (covering with plastic wrap) enhances absorption.

Must be removed thoroughly before injections.

2. Injectable Anaesthetics

Injectable anaesthetics provide deeper and longer-lasting numbing, often used for nerve blocks or direct infiltration.

Common Injectable Local Anaesthetics

Lidocaine 1% or 2% ~ Most commonly used; acts within minutes and lasts 1-2 hours.

Xylocaine (Lidocaine with Epinephrine) ~The addition of epinephrine prolongs numbing and reduces bleeding.

Mepivacaine ~Similar to lidocaine but longer-lasting, sometimes preferred for nerve blocks.

Use in Aesthetics:

Added to dermal fillers (some already contain lidocaine).

Directly injected before treatments like PDO threads, minor excisions, or lip fillers for extra comfort.

Used in nerve blocks to completely anaesthetise specific areas.

Lidocaine with Epinephrine ~Caution in Cardiac Patients

Epinephrine (adrenaline) is added to lidocaine to reduce bleeding and prolong the anaesthetic effect by constricting blood vessels. However, it can cause side effects, particularly in patients with heart conditions.

Potential Side Effects:

Increased heart rate (tachycardia)**,** Elevated blood pressure**,** Anxiety or restlessness

Dizziness or palpitations, In rare cases, cardiac arrhythmias

Contraindications & Cautions:

Patients with cardiovascular disease (e.g., hypertension, arrhythmias, recent heart attack) should avoid lidocaine with epinephrine.

Patients on beta-blockers or MAO inhibitors may experience an exaggerated response to epinephrine.

In cardiac patients, consider plain lidocaine without epinephrine or using the lowest effective dose.

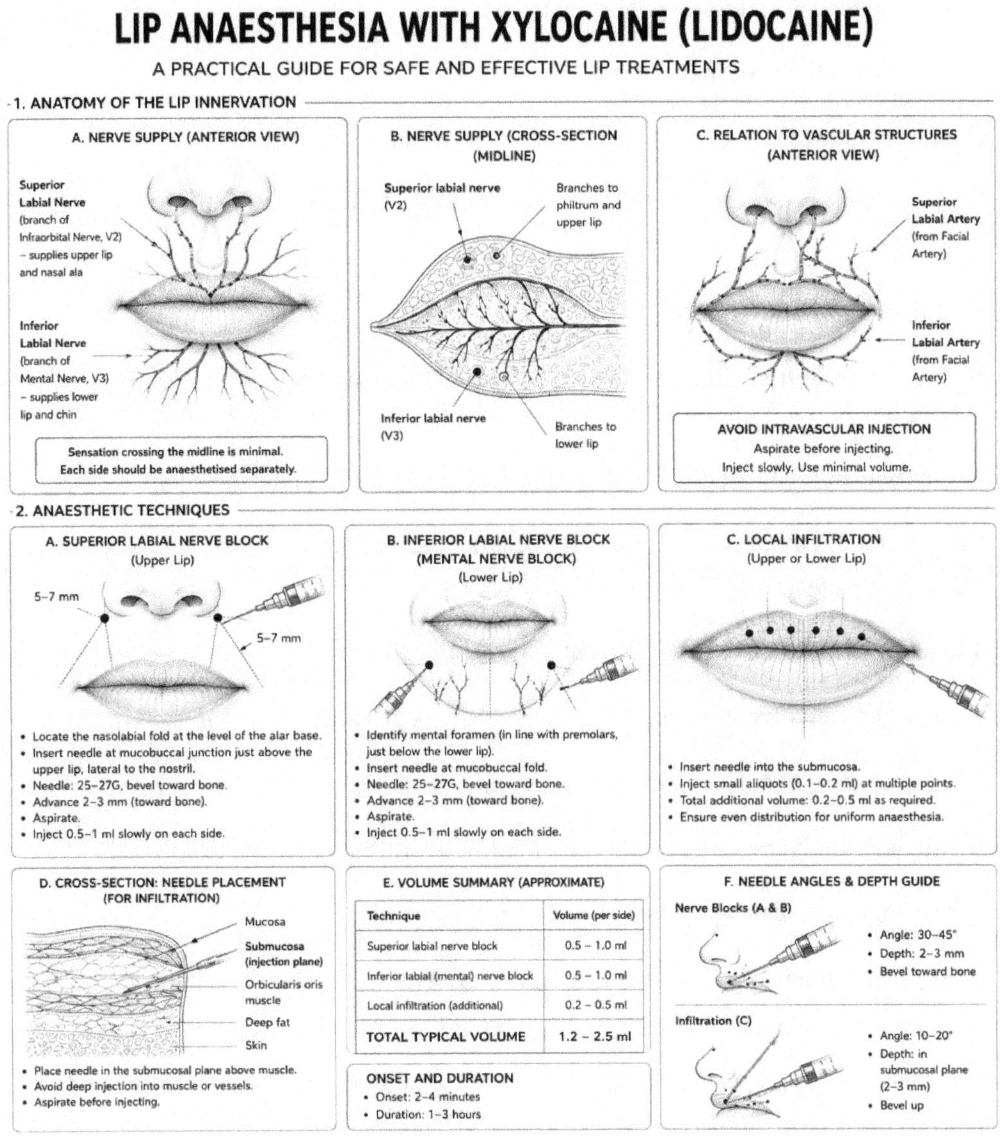

3. Caine Poisoning - Local Anaesthetic Toxicity

Overdosing on local anaesthetics (lidocaine, tetracaine, benzocaine) can lead to systemic toxicity, known as Local Anaesthetic Systemic Toxicity (LAST).

Symptoms to Watch For:

Mild Toxicity:

Dizziness, light-headedness, Numbness around the mouth or tongue

Ringing in the ears (tinnitus), Blurred vision

Severe Toxicity (Emergency):

Confusion, slurred speech, Muscle twitching, tremors, Seizures

Irregular heartbeat or bradycardia (slow heart rate), Loss of consciousness, Respiratory depression

Prevention & Management:

Dose Calculation is Key ~ Ensure the total amount injected stays within safe limits (Max safe dose: 4.5 mg/kg for plain lidocaine, 7 mg/kg with epinephrine).

Aspiration Before Injection ~Prevents accidental intravascular injection.

Emergency Protocols ~ If toxicity occurs, administer IV lipid emulsion therapy immediately and provide advanced cardiac support.

4. Nerve Blocks and Their Facial Locations

Nerve blocks involve injecting anaesthetic near specific nerves to numb a large area.

Common Nerve Blocks in Aesthetic Medicine

1. **Infraorbital Nerve Block** ~ Numbs the lower eyelid, upper lip, and mid-face.

2. **Mental Nerve Block** ~Numbs the lower lip and chin.

3. **Supratrochlear & Supraorbital Nerve Blocks** ~ Numbs the forehead and upper face.

4. **Inferior Alveolar Nerve Block** ~Used for deep numbing of the lower jaw and lips.

Benefits of Nerve Blocks:

More effective than topical anaesthetics for procedures like lip injections.

Reduces swelling and distortion caused by direct local anaesthetic infiltration.

5. Inhalation Anaesthetics

Penthrox (Methoxyflurane) -(The Green Whistle)•

An inhaled analgesic commonly used in emergency settings and minor procedures. It provides rapid pain relief without needing an IV or injection.

How does it make you feel?

Mild euphoria or lightheadedness.

Relaxed, but still conscious.

Some report dizziness or nausea in higher doses.

Longevity & Usage:

Onset within minutes, Effects last about 30~45 minutes.

Single-use; discarded after 1 dose.

Precautions:

Avoid in patients with respiratory issues or kidney problems.

Not recommended for repeated use due to potential toxicity.

Driving After Use: Wait at least 24 hours before driving, as it may impair reflexes and judgment.

6. Nitrous Oxide (Laughing Gas) A colourless, sweet-smelling gas used for mild sedation and pain relief. Often combined with oxygen and administered through a mask.

How does it make you feel?

Light-headed, giggly, or euphoric.

Relaxed but still responsive, May cause dizziness or a floating sensation.

Longevity & Usage:

Rapid onset (within seconds).

Effects wear off within 5~10 minutes after stopping inhalation.

Precautions:

Avoid in patients with severe respiratory conditions or vitamin B12 deficiency.

May cause nausea in some people.

Driving After Use: Wait at least 30 minutes to 1 hour before driving., Effects dissipate quickly, but some may still feel slightly groggy.

Choosing the right anaesthetic depends on the procedure, pain level, and patient tolerance. A combination of topical, injectable, and inhalation options can optimise comfort while ensuring safety.

NERVES OF THE FACE – ANATOMY AND ANAESTHETIC BLOCKS

1. NERVES OF THE FACE (SENSORY)

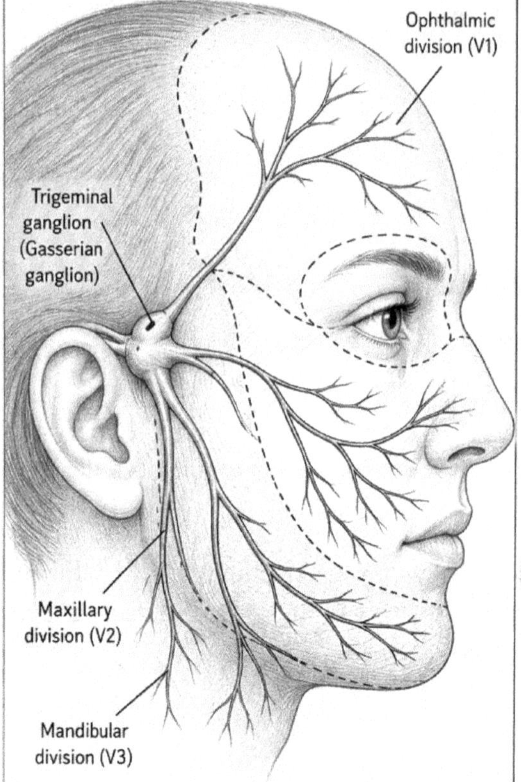

V1 Ophthalmic – Forehead, scalp (anterior), upper eyelid, dorsum of nose

V2 Maxillary – Midface, lower eyelid, side of nose, upper lip, cheek, upper teeth/gums

V3 Mandibular – Lower face, lower lip, chin, jaw, lower teeth/gums, part of ear/temple

CLINICAL NOTES

- Use aspirating syringe to avoid intravascular injection.
- Inject 0.5–1.0 ml of local anaesthetic slowly at each site.
- Bilateral blocks may be required for midline procedures.
- Always respect anatomical landmarks and avoid excessive depth.

2. ANAESTHETIC INJECTION SITES AND AREAS NUMBED

A. SUPRAORBITAL NERVE BLOCK (V1)

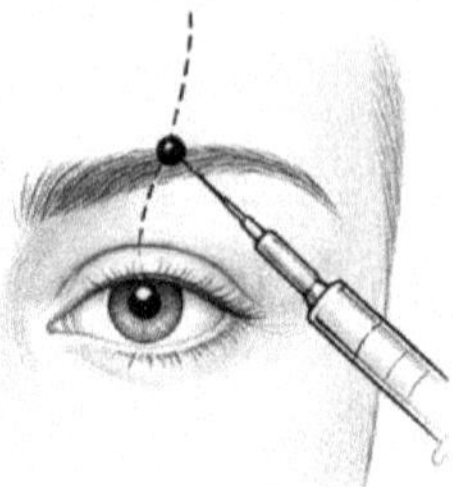

Injection site:
At supraorbital notch/foramen (approximately in line with the pupil, just above the orbital rim).

Numbs:
Forehead, scalp (anterior), upper eyelid.

B. INFRAORBITAL NERVE BLOCK (V2)

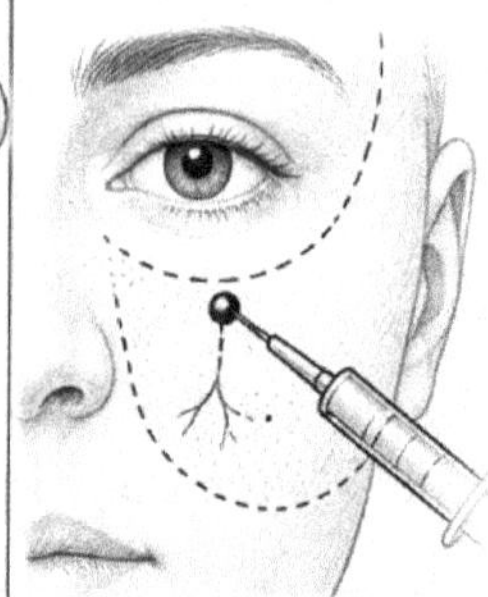

Injection site:
At infraorbital foramen (approximately 1 cm below the infraorbital margin, in line with the pupil).

Numbs:
Lower eyelid, side of nose, upper lip, cheek, upper teeth and gums.

C. MENTAL NERVE BLOCK (V3)

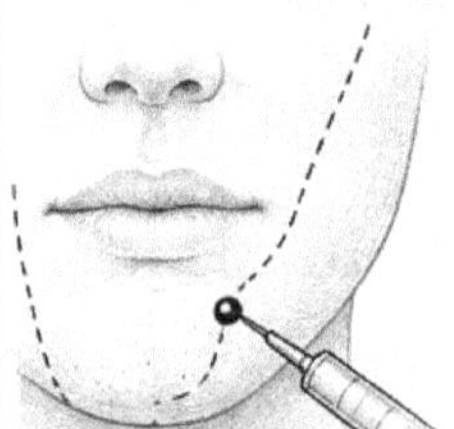

Injection site:
At mental foramen (approximately in line with the premolar teeth, on the lower border of the mandible).

Numbs:
Lower lip, chin, lower teeth and gums.

3. SUMMARY TABLE

NERVE (BRANCH)	INJECTION SITE (LANDMARK)	AREA NUMBED
Supraorbital nerve (V1)	Supraorbital notch/ foramen (above the orbital rim, in line with the pupil)	Forehead, scalp (anterior), upper eyelid
Infraorbital nerve (V2)	Infraorbital foramen (1 cm below infraorbital margin, in line with the pupil)	Lower eyelid, side of nose, upper lip, cheek, upper teeth and gums
Mental nerve (V3)	Mental foramen (in line with premolar teeth, on the lower border of mandible)	Lower lip, chin, lower teeth and gums

Chapter 62: Bruising & Cosmetic Procedures: What to Expect & How to Manage It

Bruising is a common side effect after injectable treatments, especially in delicate areas like the lips, under-eyes, and forehead. While not everyone bruises, certain factors increase the risk. Here's how to minimize, treat, and camouflage bruises effectively.

Am I Going to Bruise?

Risk Factors for Bruising:

• Thin or fragile skin (more common in mature skin)

• Use of blood thinners (aspirin, ibuprofen, fish oil, alcohol, etc.)

• History of easy bruising or bleeding disorders

• Highly vascular areas (e.g., lips and under-eyes)

• Aggressive injection technique (needle vs. cannula)

If you're prone to bruising, let your injector know beforehand!

What to Stop Using Before Treatment (Prevention Tips)

Avoid These for at Least 5-7 Days Before Treatment:

• Blood Thinners & NSAIDs (Aspirin, Ibuprofen, Naproxen)

• Alcohol (Increases blood vessel dilation)

• Omega-3 Supplements (Fish oil, flaxseed oil)

• Vitamin E & Herbal Supplements (Ginkgo, Garlic, Ginseng, St. John's Wort)

• Caffeine (Reduces platelet function)

Consider Taking Before Treatment:

• Arnica Tablets or Gel – Helps minimize bruising & swelling

• Bromelain (Pineapple Enzyme) – Anti-inflammatory properties

How to Prevent Bruising on the Day of Treatment

Hydrate well & eat before your appointment (to stabilize blood sugar)

Avoid strenuous exercise before & after

Apply ice packs immediately post-treatment

Use a cannula where possible (less trauma to blood vessels)

How to Treat Bruises (Post-Treatment Care)

First 24 Hours:

• Cold Compress (10 min on, 10 min off) – Reduces swelling & bleeding under the skin

• Avoid touching or massageing the area (unless instructed)

• Keep your head elevated (reduces blood pooling)

After 48 Hours:

• Warm Compresses – Improves circulation & speeds up healing

• Arnica Gel or Cream – Apply directly to bruised areas

• Bromelain Supplements – Continue to help with inflammation

• Vitamin K Cream – Strengthens capillaries & fades bruises

How to Camouflage a Bruise with Makeup

Step-by-Step Concealing Process:

Apply Lipstick/Color Corrector First

• For Purple/Blue Bruises: Use red or orange-toned lipstick

• For Green/Yellow Bruises: Use peach or salmon tones

Set with Translucent Powder

• Prevents smudging & ensures longevity

Apply Full-Coverage Concealer/Foundation

• Use a thick, high-pigment concealer like Dermablend or Kryolan

Final Setting Powder or Spray

• Camouflage powder locks in coverage for the day

Iron Staining (Hemosiderin Staining) from Bruising Around the Eyes: Causes & Treatment

Iron staining, also known as hemosiderin staining, occurs when red blood cells break down after a bruise, leaving iron deposits in the skin. This can result in persistent yellow-brown or grayish discoloration, particularly around the under-eyes, where the skin is thin and prone to pigmentation issues.

Why Does Iron Staining Happen?

Occurs when blood leaks into tissues from damaged capillaries

Hemosiderin (iron-containing pigment) is left behind as the body breaks down the bruise

More common in individuals with fair or thin skin

Can be prolonged if poor circulation slows clearance

How to Treat Iron Staining Around the Eyes

Key Approach: Break down iron deposits, improve circulation, and speed up cell turnover.

Topical Treatments to Fade Staining

Vitamin C Serum – Antioxidant properties help brighten the skin and reduce discoloration (e.g., Skinceuticals C E Ferulic, Medik8 C-Tetra).

Iron-Chelating Creams (Lactoferrin or EDTA-based) – Help remove iron buildup in the skin (e.g., iS Clinical C Eye Serum, Dermaceutic Mela Cream).

Retinol (Vitamin A) or Peptides – Stimulates collagen renewal and fades pigmentation (e.g., Medik8 Crystal Retinal, SkinCeuticals A.G.E. Eye Complex).

Arnica & Bromelain Creams – Reduce inflammation & improve circulation (e.g., Arnicare Gel, Auriderm XO Cream).

AMERIGEL Care Lotion with Oakin® (oak extract) has been shown to help resolve Hemosiderin Staining through its unique formulation. The Care Lotion's fast absorbing formulation penetrates through the outer layers of skin allowing the oak extract to bond with the accumulated Iron deposits, helping the body to break down and naturally reabsorb the smaller iron particles. This process continues with every application of AMERIGEL Care Lotion until the deposits have been fully dissolved.

In-Clinic Treatments for Faster Results

Q-Switched or Picosecond Laser – Targets hemosiderin pigment directly to break it down.

Chemical Peels (Low Strength TCA, Mandelic, or Lactic Acid) – Speeds up skin cell turnover and fades staining.

Microneedling with PRP or Vitamin C Infusion – Stimulates collagen remodeling and reduces stubborn pigmentation.

At-Home Skincare Routine for Long-Term Improvement

Daily SPF 50+ (Essential!) – Prevents further pigmentation (e.g., ISDIN Eryfotona Ageless, EltaMD UV Clear).

Hydration & Lymphatic Drainage Massage – Improves circulation, reducing stagnant pigmentation.

Healthy Diet (Iron-Rich Foods + Vitamin C) – Supports blood vessel health & skin regeneration.

How Long Does Iron Staining Last?

Mild cases: Fades within a few weeks with proper skincare.

Moderate cases: Can persist for months without intervention.

Severe cases: May require laser or professional treatments to fully resolve.

Final Thoughts

Iron staining after bruising is stubborn but treatable.

Early intervention with Vitamin C, retinol, and gentle exfoliation helps speed up recovery.

If discoloration persists beyond 3 months, consider laser or peels for faster resolution.

Chapter 63: Dangers of Injectables: Understanding Vascular Occlusion and Its Risks

Injectable treatments such as dermal fillers can provide beautiful, natural-looking results when performed by a skilled injector. However, like any medical procedure, there are risks, with vascular occlusion (VO) being one of the most serious. A vascular occlusion occurs when filler accidentally enters or compresses a blood vessel, blocking blood flow to the surrounding tissues. If untreated, this can lead to necrosis (tissue death) or, in rare cases, blindness.

Blindness (Rare but Serious Complication)

If filler is injected into a blood vessel that supplies the eye (such as the supratrochlear or ophthalmic artery), it can cause sudden blindness. There is no current medical treatment to reverse filler-induced blindness, making prevention and immediate action critical.

Ophthalmic Artery Occlusion (Filler Blindness)

Emergency Recognition and Immediate Management

Filler-induced blindness is one of the most devastating complications in aesthetic medicine. It occurs when filler enters a facial artery and travels retrograde into the ophthalmic circulation, obstructing blood flow to the retina or optic nerve.

Visual loss can occur within seconds and should be treated as a **medical emergency**.

Recognising Ophthalmic Occlusion

Symptoms usually occur immediately or within minutes of injection.

Visual Symptoms

- Sudden loss of vision, Blurred vision, Partial visual field loss
- "Curtain coming down" effect, Flashes of light, Double vision, Eye pain

Clinical Signs

- Ptosis (drooping eyelid), Fixed or dilated pupil, Ophthalmoplegia
- Reduced visual acuity, Relative afferent pupillary defect

Associated Skin Signs

May occur with: Glabellar occlusion, Forehead occlusion, Nasal occlusion, Temple occlusion

Look for:

- Blanching, Livedo reticularis, Dusky skin

Areas Most Commonly Associated with Blindness

Highest Risk Areas

Glabella, Nose , Forehead, Temple

These areas communicate directly with the ophthalmic circulation through:

- Supratrochlear artery, Supraorbital artery, Dorsal nasal artery, Angular artery

Immediate Management Protocol

Step 1 – STOP

Stop injecting immediately.

Record: Time of onset, Vision changes, Pupil response, Ocular motility, Visual acuity

Document everything.

Step 2 – Call for Help

Activate emergency pathways immediately.

Contact:

- Ophthalmologist, Emergency Department
- Stroke team according to local protocols

Do not adopt a "wait and see" approach.

Step 3 – Begin High-Dose Hyaluronidase

Recent Australian ophthalmology guidance increasingly supports aggressive bedside reperfusion attempts.

Suggested Protocol

Inject: **1500 IU Hyaluronidase**

into: Supratrochlear foramen, Supraorbital foramen

Flood the suspected arterial territory.

Repeat every: **10–15 minutes**

for at least: **4 cycles**

or until improvement occurs.

Step 4 – Ocular Massage

Firm intermittent ocular massage.

Suggested: 5–15 seconds compression, Repeated cycles

May help dislodge embolic material.

Step 5 – Lower Intraocular Pressure

Where appropriate and available:

Timolol 0.5%

One drop in affected eye.

Acetazolamide

500 mg orally or intravenously.

These measures attempt to improve retinal perfusion.

Step 6 – Transfer Urgently

Transfer urgently to a centre capable of:

- Ophthalmology review, CT brain
- CT angiography, Orbital imaging

Imaging should not delay treatment.

Retrobulbar Hyaluronidase

Current Australian recommendations indicate:

Retrobulbar hyaluronidase should only be performed by appropriately trained medically qualified clinicians experienced in orbital procedures.

It is **not** considered a first-line bedside treatment for most injectors.

What Should Be in Every Filler Blindness Crash Kit?

Drugs

- Hyaluronidase (minimum 6 vials), Timolol 0.5%, Acetazolamide 500 mg, Normal saline

Equipment

- Visual acuity chart, Penlight, Occluder card, 27G needles, 25G cannulas
- Emergency contact list, Printed blindness protocol

The First 15 Minutes

1. Stop treatment.
2. Assess vision.

3. Assess pupils.
4. Assess ocular movements.
5. Activate emergency referral.
6. Begin supratrochlear/supraorbital hyaluronidase.
7. Perform ocular massage.
8. Repeat hyaluronidase every 10–15 minutes.
9. Lower intraocular pressure if appropriate.
10. Transfer urgently.

Clinical Pearl

The supratrochlear and supraorbital foramina have become important bedside landmarks in current Australian protocols because they provide direct access to vessels supplying the ophthalmic circulation. Every injector should know how to locate these landmarks before they ever encounter a vascular emergency.

Warning

No protocol has been proven to reliably reverse filler-induced blindness. Prevention remains the most effective treatment.

The safest injector is not the one who knows how to manage blindness—the safest injector is the one who understands anatomy well enough to avoid causing it.

Stroke (Extremely Rare but Possible)

If filler enters the brains blood supply, it could cause neurological damage.

Signs of a Vascular Occlusion (VO)

Immediate Signs (During or Immediately After Injection):

Blanching (White or Gray Skin) " Lack of blood flow makes the skin look pale, gray, or mottled in the affected area.

No Blood Return When Pressing (Capillary Refill Delay) When pressing on the skin, it does not turn pink again within 2-3 seconds.

Sudden, Severe Pain Patients often describe it as a burning, intense pain that worsens over time.

Cold Skin Temperature . The skin may feel unusually cold compared to surrounding areas.

Signs of Necrosis (Hours to Days After Injection):

Increasing Pain and Skin Darkening The area may turn dusky, purple, or black as tissue begins to die.

Blistering or Ulceration . If untreated, the skin may form blisters and break down, leading to permanent scarring.

Delayed Wound Healing or Open Wounds .If tissue necrosis progresses, open wounds and deep scarring can develop.

What to Do If You Have These Signs?

1. Seek Immediate Help From Your Injector

Contact your injector IMMEDIATELY if you experience pain, blanching, or delayed capillary refill.

2. Apply a Warm Compress (NOT Ice)

Warmth helps dilate blood vessels and improve circulation.

Avoid ice, as it can further constrict blood flow.

3. Massage the Area Firmly (If Advised by a Professional)

Sometimes, gentle massage may help disperse the filler if the occlusion is caused by compression rather than direct arterial blockage.

4. Take Aspirin (If Advised by Your Practitioner)

Aspirin can thin the blood and improve circulation in partially blocked vessels. Only take if recommended by your injector.

How a Practitioner Will Treat a Vascular Occlusion

1. Hyaluronidase (Hyalase) Injections If an occlusion is caused by hyaluronic acid (HA) fillers, your practitioner will immediately inject hyaluronidase to dissolve the filler and restore blood flow.

2. High-Dose Hyaluronidase Repeated Every Hour (If Needed) The dose and frequency depend on the severity of the occlusion.

3. Nitroglycerin (GTN) Creams May be applied to help dilate blood vessels.

4. Oxygen Therapy (Hyperbaric Oxygen, If Available. Helps deliver oxygen to tissues at risk of necrosis.

5. Blood Thinners (If Necessary) Low-dose aspirin or anticoagulants may be used to improve circulation.

6. Follow-Up Monitoring :The practitioner will check the area for several days to ensure recovery and prevent long-term damage.

Preventing Vascular Occlusions : What Skilled Injectors Do

Knowledge of Facial Vascular Anatomy A skilled injector understands where major arteries are located and avoids high-risk areas.

Aspiration Before Injection Pulling back on the syringe before injecting can sometimes detect if a blood vessel has been entered.

Slow Injection Technique Injecting filler slowly reduces pressure and the risk of arterial blockage.

Using Cannulas in High-Risk Areas Cannulas reduce the risk of vascular occlusion because they bluntly push vessels aside instead of penetrating them.

Using the Correct Type of Filler Some fillers are more cohesive and less likely to spread into vessels.

Conclusion: Taking Occlusions Seriously

Vascular occlusions are rare but serious and can lead to skin necrosis or blindness if untreated.

Early signs include blanching, severe pain, and delayed capillary refill.

Immediate action is critical, including seeking an experienced injector, applying warmth, and using hyaluronidase for HA fillers.

Choosing a highly skilled, medically trained injector significantly reduces risks.

The best treatment for a vascular occlusion is prevention and early recognition. Knowing the signs can save your skin and vision.

FACIAL VASCULATURE CONNECTED TO THE OPHTHALMIC ARTERY

The facial arteries have connections to the ophthalmic artery through tiny anastomoses around the orbit. Injections in these areas can lead to retrograde flow of filler into the ophthalmic artery and may cause blindness.

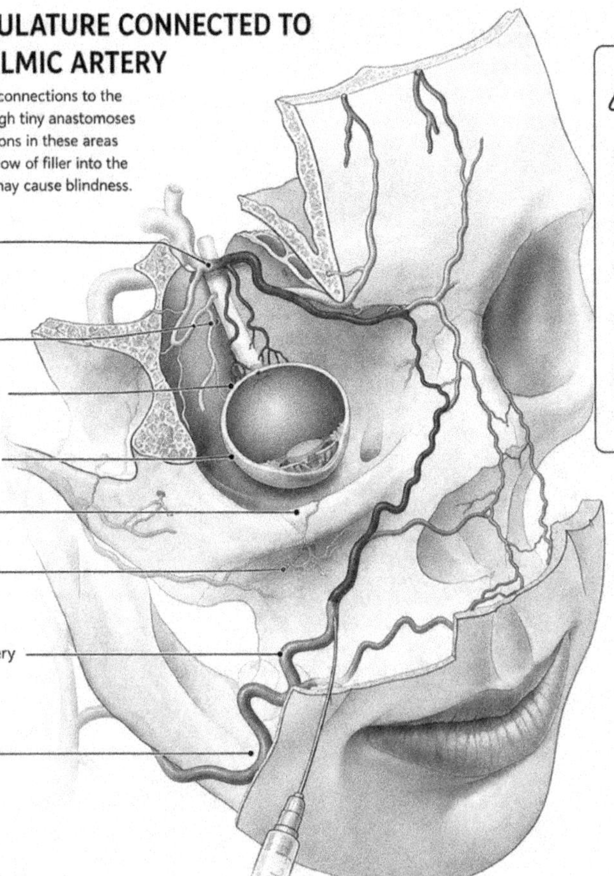

THE RISK: HOW INJECTIONS CAN CAUSE BLINDNESS

If filler or other injectable material is accidentally injected into a facial artery, it can travel backward (retrograde) through connections (anastomoses) to the ophthalmic artery.

↓

The material can then enter the **central retinal artery**, blocking blood flow to the retina and causing sudden, permanent blindness.

THE PATHWAY: HOW INJECTIONS CAN LEAD TO BLINDNESS

1 Injection into Facial Artery

Filler is accidentally injected into a facial artery (e.g., angular or superior labial artery).

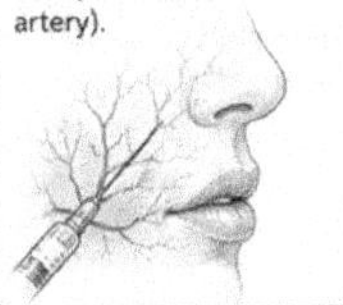

→

2 Retrograde Flow

The filler travels backward through an anastomosis to the ophthalmic artery.

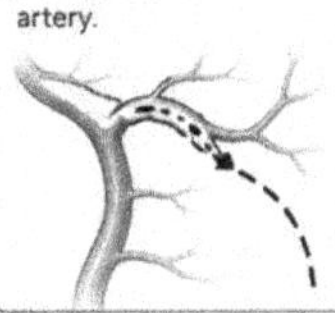

→

3 Entry into Ophthalmic Artery

The filler continues into the ophthalmic artery.

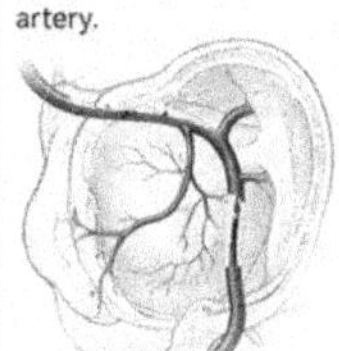

→

4 Central Retinal Artery Occlusion

The filler blocks the central retinal artery, cutting off blood supply to the retina.

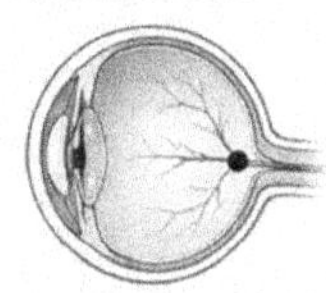

→

5 Sudden, Permanent Blindness

Retinal ischemia occurs, leading to irreversible vision loss.

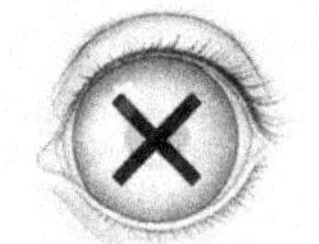

FOREHEAD VASCULAR OCCLUSION

CASE ANALYSIS

BEFORE

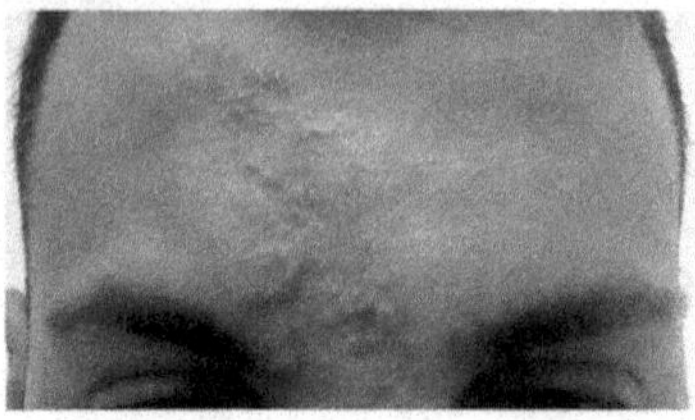

AFTER (3 MONTHS)

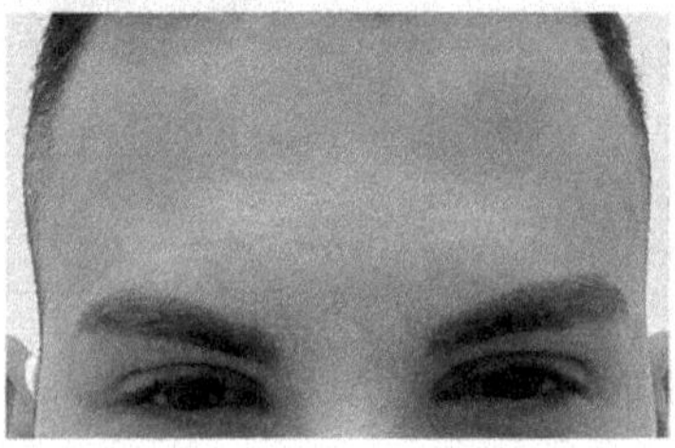

WHICH ARTERY WAS AFFECTED?

Most likely: SUPRAORBITAL ARTERY (branch of the ophthalmic artery).

The pattern of ischemia, inflammation and subsequent scarring is classic for occlusion of the supratrochlear/ supraorbital vascular plexus.

Rationale:

- Central upper forehead involvement (midline to paramedian)
- Significant initial inflammation
- Risk area supplied by supratrochlear and supraorbital arteries
- High anastomotic connection to the ophthalmic circulation → risk of visual complications

Likely scenario:

Inadvertent intra-arterial injection or compression of the supratrochlear or supraorbital artery leading to retrograde filler embolization and cutaneous ischemia.

ARTERIAL SUPPLY OF THE FOREHEAD
(Anterior View)

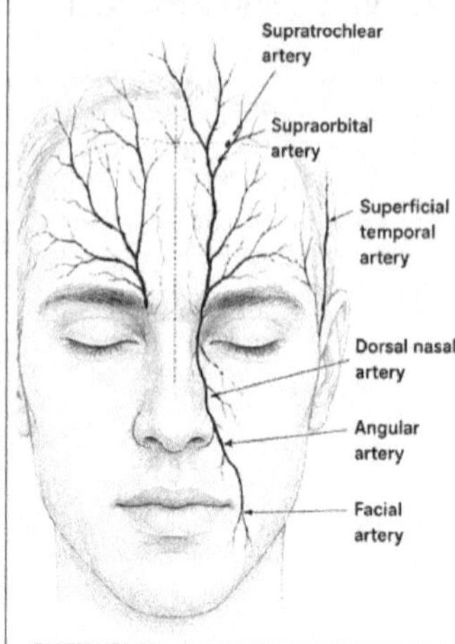

The supratrochlear and supraorbital arteries anastomose with branches of the superficial temporal artery laterally and with the dorsal nasal and angular arteries medially.

FOREHEAD GÄCKEL (GABELA) VESSELS

The glabellar region has a rich subdermal vascular network with extensive anastomoses.

Key Vessels:

- Supratrochlear arteries (medial superior)
- Supraorbital arteries (lateral superior)
- Dorsal nasal artery (midline inferior)
- Angular arteries (medial inferior)
- Superficial temporal artery (lateral)

These vessels form a dangerous anastomotic plexus, allowing:

- **Retrograde flow to the ophthalmic artery**
- Potential embolization to the central retinal artery → blindness

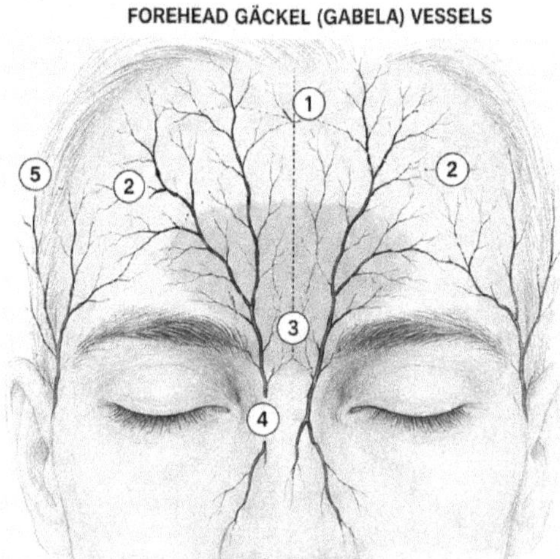

KEY

1. Supratrochlear arteries
2. Supraorbital arteries
3. Dorsal nasal artery
4. Angular arteries
5. Superficial temporal artery

High-risk glabellar zone (danger triangle)

Injections in this zone carry high risk of vascular occlusion and visual loss.

SIGNS OF FOREHEAD VASCULAR OCCLUSION

- Immediate severe pain
- Blanching / pallor
- Mottling or livedo reticularis
- Delayed capillary refill
- Burning or throbbing sensation
- Potential progression to necrosis
- Visual changes (if embolization occurs): blurred vision, loss of vision, eye pain

MANAGEMENT (IMMEDIATE)

1. Stop injection immediately
2. Aspirate if possible
3. Hyaluronidase – high dose, multiple sites
4. Warm compresses
5. Massage gently
6. Consider aspirin (if not contraindicated)
7. Nitroglycerin paste (2%)
8. Monitor closely
9. Urgent ophthalmology referral if any visual symptoms

PRACTICE PEARLS

- Avoid deep bolus injections in the glabella and upper forehead.
- Use small aliquots, low pressure, and aspirate.
- Stay superficial in the central forehead.
- Understand the vascular map – this area is NOT safe.
- When in doubt – don't inject.

THE FOREHEAD AND GLABELLA ARE HIGH-RISK ZONES DUE TO DENSE VASCULAR ANASTOMOSES AND CONNECTIONS TO THE OPHTHALMIC CIRCULATION.

Anatomy knowledge, caution and technique prevent devastating complications.

Temple Vascular Occlusion – Recognition and Management

The temple is one of the most anatomically complex and potentially dangerous areas of the face to inject. While temple augmentation can restore youthful contours and improve facial harmony, injectors must have a thorough understanding of the vascular anatomy to minimise the risk of vascular occlusion.

Although vascular occlusion in the temple is uncommon, it can have devastating consequences including skin necrosis, scalp necrosis, and blindness.

Why Is the Temple a High-Risk Area?

Several important arteries pass through the temple and communicate with vessels supplying the eye.

These include:

- Superficial Temporal Artery
- Frontal Branch of the Superficial Temporal Artery
- Parietal Branch of the Superficial Temporal Artery
- Middle Temporal Artery, Zygomatico-Orbital Artery, Sentinel Vein

The frontal branch is particularly important because it communicates with the supraorbital and supratrochlear vessels, which ultimately connect to the ophthalmic circulation.

This means filler inadvertently injected into a temporal artery may potentially travel retrograde toward the eye and then forward into the retinal circulation.

Key Temple Arteries

Superficial Temporal Artery

The superficial temporal artery is a terminal branch of the external carotid artery.

It emerges just in front of the ear and divides into:

Frontal Branch

Supplies: Forehead, Anterior scalp, Hairline

Occlusion may cause: Forehead blanching, Hairline pain, Scalp pain, Delayed scalp necrosis, Hair loss (alopecia)

Parietal Branch

Supplies: Lateral scalp, Temporal scalp

Occlusion may cause: Temporal scalp pain, Scalp blanching, Hair loss, Delayed scalp necrosis

Middle Temporal Artery

Located deeper within the temporal fascia.

Supplies: Temporal muscle, Deep temporal tissues

Occlusion may present with: Deep temporal pain, Pressure sensation, Local tissue compromise

Zygomatico-Orbital Artery

Travels toward the lateral orbital rim.

Potential symptoms include: Lateral orbital pain, Periorbital blanching, Visual disturbance if connected to ophthalmic circulation

Recognising Temple Vascular Occlusion

Immediate Signs

The earliest sign is usually:

Sudden Severe Pain

The patient may describe: Burning, Sharp pain, Pressure, Headache-like discomfort

Pain is often disproportionate to the injection.

Blanching

Look for: White patches, Mottled skin, Delayed capillary refill

Blanching may occur in: Temple, Forehead, Hairline, Scalp

Colour Changes

The skin may become: Pale, Dusky, Purple, Grey

Livedo reticularis may develop within minutes to hours.

Visual Symptoms

Any visual symptom is an emergency.

Symptoms include:

- Blurred vision, Loss of vision, Flashing lights, Curtain effect, Double vision

Stop treatment immediately and initiate emergency protocols.

Delayed Signs

Over the next 24–72 hours patients may develop:

- Increasing pain, Darkening skin, Crusting, Ulceration, Scalp tenderness, Hair loss

Alopecia can occur weeks later due to interruption of blood supply to hair follicles.

Which Artery Is Likely Affected?

Clinical Sign	Likely Vessel
Forehead blanching	Frontal branch of superficial temporal artery
Hairline pain	Frontal branch
Scalp pain and blanching	Parietal branch
Lateral orbital blanching	Zygomatico-orbital artery
Deep temple pain	Middle temporal artery
Visual symptoms	Communication with ophthalmic circulation

Temple Blindness Risk

The greatest fear with temple injection is inadvertent entry into a vessel communicating with the ophthalmic artery.

Warning signs include: Sudden visual loss, Eye pain, Ptosis, Ophthalmoplegia, Dilated pupil

Visual symptoms following filler injection should always be treated as an ophthalmic emergency.

Prevention

Temple treatments should be performed with meticulous anatomical knowledge.

Safety principles include:

✓ Slow injection, Small aliquots, Minimal pressure

✓ Constant movement if using a cannula, Awareness of superficial and deep vascular layers

✓ Knowledge of the danger zone around the sentinel vein, Careful patient monitoring throughout treatment

Clinical Pearl

One of the most overlooked signs of temple vascular compromise is **scalp pain**.

A patient complaining that "my scalp hurts when I touch my hair" following temple filler should raise immediate suspicion for involvement of the frontal or parietal branches of the superficial temporal artery. Early recognition may prevent scalp necrosis and permanent hair loss.

ARTERIES OF THE TEMPLE
(Right Side)

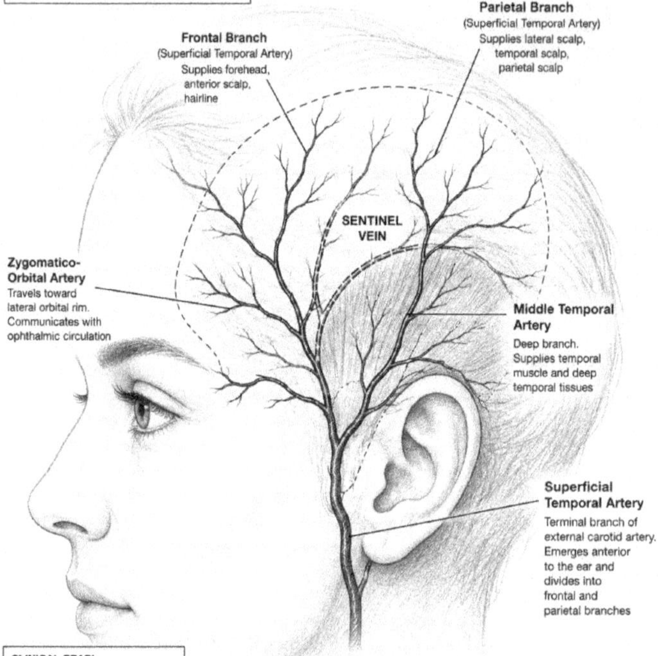

KEY ARTERIES

1. **Superficial Temporal Artery** Main artery that emerges anterior to the ear and divides into frontal and parietal branches.
2. **Frontal Branch (STA)** Supplies forehead, anterior scalp, and hairline.
3. **Parietal Branch (STA)** Supplies lateral scalp and temporal scalp.
4. **Middle Temporal Artery** Deep branch supplying temporal muscle and deep tissues.
5. **Zygomatico-Orbital Artery** Travels toward the lateral orbital rim and communicates with ophthalmic circulation.
6. **Sentinel Vein** Superficial vein that runs in the temporal region. Important landmark to avoid.

AREAS AT RISK IF ARTERY OCCLUDED

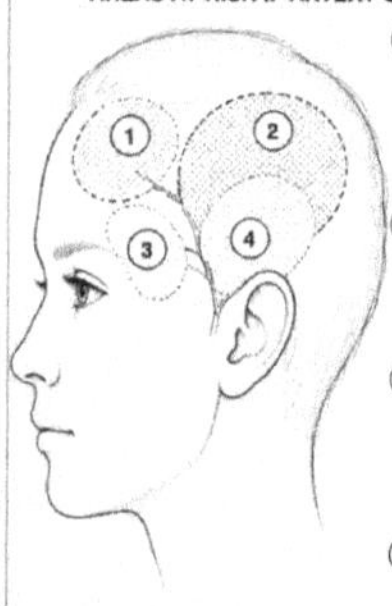

1. **Frontal branch occlusion** → Forehead blanching, hairline pain, scalp necrosis, hair loss
2. **Parietal branch occlusion** → Scalp pain, blanching, necrosis, hair loss
3. **Zygomatico-orbital artery occlusion** → Lateral orbital blanching, pain, potential visual risk
4. **Middle temporal artery occlusion** → Deep temple pain, tissue compromise

CLINICAL PEARL
Sudden severe pain during injection, blanching, or scalp tenderness are early signs of vascular compromise. Act immediately.

Always aspirate, inject slowly, use minimal pressure, small aliquots, and stay in the safest planes.

VASCULAR OCCLUSION FROM CHIN FILLER
Potential Impact on Tongue & Floor of Mouth

Chin filler can inadvertently enter arterial supply and cause retrograde embolization leading to ischemia and necrosis of the tongue and floor of mouth.

PATHWAYS OF OCCLUSION

1. Filler injected into the mental artery or inferior labial artery
2. Retrograde flow into the submental artery
3. Embolization into the submental and lingual arteries
   → occlusion of tongue and floor of mouth

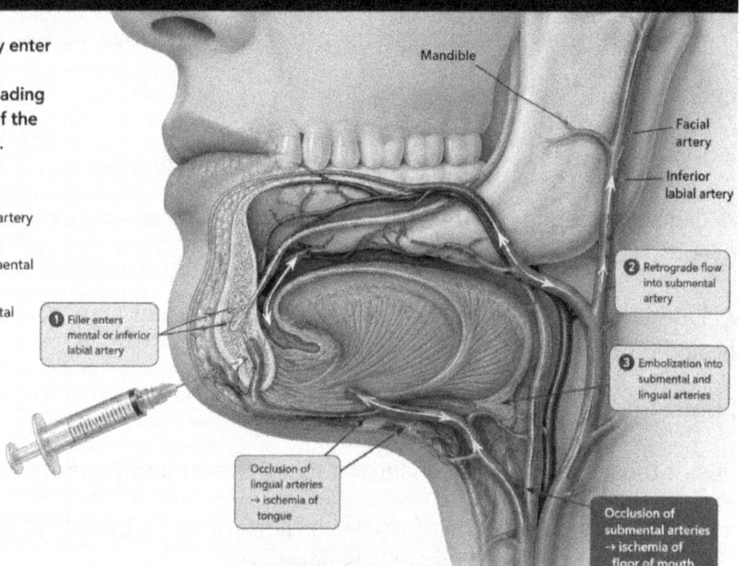

CLINICAL SIGNS
- Severe tongue pain, heaviness
- Swelling, discoloration (mottled, purple)
- Difficulty speaking or swallowing
- Floor of mouth swelling
- Potential necrosis if not treated immediately

RISK: TISSUE NECROSIS
Rapid recognition and treatment is critical to prevent permanent damage.

FACIAL SAFETY ZONES MAP

VASCULAR RISK AREAS FOR FACIAL INJECTION

RISK LEVELS

HIGH RISK
Areas with dense vascular anastomoses and direct connections to the ophthalmic circulation.

MODERATE RISK
Areas with significant arterial branches. Use caution.

CAUTION
Thin skin, proximity to important vessels. Higher risk if injected incorrectly or too deeply.

RELATIVELY SAFER
Areas with fewer large vessels and safer planes when proper technique is used.

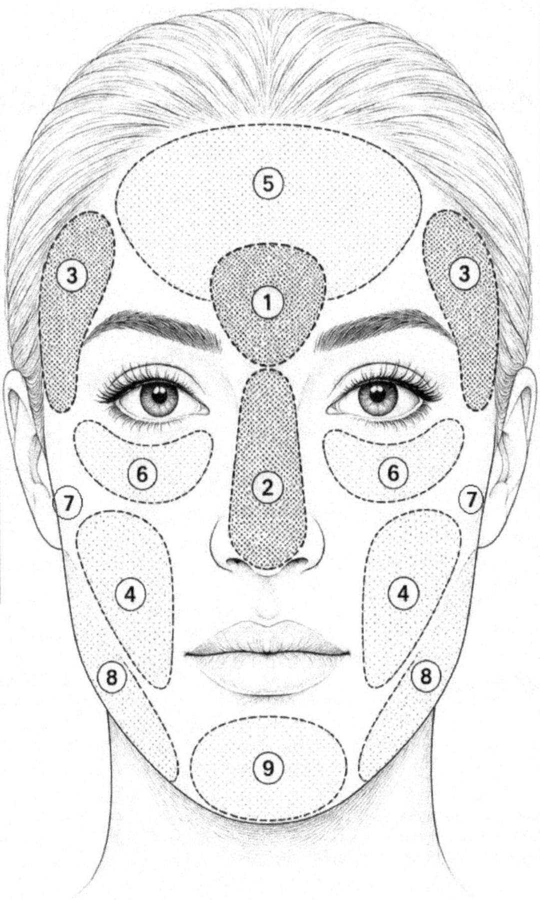

RISK ZONES LEGEND

1. **GLABELLA**
   Very high risk of vascular occlusion. Rich anastomoses with supraorbital, supratrochlear and ophthalmic vessels.
2. **NOSE**
   Very high risk. Dorsal nasal, angular and lateral nasal arteries have direct connections to the ophthalmic circulation.
3. **TEMPLES**
   High risk. Superficial temporal artery branches communicate with the ophthalmic system.
4. **NASOLABIAL FOLDS**
   Moderate risk. Facial artery branches (angular, superior and inferior labial arteries). Use caution with depth and technique.
5. **FOREHEAD**
   Moderate risk. Supratrochlear and supraorbital arteries course in this area. Stay superficial.
6. **TEAR TROUGH**
   Caution. Thin skin and proximity to infraorbital vessels. High risk if injected incorrectly or too deeply.
7. **LATERAL CHEEKS**
   Relatively safer. Fewer large arteries. Use appropriate planes and technique.
8. **JAWLINE / PRE-JOWL**
   Relatively safer. Fewer major vessels laterally. Avoid facial artery as it crosses the anterior masseter.
9. **CHIN**
   Relatively safer. Avoid mental artery and labiomental crease. Inject on bone / periosteum with caution.
10. **NECK (NOT SHOWN)**
    High caution. Carotid artery, external jugular vein, and multiple branches. Only treat with advanced anatomy knowledge.

HIGH-RISK COMPLICATIONS

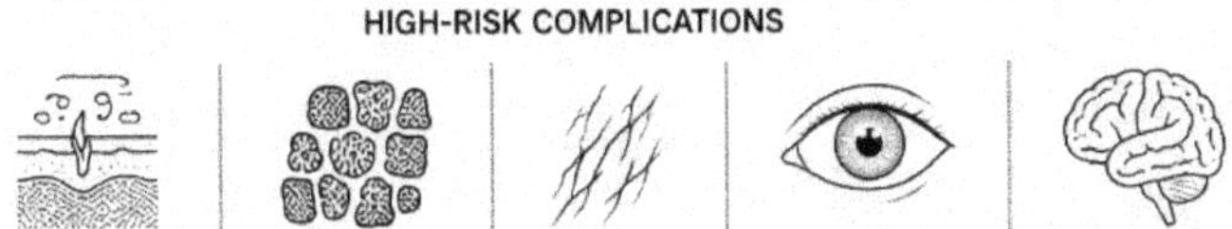

VASCULAR OCCLUSION | SKIN NECROSIS | SCARRING | VISUAL LOSS / BLINDNESS | STROKE (RARE)

KEY SAFETY PRINCIPLES

- Know your anatomy inside out.
- Aspirate before injecting with a needle.
- Use small aliquots (0.1 ml or less).
- Inject slowly with low pressure.
- Use cannula in high-risk areas when appropriate.
- Constantly monitor your patient.
- Stop immediately if pain, blanching or visual changes occur.
- When in doubt – don't inject.
- Treat complications immediately.

EARLY WARNING SIGNS

- Sudden severe pain
- Blanching / pallor
- Mottling or livedo
- Delayed capillary refill
- Burning or throbbing
- Visual changes

THERE ARE NO COMPLETELY "SAFE" AREAS.
Every injection carries risk. Your knowledge, technique, judgment and respect for anatomy protect your patients.

SAFETY FIRST
Anatomy • Technique • Respect
that's what keeps your patient safe.

CANNULA VS NEEDLE PLANES

KNOW THE PLANES. RESPECT THE ANATOMY. MAXIMIZE SAFETY.

Both needles and cannulas have a place in aesthetic medicine. Understanding their differences, ideal planes, and tissue behavior is key to safe and predictable results.

NEEDLE
POINT IN – POINT OUT

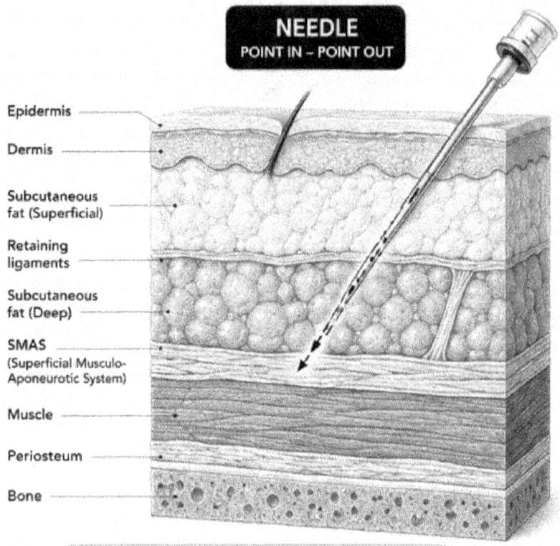

- Sharp tip creates an entry and exit point
- Higher risk of intravascular injection and bruising
- Best for precise, small-volume, or fibrous areas
- More trauma to tissues and vessels

CANNULA
BLUNT TIP – SIDE PORT

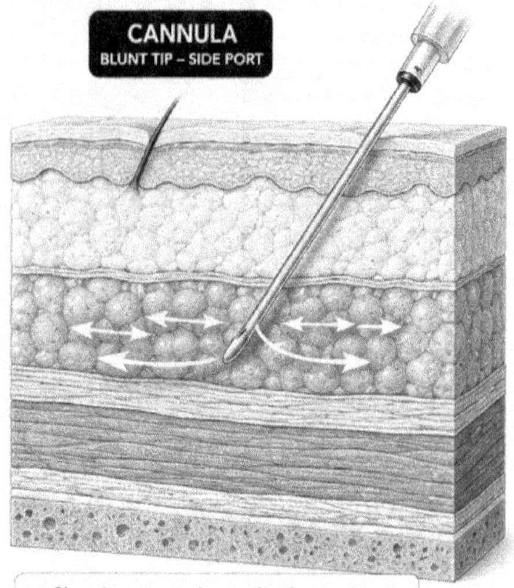

- Blunt tip separates tissue rather than cutting
- Lower risk of vascular injury and bruising
- Ideal for larger areas and volume distribution
- Fewer entry points, less trauma, more comfort

WHERE EACH IS BEST USED

NEEDLE – Best For:

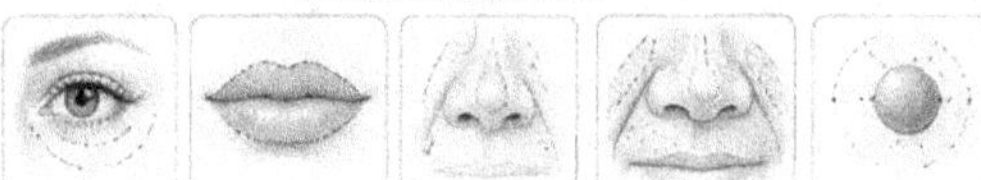

Tear trough (fine, precise placement) · Lip borders & definition · Superficial lines (Perioral, fine wrinkles) · Fibrous areas (nasolabial fold, marionette lines) · Small-volume precision placement

CANNULA – Best For:

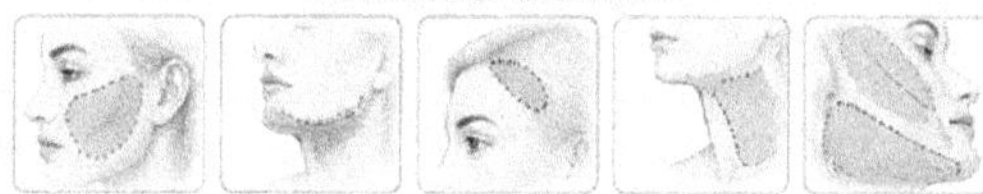

Cheeks (Volume & lift) · Jawline (Contour & definition) · Temples (Volume restoration) · Neck (Contour & lines) · Large areas (General volume distribution)

PLANES OF INJECTION: WHERE TO PLACE PRODUCT

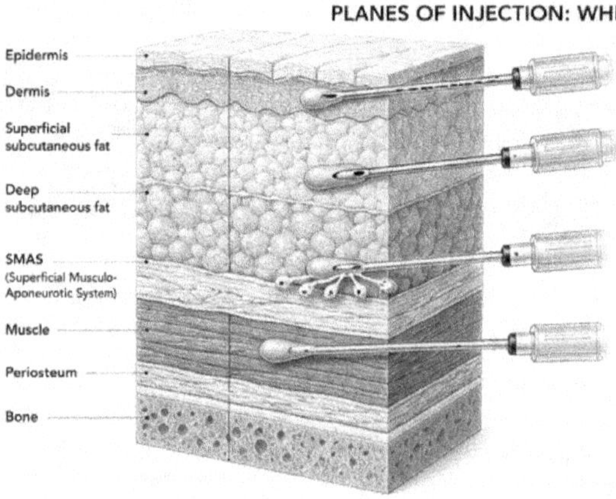

PLANE	DEPTH	BEST FOR	INSTRUMENT
INTRADERMAL / SUPERFICIAL DERMIS	0–1 mm	Skin quality, fine lines, microdroplets, hydration	NEEDLE (30–32G)
SUPERFICIAL SUBCUTANEOUS FAT	1–3 mm	Fine lines, texture, superficial volume	NEEDLE (30–27G)
DEEP SUBCUTANEOUS FAT	3–10 mm	Cheeks, midface volume, soft tissue augmentation	CANNULA (25G–22G)
SUB-SMAS PLANE	Deep to SMAS	Lift, structural support, jawline, chin	CANNULA (25G – 19G)
SUPRAPERIOSTEAL (OVER BONE)	On bone	Chin, jawline, temples (bony scaffold support)	NEEDLE or CANNULA*

*Cannula can be used on bone with caution and only with appropriate technique.

FACIAL ARTERIES – LAYER BY LAYER

UNDERSTANDING VASCULAR DEPTH FOR SAFER INJECTION

1. DEEP LAYER
(DEEP TO MUSCLE)

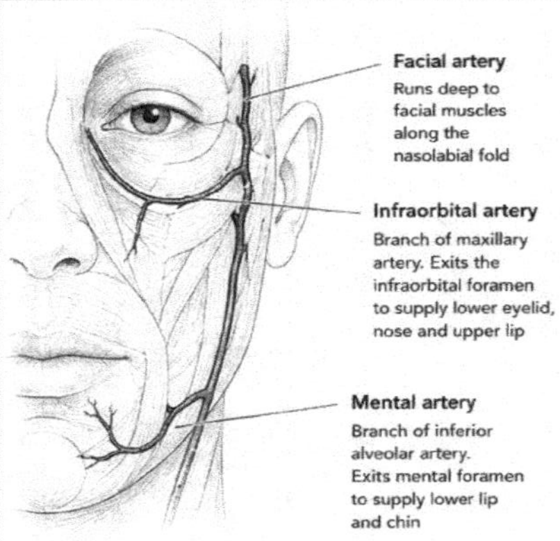

KEY ARTERIES (DEEP LAYER)

- Facial artery
- Infraorbital artery
- Mental artery

CLINICAL RELEVANCE

- Deep injections near the nasolabial fold, nose and chin carry risk due to proximity to major arterial trunks.
- Retrograde flow can lead to occlusion of ophthalmic circulation and blindness.

2. MID LAYER
(WITHIN MUSCLE / SUPERFICIAL TO MUSCLE)

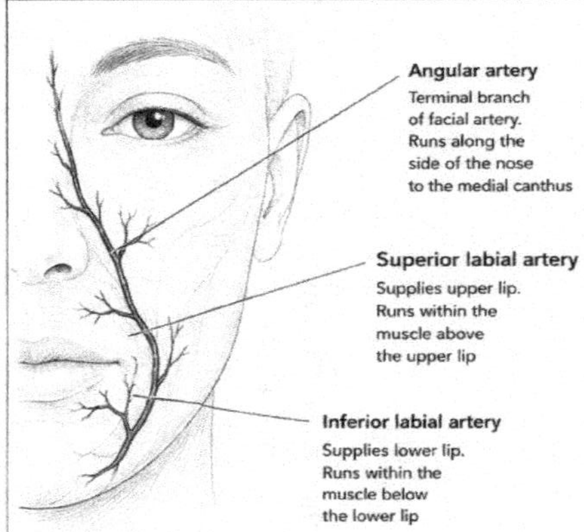

KEY ARTERIES (MID LAYER)

- Angular artery
- Superior labial artery
- Inferior labial artery

CLINICAL RELEVANCE

- Mid-layer bolus injections in the perioral and nasal areas can compromise arterial branches.
- High risk of skin necrosis of lips, nose and medial cheek.

3. SUPERFICIAL LAYER
(SUPERFICIAL TO MUSCLE)

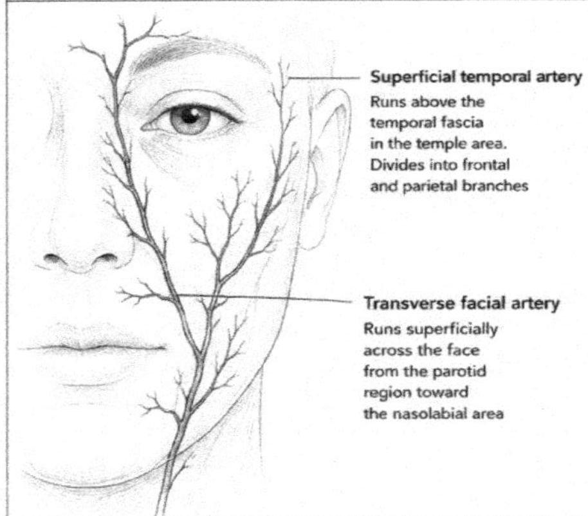

KEY ARTERIES (SUPERFICIAL LAYER)

- Superficial temporal artery
- Transverse facial artery

CLINICAL RELEVANCE

- Superficial injections in the temple and lateral face can occlude these vessels.
- Risk of skin necrosis, alopecia and poor healing.

WHY DEPTH MATTERS

The same injection placed at different depths can carry very different risks. Know the layers. Respect the anatomy. Inject with knowledge and caution.

GENERAL SAFETY PRINCIPLES

- Aspirate
- Use small aliquots
- Inject slowly with low pressure
- Constantly monitor
- STOP — Stop immediately if pain or blanching

Chapter 64: Lumps, Nodules, Granulomas and Biofilms

Not Every Lump Is a Granuloma

One of the most common reasons patients return to a clinic after having injectable treatments is because they have discovered a lump.

Naturally, this can cause anxiety.

The patient immediately assumes something has gone wrong, while the injector begins running through a list of possible causes.

Is it filler?

Is it collagen?

Is it inflammation?

Is it infection?

The truth is that not all lumps are created equal.

Over the years, I have heard many injectors, patients, and even practitioners use the terms lump, nodule, granuloma and biofilm interchangeably. In reality, these are very different conditions with different causes and different management strategies.

Understanding the difference is one of the most important skills an injector can develop.

The first step is not treatment. The first step is diagnosis.

Simple Lumps

The most straightforward explanation is often the correct one.

Sometimes a lump is simply product that can be seen or felt beneath the skin.

This may occur because too much product was placed in one location, the filler was injected too superficially, the patient has particularly thin skin, or the product has not yet integrated into the surrounding tissues.

These lumps are usually soft, painless and non-inflammatory.

The skin appears normal and the patient often notices them within days or weeks of treatment.

In many cases they improve with time as the product settles and integrates.

With hyaluronic acid fillers, they may also be related to migration or overcorrection.

Fortunately, these types of lumps are generally the easiest to manage.

Nodules

A nodule is different.

Nodules are typically firmer and more defined than simple lumps and may develop weeks, months or even years after treatment.

Some are completely non-inflammatory and simply represent concentrated product or collagen. Others become tender, swollen and inflamed.

When inflammation is present, the diagnosis becomes more complex.

The injector must consider delayed inflammatory reactions, infection, biofilm formation, foreign body responses and other causes.

This is where careful assessment becomes essential.

Not every firm lump is a granuloma.

In fact, true granulomas are relatively uncommon.

What Is a Granuloma?

A granuloma is a chronic inflammatory response created by the immune system.

When the body identifies a substance it cannot easily remove, it may attempt to isolate it by surrounding it with specialised inflammatory cells.

This process creates what is known as a granuloma.

True granulomas are rare and often overdiagnosed.

Historically, many delayed lumps were labelled granulomas when they were actually inflammatory nodules, localised collagen deposits or biofilm-related reactions.

The distinction matters because the treatment approach may be very different.

A granuloma is not simply a lump.

It is a specific immune response.

The Sculptra Story

No discussion about granulomas would be complete without talking about Sculptra.

For many years, Sculptra developed a reputation for causing granulomas.

Even today, some injectors remain hesitant to use it because of stories they heard during the early years of its introduction.

The reality is far more nuanced.

Sculptra is not a traditional filler. It is a collagen stimulator composed of Poly-L-Lactic Acid (PLLA) particles suspended in sterile water.

Unlike hyaluronic acid fillers that create immediate volume, Sculptra works by stimulating the body's own collagen production over time.

When it first entered the aesthetic market, practitioners were still learning how to use it effectively.

Early treatment protocols frequently involved lower dilution volumes and shorter reconstitution times than we commonly use today. Injection techniques were also evolving.

As a result, PLLA particles could occasionally cluster together rather than being dispersed evenly throughout the tissue.

When collagen subsequently formed around these concentrated pockets of particles, patients sometimes developed palpable lumps.

Many of these lumps were labelled granulomas.

As our understanding improved, it became clear that many were not true granulomas at all.

Instead, they were often areas of localised collagen production, product aggregation or inflammatory nodules caused by uneven particle distribution.

In other words, the body's collagen-building response had become concentrated in one area rather than being spread evenly through the tissue.

This understanding changed the way practitioners approached treatment.

Dilution protocols increased.

Reconstitution times became longer.

Injection techniques improved.

Patient selection improved.

And perhaps most famously, massage became part of routine aftercare.

Many injectors still teach the traditional Rule of 5s:

Massage for 5 minutes

5 times per day

For 5 days

The goal is simple: to encourage even particle distribution and minimise the risk of localised collagen accumulation.

Today's Sculptra treatments bear little resemblance to those performed twenty years ago.

Modern protocols often use significantly larger dilution volumes with the addition of lidocaine for patient comfort. Combined with improved training and greater understanding of facial anatomy, the incidence of nodules has reduced dramatically.

In my own experience, Sculptra remains one of the most rewarding treatments in aesthetic medicine when used correctly.

The lesson is not that Sculptra caused problems.

The lesson is that technique matters.

Many complications that become associated with products are often complications of placement, dilution, distribution and education rather than the product itself.

Biofilms

Biofilms are perhaps one of the most misunderstood complications in aesthetic medicine.

A biofilm occurs when bacteria form a protective community around themselves, creating a microscopic shield that makes them difficult for both the immune system and antibiotics to eliminate.

Think of it as a bacterial fortress.

The most challenging aspect of biofilms is that they may remain completely dormant for months or even years.

A patient may have no symptoms whatsoever until something triggers the bacteria to become active.

This trigger may be dental treatment, illness, trauma, vaccination, immune activation or further injectable treatments.

The patient suddenly develops swelling, tenderness or recurring inflammatory nodules.

The symptoms improve.

Then they return.

This recurring cycle is often one of the clues that suggests a biofilm may be present.

Unlike simple lumps or collagen accumulation, biofilms tend to have a fluctuating and unpredictable nature.

The Art of Diagnosis

When a patient presents with a lump, the most important question is not how to treat it.

The most important question is what it actually is.

A simple lump caused by product accumulation is very different from a delayed inflammatory nodule.

A delayed inflammatory nodule is different from a granuloma.

A granuloma is different from a biofilm.

Each requires a different management strategy.

The injector who immediately assumes every lump is a granuloma may create unnecessary anxiety and potentially inappropriate treatment.

The injector who understands the difference between product, collagen, inflammation and infection is far more likely to achieve a successful outcome.

Nita's Clinical Pearl

After more than three decades in aesthetics, I have learned that most complications are not caused by the product itself.

They are caused by technique, diagnosis, or misunderstanding.

Not every lump is a granuloma.

Not every nodule is infected.

Not every Sculptra lump is a granuloma.

The secret is learning to recognise the difference.

Because in aesthetics, the correct diagnosis is often the most important treatment of all.

.

Chapter 65: Medical Emergencies Beyond Fillers

When new injectors attend aesthetic training courses, most of the focus is placed on vascular occlusion, blindness, infection and other filler-related complications. These are important topics and every injector should understand them thoroughly.

However, after more than 30 years in nursing and aesthetic medicine, I can tell you that some of the most common emergencies you will encounter have absolutely nothing to do with the product you injected.

They are reactions to fear, anxiety, needles, medications, underlying medical conditions or simply the body's normal physiological response to stress.

The first time a patient suddenly turns pale, loses consciousness, begins hyperventilating or tells you they feel as though they are dying, it can be confronting.

The good news is that most of these situations can be managed successfully if you remain calm, think clearly and assess the patient systematically.

The golden rule is simple:

Stay calm. Your patient will take their emotional cues from you.

Vasovagal Episodes

The most common medical emergency in aesthetic practice is not vascular occlusion.

It is a vasovagal episode.

A vasovagal reaction occurs when the vagus nerve is overstimulated, causing a sudden drop in heart rate and blood pressure. As blood flow to the brain decreases, the patient becomes dizzy, nauseated and may faint.

The trigger may be surprisingly simple.

Some patients are frightened of needles.

Others have not eaten.

Some become anxious at the sight of blood.

Occasionally the emotional anticipation of treatment is enough to trigger a response.

Patients often tell you they feel hot, dizzy or nauseated. They may suddenly become pale, clammy and sweaty. Vision may blur and hearing may become muffled. If the reaction progresses, the patient may briefly lose consciousness.

Fortunately, most vasovagal episodes resolve quickly when recognised early. Placing the patient flat, elevating the legs and providing reassurance is often all that is required.

While the event can be alarming, it is usually benign and self-limiting.

Panic Attacks

Panic attacks can be one of the most dramatic situations encountered in cosmetic practice.

The patient may genuinely believe they are dying.

They may experience chest tightness, palpitations, dizziness, trembling, sweating and an overwhelming sense of fear.

Some patients are convinced they are having a heart attack.

Others feel they cannot breathe.

The symptoms are very real to the patient and should never be dismissed.

One of the most important skills an injector can develop is the ability to recognise anxiety while still maintaining a high index of suspicion for genuine medical emergencies.

Patients need reassurance, calm communication and a sense of safety.

I have learned that the phrase:

"You are safe. I'm here with you."

is often far more effective than repeatedly telling someone to calm down.

Most panic attacks settle within minutes when the patient feels supported and understood.

Hyperventilation

Hyperventilation often accompanies anxiety and panic attacks.

As breathing becomes rapid and shallow, excessive carbon dioxide is expelled from the body. This alters blood chemistry and creates symptoms that can feel frightening.

Patients may complain of dizziness, tingling around the mouth, numb fingers, muscle cramps, chest tightness and the sensation that they cannot get enough air.

Ironically, they are usually receiving plenty of oxygen.

What they need is slower breathing.

Speaking calmly, encouraging slow controlled breaths and providing reassurance are often the most effective interventions.

Once breathing normalises, symptoms usually resolve quickly.

Syncope (Fainting)

Syncope is a temporary loss of consciousness caused by reduced blood flow to the brain.

In aesthetic practice it most commonly occurs as the result of a vasovagal reaction.

Although the sight of a patient fainting can be frightening for an inexperienced injector, most episodes are brief and resolve rapidly.

The priority is always patient safety.

Protect the patient from injury, maintain a clear airway and monitor recovery carefully.

Any patient who does not recover promptly, experiences prolonged unconsciousness or demonstrates abnormal neurological signs requires urgent medical assessment.

Anaphylaxis

Of all the medical emergencies that may occur in an aesthetic clinic, anaphylaxis is perhaps the one that most practitioners fear.

Fortunately, it is rare.

However, because it develops rapidly and can become life-threatening within minutes, every injector must be prepared to recognise it and respond immediately.

Anaphylaxis is a severe allergic reaction involving multiple body systems. Unlike a simple local allergic response that may cause redness, itching or swelling at the injection site, anaphylaxis affects the entire body and can compromise the airway, breathing and circulation.

Potential triggers in aesthetic practice include local anaesthetic agents, topical preparations, antiseptics, latex, medications and, in rare cases, products used during emergency management itself.

One such product is hyaluronidase.

Hyaluronidase has become one of the most important medications in modern aesthetics. It allows injectors to dissolve hyaluronic acid fillers and plays a critical role in the management of vascular occlusion.

Ironically, while it can save tissue and prevent devastating complications, it can also occasionally cause allergic reactions.

Historically, patients with significant bee or wasp venom allergies have been considered at increased risk of hypersensitivity reactions because bee and wasp venom naturally contain hyaluronidase enzymes. Although most patients with insect sting allergies tolerate hyaluronidase without difficulty, this history should always form part of your medical assessment.

Every injector should ask about:

• Previous reactions to hyaluronidase

• Bee sting allergies

• Wasp sting allergies

• Previous episodes of anaphylaxis

• Severe medication allergies

• Hospital admissions for allergic reactions

The earliest signs of anaphylaxis are often subtle.

Patients may report that they feel strange, itchy, flushed or unwell. Swelling may develop around the lips, tongue or throat. Breathing may become difficult. Wheezing can occur. The patient may become pale, anxious or confused.

As the reaction progresses, blood pressure may fall rapidly, leading to collapse and loss of consciousness.

One of the most valuable lessons I learned during my nursing career is to listen carefully when a patient says:

"I don't feel right."

Those four words should never be ignored.

Anaphylaxis is a medical emergency requiring immediate recognition, activation of emergency procedures, administration of emergency treatment according to current guidelines and urgent medical assistance.

Every clinic should maintain current emergency protocols, emergency medications and regular staff training.

True anaphylaxis is uncommon, but preparedness saves lives.

Seizures

Although uncommon in aesthetic medicine, seizures can occur unexpectedly.

Some patients have a known seizure disorder. Others may have never experienced a seizure before.

Witnessing a seizure for the first time can be confronting, but the priorities remain straightforward.

Protect the patient from injury.

Do not attempt to restrain them.

Do not place anything in their mouth.

Monitor the duration of the seizure and ensure the airway remains clear once the event has ended.

Most seizures stop spontaneously within a few minutes. However, prolonged seizures, repeated seizures or failure to recover normally require urgent medical intervention.

Being Prepared

The reality is that most medical emergencies encountered in aesthetics are not caused by filler.

They are caused by fear, physiology, anxiety, allergies or underlying medical conditions.

Every clinic should have emergency protocols, emergency medications, a blood pressure monitor, pulse oximeter, emergency contact numbers and staff who know exactly what to do when something goes wrong.

Good injectors know anatomy.

Great injectors know emergency management.

Nita's Clinical Pearl

Patients rarely remember the exact product you used or the number of units you injected.

What they remember is how safe they felt in your care.

When an unexpected event occurs, your calmness becomes their confidence.

The syringe may be your tool, but reassurance, preparedness and clinical judgement are often your most important treatments.

Chapter 66: When Things go Wrong Emotionally

The Complications Nobody Warns You About

When injectors think about complications, they usually think about vascular occlusions, bruising, swelling, infection or nodules.

Yet some of the most challenging situations you will encounter have nothing to do with anatomy, products or technique.

They are emotional.

No one teaches you what to do when a patient bursts into tears during a consultation.

No one teaches you how to respond when a patient who loved their treatment yesterday suddenly hates it today.

No one teaches you how to manage anger, disappointment, anxiety or unrealistic expectations.

Yet these situations occur every day in aesthetic practice.

Because aesthetic medicine is not just about faces.

It is about feelings.

Every patient who sits in your chair brings more than wrinkles, volume loss or skin concerns.

They bring their life experiences, They bring their insecurities, They bring their hopes.

Sometimes they are celebrating a new chapter.

Sometimes they are trying to recover from a difficult one.

And occasionally, what they are really seeking has very little to do with the treatment itself.

The Emotional Investment

Most patients have thought about a treatment long before they book an appointment.

They have looked in mirrors, Compared themselves to old photographs, Studied social media images.

Imagined how they will feel after treatment.

By the time they arrive, they have often attached an emotional expectation to the outcome.

They imagine feeling younger., More confident, More attractive, More visible, More themselves.

The challenge is that cosmetic treatments can improve appearance, but they cannot solve every problem in a person's life.

A patient may look refreshed but still be grieving.

They may look younger but still feel lonely.

They may have beautiful results and still struggle with confidence.

When the emotional expectation is bigger than the physical result, disappointment can occur.

Not because the treatment failed.

But because the treatment was expected to do more than it possibly could.

The Patient Who Cries

Sometimes the tears arrive unexpectedly.

A simple question such as, "How have you been?" can open a door to something much deeper.

A patient may tell you about a divorce, the loss of a parent, a health scare, retirement, relationship breakdown or a difficult life transition.

At that moment, the consultation is no longer about filler or Botox.

It becomes about connection.

One of the greatest mistakes practitioners make is feeling they need to fix the emotion.

You don't.

Most people simply want to be heard.

Listen, Allow silence, Show empathy.

Often your presence is more valuable than your advice.

Patients rarely forget how they were treated when they were vulnerable.

The Patient Who Regrets Treatment

Few things create more anxiety for an injector than hearing the words:

"I don't like it."

The immediate reaction is often panic.

But not every complaint indicates a poor result.

Sometimes patients are simply adjusting to change.

Human beings become very attached to familiarity.

Even positive changes can feel strange at first.

This is particularly common following treatments that alter facial proportions such as lips, chin, cheeks or jawline enhancement.

The patient sees something different in the mirror and their brain needs time to catch up.

This adjustment period is completely normal.

The key is not to become defensive.

Listen carefully, Ask questions.

Determine whether the concern is emotional, aesthetic or clinical.

Sometimes intervention is required.

Sometimes reassurance is required.

And sometimes the best treatment is simply time.

The Angry Patient

Every injector will eventually encounter an angry patient.

The natural temptation is to immediately explain, defend or justify.

Unfortunately, that rarely helps.

People generally calm down when they feel heard.

They become more frustrated when they feel dismissed.

Allow the patient to speak, Listen without interruption, Acknowledge their concerns.

This does not mean admitting fault.

It simply means recognising their experience.

There is a significant difference between saying:

"I can see this has been upsetting for you."

and

"That's not what happened."

One opens communication. The other usually closes it.

The Patient Who Blames You

Occasionally, a patient will direct all of their frustration towards the practitioner.

Perhaps their expectations were unrealistic.

Perhaps they were influenced by social media.

Perhaps they expected perfection.

Whatever the reason, you may find yourself carrying responsibility for emotions that were never yours to begin with.

This is where professionalism becomes essential.

Stay calm, Remain objective, Avoid emotional reactions.

And most importantly, document everything.

Photographs, Consultation notes, Consent forms, Treatment plans.

These records protect both practitioner and patient.

Good documentation is not just a legal safeguard.

It is an important part of good clinical care.

The Patient Who Becomes Fixated

Some patients become focused on tiny imperfections that nobody else can see.

You correct one concern and another appears.

Then another. And another.

No result ever feels good enough.

These patients are not pursuing improvement.

They are pursuing perfection, Perfection is impossible.

The more you chase it, the further away it becomes.

This is where boundaries matter.

Learning when not to treat is just as important as learning how to treat.

Sometimes the most ethical decision is to put the syringe down.

Managing Your Own Emotions

Difficult consultations affect practitioners too.

There will be patients who keep you awake at night.

Conversations you replay in your head.

Outcomes you analyse repeatedly.

Moments where you question yourself.

That is part of caring.

However, there is an important difference between empathy and responsibility.

Empathy allows us to understand another person's experience.

Responsibility suggests we must solve it.

You cannot carry every patient's emotional burden.

Nor should you.

The ability to care deeply while maintaining healthy professional boundaries is one of the most valuable skills an injector can develop.

The Treatment Room Confessional

Over time, many injectors discover that the treatment room becomes something unexpected.

A confessional, A safe space, A place where people tell the truth.

Perhaps it is because aesthetic practitioners spend time listening.

Perhaps it is because touch creates trust.

Perhaps it is because when people decide to change something about their appearance, they are often navigating change in other parts of their lives as well.

Whatever the reason, aesthetic medicine frequently involves much more than aesthetics.

We may be treating a face, But there is always a person attached to it, And that person arrives with a story.

Nita's Clinical Pearl

Not every complication can be seen in a mirror.

Some of the most important moments in aesthetic practice occur long before the syringe touches the skin.

Listen carefully, Treat people with kindness, Maintain healthy boundaries..

And remember that while you may improve someone's appearance, what they often remember most is how you made them feel.

Sometimes feeling seen is the most powerful treatment of all.

Chapter 67: Botulinum Toxin A Side Effects ,Causes, Prevention, and Treatment

Botulinum toxin A injections (Botox, Dysport, Xeomin, Daxxify) are generally safe and well-tolerated when performed by an experienced injector. However, like any medical treatment, side effects can occur. While most are temporary, some can impact facial function and require management.

Common Botulinum Toxin A Side Effects

1. Blurred Vision & Dry Eyes

Occurs when botulinum toxin A diffuses into nearby muscles, affecting the orbicularis oculi or eye muscles responsible for blinking and tear production.

Patients may experience difficulty focusing, dry eyes, or excessive tearing.

Treatment:

Lubricating eye drops (artificial tears)

Warm compresses

Wait for botulinum toxin A to wear off (typically 4-6 weeks for mild cases)

2. Brow Ptosis (Heavy Brows or Droopy Eyebrows)

Caused by excessive botulinum toxin A in the frontalis (forehead muscle) without balancing the opposing depressor muscles.

Results in a heavy, tired-looking forehead with reduced eyebrow elevation.

Treatment:

Frown muscle (glabellar complex) botulinum toxin A can be adjusted to slightly lift the brows.

Taping techniques or facial exercises may help stimulate muscle activity.

Wait for botulinum toxin A to wear off (usually 6-8 weeks for improvement).

To avoid this: A skilled injector will ensure the correct dose and placement to maintain natural eyebrow movement.

3. Eyelid Ptosis (Drooping Eyelid)

Occurs when botulinum toxin A diffuses into the levator palpebrae muscle, which lifts the upper eyelid.

More common when treating glabellar frown lines.

Treatment:

Apraclonidine (Iopidine) 0.5% Eye Drops .Temporarily lifts the eyelid by activating Mullers muscle.

Time : The effect gradually improves over 4-6 weeks as botulinum toxin A wears off.

To avoid this: The injector should place botulinum toxin A at the correct depth and avoid excessive dosing near the upper eyelid muscles.

4. Painful Welts & Histamine Reaction

Some patients experience raised, red, itchy welts at the injection site due to a localized histamine response.

Can be mistaken for an allergic reaction but is usually mild.

Treatment:

Cold compresses

Oral antihistamines (Zyrtec, Claritin)

Topical arnica or aloe vera for soothing

If symptoms persist or worsen, seek medical advice.

5. Headaches After Botulinum Toxin A Injections

Some patients experience mild headaches after treatment, likely due to:

Temporary muscle tension changes, Needle trauma, Dehydration

Treatment:

Drink plenty of water.

Take mild pain relievers like paracetamol (acetaminophen) Avoid ibuprofen or aspirin to reduce bruising risk.

Apply a cool compress to the forehead. Headaches usually resolve within 24-48 hours.

6. Crooked Smile or Facial Asymmetry

Can occur when botulinum toxin A affects nearby muscles unintentionally.

Most commonly happens when treating:

DAO (Depressor Anguli Oris) for downturned mouth. Can lead to an uneven smile.

Masseter injections (jaw slimming).Can cause one side of the mouth to feel weaker when smiling.

Treatment:

Massage the area to encourage muscle recovery.

Neuromodulator like botulinum toxin A can be adjusted or corrected by balancing the other side.

Effects wear off in 6-12 weeks.

7. Masseter Bulge (Uneven Jawline or Lumps After Masseter Botulinum Toxin A Injections)

In some cases, one part of the masseter muscle compensates, creating an uneven bulge or hollowing.

Happens when botulinum toxin A isn't evenly distributed or when injection sites are incorrect.

Treatment:

Follow-up botulinum toxin A injections to balance the muscle activity.

Facial exercises to strengthen the weaker side. Massage to help smooth out the muscle contraction pattern.

To prevent this: A skilled injector will analyze facial symmetry and muscle dynamics before treatment.

8. Difficulty Smiling After Masseter Botulinum Toxin A Injections

If botulinum toxin A diffuses into the risorius muscle, patients may have trouble lifting the corners of the mouth when smiling. The smile may feel restricted or unnatural.

Treatment:

Massage and facial exercises to encourage nerve activation.

Wait 6-8 weeks for muscle function to return.

In rare cases, a small amount of additional botulinum toxin A can be placed strategically to rebalance the movement.

How Long Do Side Effects Last?

Most botulinum toxin A side effects are temporary and resolve within weeks to a few months as the toxin naturally wears off.

Side Effect Expected Duration Treatment Options

Blurred Vision / Dry Eyes 4-6 weeks Lubricating eye drops, warm compresses

Brow Ptosis (Heavy Brows) 6-8 weeks Botulinum toxin A adjustment, brow taping

Eyelid Ptosis (Droopy Eyelid) 4-6 weeks Apraclonidine eye drops

Painful Welts / Histamine Reaction 24-48 hours Antihistamines, cold compress

Headaches 24-48 hours Hydration, paracetamol, ice packs

Crooked Smile / Facial Asymmetry 6-12 weeks Massage, follow-up adjustments

Masseter Bulge 6-12 weeks Massage, additional botulinum toxin A correction

Smiling Difficulty After Masseter Botulinum Toxin A Injections 6-8 weeks Facial exercises, time

Severe or prolonged side effects should always be evaluated by a qualified injector.

Conclusion: Are Botulinum Toxin A Side Effects Serious?

Most botulinum toxin A side effects are minor, temporary, and self-resolving. Serious complications like ptosis, asymmetry, or masseter bulging can be managed with follow-up treatments. Choosing an experienced injector reduces the risk of side effects. If side effects occur, knowing what to do can help manage them effectively. The key to a successful botulinum toxin. A experience is proper technique, patient selection, and realistic expectations.

Chapter 68: Filler Migration: Causes, Anatomy, Prevention, and Solutions

What Is Filler Migration?

Filler migration occurs when dermal filler moves from the intended injection site to an adjacent or unintended area. This can cause aesthetic concerns (such as uneven swelling, puffiness, or unnatural contours) and, in some cases, functional issues (like obstructed lymphatic drainage under the eyes).

While migration can happen with any type of filler, it is most commonly seen with hyaluronic acid (HA) fillers, which are more mobile compared to thicker, more cohesive fillers like calcium hydroxyapatite (Radiesse) or poly-L-lactic acid (Sculptra).

Why Does Filler Migration Happen?

Filler migration can occur due to several anatomical, injection technique, and product-related factors:

1. Incorrect Placement in High-Movement Areas

Fillers injected into areas that experience frequent movement (e.g., lips, perioral region, under-eyes) are more likely to disperse over time.

The orbicularis oris (around the mouth) and orbicularis oculi (around the eyes) are constantly contracting, which can cause fillers to move or spread.

2. Poor Injection Depth

Superficial injection (too close to the skin surface) can allow the filler to move more easily compared to deep injections placed near the periosteum (bone layer).

Example: If cheek filler is injected too close to the surface, it may drift downward into the lower face due to gravity and facial movement.

3. Overfilling or Overcorrection

Injecting excessive filler into one area increases the risk of it spreading beyond the intended site.

This is particularly problematic in the lips, where an overfilled vermillion border can lead to the duck lip effect or migration into the white roll of the lip.

4. Soft Gel-Like Fillers

Softer, less crosslinked fillers (e.g., those used for lip augmentation or tear troughs) have a higher tendency to migrate compared to more structured, cohesive fillers used for deep structural support.

Some filler brands, such as those using Vycross technology (e.g., Juvederm Volbella, Volift, Voluma), may integrate well but can also be more prone to migration over time.

5. Muscle Activity & Gravity

Frequent muscle movement (e.g., talking, chewing, smiling) can push filler away from the intended site.

Gravity plays a role in downward migration, particularly in areas like the temples and cheeks, where misplaced filler can drift lower.

6. Lymphatic Blockage & Fluid Retention

The under-eye region is particularly prone to filler migration because the lymphatic drainage system is delicate.

If filler is injected too superficially or too close to lymphatic channels, it can trap fluid, leading to chronic puffiness or festoon-like swelling.

7. Repeated Treatments Without Full Dissolution

Over time, multiple layers of filler build up, creating an unnatural, doughy appearance.

Filler that was not fully dissolved from previous treatments may continue migrating even after new injections.

Where Does Filler Migrate?

1. Temple Filler Moving to the Cheek

If temple filler is injected too superficially, it can drift downward into the cheek over time.

This occurs because the temporalis muscle and fascia are connected to the zygomatic (cheek) region, allowing movement between these compartments.

2. Under-Eye Filler Causing Puffy Eyes

When filler is placed too superficially in the tear trough, it can obstruct lymphatic drainage, leading to persistent swelling and fluid retention.

This is often seen when soft fillers (like Volbella or Belotero Balance) are placed in the wrong tissue plane.

3. Lip Filler Spreading Beyond the Lip Border

Overfilled lips may push filler beyond the vermillion border, causing a duck lip or filler Mustache appearance.

This often occurs when filler is injected too superficially or in excessive amounts, leading to migration into the white roll or perioral area.

4. Nasolabial Fold Filler Spreading Laterally

Fillers injected into the nasolabial folds (smile lines) can sometimes spread outward, creating a bloated or widened appearance.

This is due to poor injection technique or placing filler too superficially.

5. Jawline Filler Moving Into the Neck

If too much filler is injected too low on the jawline, it may spread into the submental (under-chin) area, leading to an unnatural fullness or heaviness in the lower face.

How to Prevent Filler Migration

1. Proper Injection Techniques

Deep injections (near bone or deeper fat compartments) reduce movement.

Avoid overfilling in soft areas (e.g., lips, tear troughs).

Use microbolus techniques-small, precise amounts instead of large boluses.

Cannula technique may help reduce migration compared to needles in certain areas.

2. Choosing the Right Filler for the Right Area

Higher G (stiff, cohesive fillers) for structural support (e.g., cheeks, jawline).

Lower G (soft, fluid fillers) for mobile areas (e.g., lips, tear troughs).

Avoid highly crosslinked, dense fillers in delicate areas (e.g., under-eyes).

3. Spacing Out Treatments

Avoid layering too much filler over old injections.

Consider hyaluronidase (filler dissolver) before re-treating a migrated area.

Solutions for Filler Migration: Hyaluronidase

If filler migration occurs, it can often be corrected using hyaluronidase, an enzyme that breaks down hyaluronic acid-based fillers.

How Hyaluronidase Works

Hyaluronidase is a naturally occurring enzyme that dissolves HA fillers within hours to days.

It can be injected in small, targeted doses to selectively remove migrated or misplaced filler.

The effects are immediate but may take up to 48 hours for full results.

In some cases, a second or third session may be needed if the filler is deeply embedded.

When to Use Hyaluronidase

Under-eye puffiness caused by migrated filler.

Lip filler that has spread beyond the lip border.

Temple or cheek filler that has drifted into unwanted areas.

Overfilled, lumpy, or asymmetrical filler placements.

Can All Fillers Be Dissolved?

Hyaluronic acid fillers (e.g., Juvederm, Restylane, Belotero, Teoxane) can be dissolved.

Non-HA fillers (e.g., Radiesse, Sculptra, Bellafill) CANNOT be dissolved and may require alternative treatments like surgical removal.

Conclusion

Filler migration is caused by poor injection technique, overfilling, anatomical movement, and soft gel-like fillers in high-motion areas.

Common migration sites include under-eyes (causing puffiness), lips (spreading beyond the vermillion border), and cheeks (dropping from the temple).

Prevention strategies include using the correct filler type, proper injection depth, and avoiding excessive product placement.

Hyaluronidase is the go-to solution for dissolving migrated hyaluronic acid fillers.

Choosing an experienced injector who understands anatomy and rheology is critical to avoiding filler migration.

When considering the use of Hyalase (hyaluronidase) in individuals with known bee or wasp sting allergies, caution is imperative due to potential cross-reactivity. Hyaluronidase is an enzyme present in both bee and wasp venoms, facilitating the spread of venom through tissues.

This structural similarity can lead to the immune system recognizing medical hyaluronidase as a foreign substance, potentially triggering allergic reactions ranging from mild skin irritation to severe anaphylaxis.

Cross-reactivity occurs when the immune system identifies structurally similar proteins from different sources as the same allergen. In this context, the hyaluronidase enzyme in insect venom shares epitopes with medical hyaluronidase, leading to potential cross-reactive allergic responses. Clinical Implications:

Risk Assessment: Before administering hyaluronidase, it's crucial to assess patients for a history of severe reactions to bee or wasp stings.

Chapter 69: The Overfilled Face

When more becomes less

Over the years, I've watched aesthetic trends constantly evolve. Lips have become fuller, cheeks more projected, and jawlines sharper and more sculpted. But alongside these trends, I've also seen something becoming increasingly common — the overfilled face.

Patients are starting to recognise it, even if they can't always explain exactly what feels wrong. They'll often say things like:

"She looks different."

"Something doesn't look right."

"She doesn't look natural anymore."

What they are often noticing is not ageing at all, but the gradual build-up of too much filler over time.

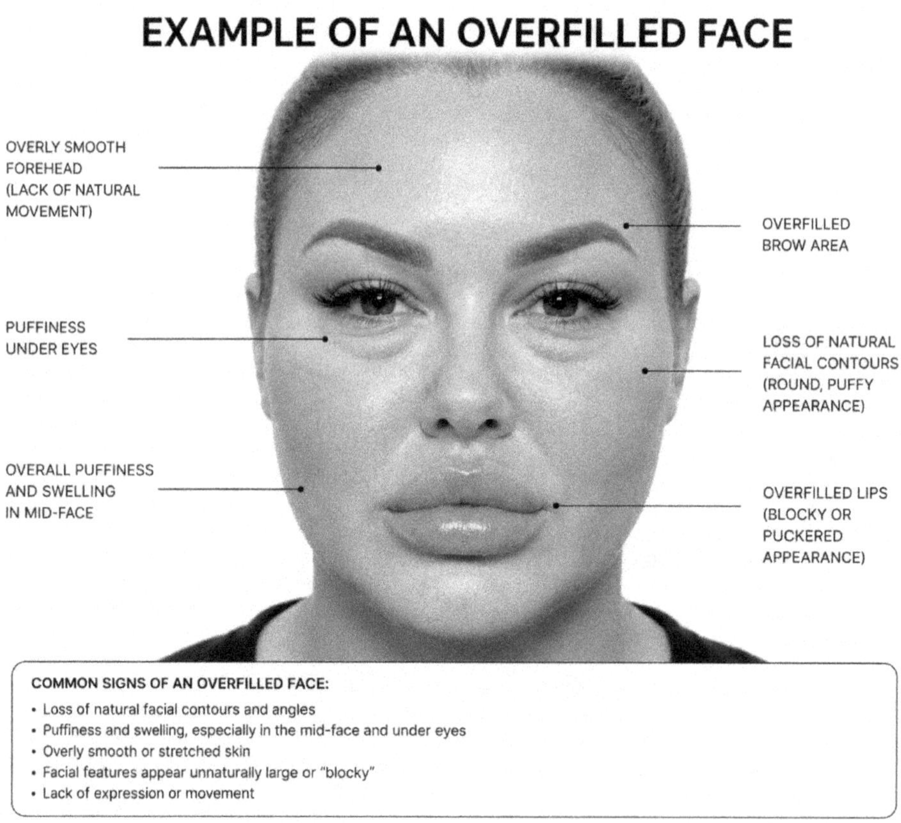

The truth is, people rarely become overfilled after one treatment. It usually happens slowly. A little filler here. A touch-up there. Another syringe a few months later. Without a long-term treatment plan, product begins to accumulate and the face gradually adapts to carrying more volume.

What once looked refreshed can eventually become excessive, but because the change happens gradually, patients often don't notice it themselves. The eye adjusts. The face becomes the new normal. And so the cycle continues.

One of the biggest mistakes in aesthetics is chasing lines in isolation. Patients understandably focus on the folds or wrinkles that bother them most — nasolabial folds, marionette lines, lip lines — but these lines are often only symptoms of deeper structural changes occurring in the face.

If you repeatedly inject directly into lines without addressing the underlying cause, you start placing bulk where bulk doesn't belong. Over time this creates heaviness, distortion, and loss of natural contour.

Filler is designed to restore lost support and volume, but when too much is used, volume eventually becomes weight. Instead of lifting the face, it can begin to drag features downward. The midface becomes puffy, the lower face heavy, and the area around the mouth thickened or swollen. Ironically, these are often the exact areas patients were hoping to improve.

One of the saddest things about overfilling is that the face actually starts to lose definition. The natural transitions between facial features soften. Contours blur. Shadows disappear. The unique character of the face becomes over-smoothed.

This is where the term "pillow face" comes from — a face that appears overly full, swollen, or inflated, without natural structure or movement. It is often mistaken for youthfulness, but true youth is not simply fullness. Youth is balance. It is proportion, softness, movement, and lightness.

Many patients believe more filler will make them look younger, but the opposite can happen. An overfilled face reflects light differently. It loses its natural contours and begins to appear heavy rather than lifted. Instead of looking refreshed, the face can start to look artificial, less refined, and in many cases, older.

Social media has played a major role in this trend. Many of the faces patients admire online are heavily filtered, edited, or photographed from highly flattering angles. What looks good in a still image does not always translate well in real life. Faces need to move naturally when we speak, laugh, smile, and express emotion.

Patients will often bring in photos requesting a certain look, but not every trend suits every face, and not every aesthetic ages well over time.

One of the most important skills in cosmetic medicine is knowing when to stop. Not every hollow needs filling. Not every line requires correction. Sometimes the best decision is to pause, reassess, allow filler to settle, or shift the focus toward improving skin quality instead.

Correcting an overfilled face can take patience. In many cases, it involves dissolving existing filler and allowing the face to return closer to its natural structure before rebuilding carefully and conservatively. This process can feel confronting for patients initially, but often the final result is softer, fresher, and far more natural.

I believe the future of aesthetics is moving away from excessive volume and toward healthier, more regenerative approaches. Better skin quality. Stronger structural support. Subtle enhancement rather than obvious alteration.

Today, I use smaller amounts of product, more strategic placement, and longer intervals between treatments. My goal is never to make someone look "done." My goal is to help them look refreshed, balanced, and still recognisably themselves.

I don't chase lines. I assess the whole face and treat what is actually causing the change. Sometimes the best treatment is not adding more filler at all.

The most beautiful results are the ones nobody can quite pinpoint. People simply say:

"You look well."

"You look refreshed."

"You look like yourself."

And to me, that is the true art of aesthetic medicine.

Chapter 70: Ozempic Face

Ozempic (semaglutide) and similar GLP-1 receptor agonists (e.g., Wegovy, Mounjaro) have revolutionized weight loss, helping thousands shed stubborn fat. However, rapid weight loss can have visible effects on the face, leading to a phenomenon known as "Ozempic Face."

This chapter explores the science behind facial fat loss, the specific fat pads affected, and how aesthetic treatments can restore a natural, youthful look.

How Weight Loss Affects the Face

Fat Redistribution & Volume Loss: Semaglutide-induced weight loss does not discriminate—it reduces fat in the face just as it does in the body.

Structural Support Weakens: With reduced deep and superficial fat pads, the face appears gaunt, hollow, and aged.

Skin Laxity Increases: Without the underlying fat to "hold up" the skin, the face can appear saggy and deflated.

Key Fat Pads Affected in Ozempic Face:

Fat Pad	Effect of Fat Loss
Buccal Fat Pad (Cheeks)	Sunken cheeks, gaunt appearance
Lateral Cheek Fat Pads	Loss of mid-face support, sagging
Temple Fat Pads	Hollow temples, skeletal look
Prezygomatic (Upper Cheek) Fat Pads	Loss of cheekbone definition
Submalar Fat Pads	Prominent nasolabial folds, deeper smile lines
Jawline & Submental Fat	Jowling and loose skin under the chin

Rapid weight loss can also accelerate skin ageing by depleting collagen and elastin, causing wrinkles and fine lines to appear more pronounced, due to reduced nutrients.

Common Symptoms of Ozempic Face

Hollowed cheeks, Sunken temples, More prominent nasolabial folds

Drooping jowls & marionette lines. Loose, crepey skin due to reduced elasticity

Which Facial Fat Pads Deplete?

Facial ageing occurs in layers, and weight loss accelerates fat depletion in both superficial and deep fat pads.

How to Restore Facial Volume & Structure

Collagen Biostimulators (Sculptra & Radiesse)

Best for: Global facial rejuvenation, natural volume restoration, collagen stimulation

Sculptra (Poly-L-Lactic Acid)

- Works by stimulating collagen production over time. Provides a gradual thickening of the skin & volume replacement
- Ideal for cheeks, temples, jawline, and overall face rejuvenation. Results last 2+ years

Radiesse (Calcium Hydroxylapatite – CaHA)

- Provides instant volume and long-term collagen stimulation
- Great for midface, jawline, and lower face definition
- Can be used in hyperdiluted form for skin tightening

Hyaluronic Acid Fillers (HA Fillers)

Best for: Immediate volume restoration, targeted fat pad replenishment

1. Cheeks & Midface – Restores lift and support

- Juvederm Voluma, Restylane Lyft, RHA4

2. Temples – Corrects hollowing and skeletal look

- Juvederm Voluma, Restylane Lyft

3. Nasolabial Folds & Marionette Lines – Softens deep creases

- Restylane Defyne, Juvederm Ultra Plus

4. Jawline Contouring – Defines and sharpens the jawline

• Juvederm Volux, Restylane Contour

Immediate improvement with HA fillers, Lasts 12-24 months depending on the product

Skin Tightening & Regenerative Treatments

If weight loss has caused loose, sagging skin, combining volume restoration with skin-tightening therapies enhances results:

1. Radiofrequency Microneedling (Morpheus8, Profound RF) – Tightens skin, improves collagen production

2. Ultrasound (Ultherapy, Sofwave) – Lifts and firms without adding volume

3. PRP (Platelet-Rich Plasma) & Exosomes – Boosts skin regeneration and elasticity

Maintaining a Youthful Look After Weight Loss

Hydrate & Support Skin Health

• Collagen supplements (marine collagen, peptides), Hyaluronic acid-based skincare (topical & ingestible), Vitamin C & Retinol for skin renewal

Regular Aesthetic Maintenance

• Touch-ups every 12-24 months, Non-invasive treatments to preserve elasticity & collagen

Balanced Weight Loss & Nutrition

• Losing weight gradually prevents extreme facial volume loss, Protein-rich diets help maintain skin firmness & muscle tone

White Fat Cells – The Missing Piece of Ozempic Face

One of the most fascinating discoveries in skin ageing research is the important role played by **white adipose tissue**, commonly known as white fat cells. For many years, we believed that youthful skin depended primarily on collagen and elastin. We now know there is a third key player—specialised white fat cells that sit beneath the skin and around hair follicles. These cells do far more than store energy.

They communicate with fibroblasts, support collagen production, regulate inflammation, assist wound healing, contribute to skin hydration, and help maintain the skin's thickness, elasticity, and overall youthful appearance.

When significant weight loss occurs, particularly with medications such as Ozempic, Wegovy, or Mounjaro, these fat cells shrink along with the deeper facial fat pads. As this support network diminishes, the skin can lose its underlying scaffold, causing it to appear thinner, looser, and less resilient.

The result is often the characteristic appearance patients describe as their face "melting"—with hollow temples, flattened cheeks, deeper folds, jowls, and a more gaunt appearance.

Research suggests that healthy skin requires a delicate balance of collagen, elastin, and white adipose tissue. Too much fat may contribute to inflammation, while too little can accelerate visible ageing.

This understanding helps explain why some patients experience dramatic facial changes after rapid weight loss and why modern treatment approaches focus not only on replacing volume but also on restoring skin quality and supporting the health of these vital fat cells.

Conclusion: Reverse Ozempic Face Without Overfilling

Restoring Ozempic Face isn't just about replacing lost fat—it's about strategically rebuilding volume while maintaining natural proportions. Sculptra & Radiesse for long-term collagen stimulation. HA Fillers for immediate, targeted volume replacement,. Skin-tightening treatments to prevent sagging. Preventative maintenance to sustain results

By approaching facial rejuvenation holistically, patients can enjoy weight loss benefits without sacrificing their youthful appearance.

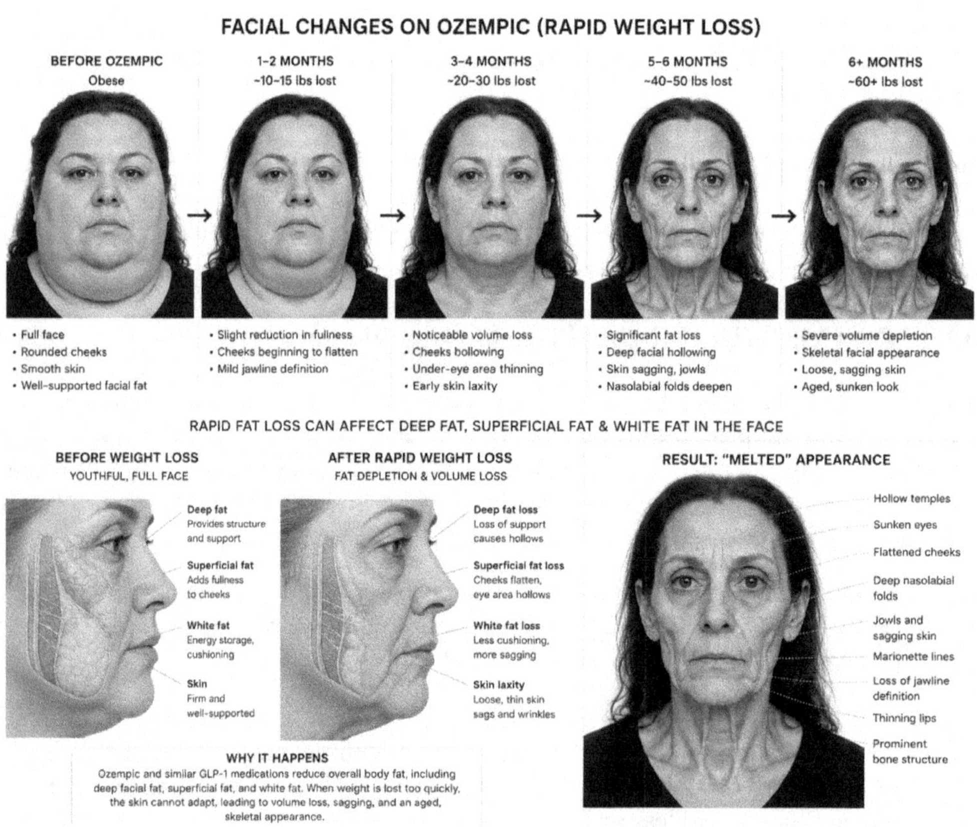

Chapter 71: Aftercare Essentials: Maximise Results, Minimise Risk

The right aftercare can make all the difference between a good result and a great one. Here's a treatment-by-treatment guide to what you should and shouldn't do after your injectable procedures.

After BOTOX/Dysport/Xeomin (Wrinkle Relaxers)

DO:

Stay upright for 4 hours

Use facial muscles (frown, smile, raise brows) to help product settle

Light walking is fine

DON'T:

No lying down or napping

Avoid strenuous exercise for 24 hours

No facial massages, saunas, or hot yoga for 48 hours

Avoid alcohol on the day of treatment

TIP: Results take 3–7 days to appear; full effect at 2 weeks.

After DERMAL FILLERS

DO:

Ice gently for 5–10 minutes at a time to reduce swelling

Sleep on your back for at least 2 nights

Keep head elevated first night

Drink plenty of water

DON'T:

No vigorous exercise for 24–48 hours

No facials or massage for 2 weeks

Don't touch, press or manipulate the area

Avoid alcohol and high-sodium foods for 24 hours

TIP: Minor swelling or bruising is common and resolves in a few days.

After SKIN BOOSTERS (e.g. Volite, NCTF 135HA)

NIGHT OF TREATMENT:

Do not apply makeup

Avoid touching or washing the area unnecessarily

Expect small papules or bumps where product was placed

NEXT DAY (AND ONWARD):

Use gentle cleanser and moisturiser

Resume makeup if no open punctures remain

Avoid harsh exfoliants or acids for 3–5 days

No sauna or vigorous exercise for 24–48 hours

TIP: Redness or papules usually subside within 24–72 hours.

After BIOSTIMULANTS (e.g. Sculptra, Lenisna, Radiesse, Juvelook)

DO:

Massage the treated areas for 5 minutes, 5 times a day, for 5 days (unless otherwise advised)

Use a clean moisturiser or oil to aid massage

Stay hydrated—biostimulants love water

DON'T:

No intense exercise or facial treatments for 1 week

Avoid alcohol, blood thinners, and anti-inflammatories for 24 hours

TIP: Collagen stimulation is gradual—results may build over 6–12 weeks and may require multiple sessions.

After PRP (Platelet-Rich Plasma)

DO:

Keep skin clean and dry for the first 12 hours

Use only gentle, non-active skincare for 2–3 days

Sleep on a clean pillowcase

DON'T:

Avoid anti-inflammatories (e.g., Nurofen, aspirin) for 5–7 days—they can blunt the healing response

No active skincare, acids, or vitamin A for 3–5 days

No makeup for 12–24 hours

Avoid sun exposure for 48 hours

TIP: Tingling, redness or pinpoint bruising is normal and settles quickly. PRP is about healing—not instant plumping.

When to ICE (and when not to)

YES—Ice After:

Filler (especially lips or tear troughs): Helps reduce swelling and bruising

Skin boosters if swollen

After any injectables to ease discomfort (short, clean applications)

NO—Do Not Ice:

After PRP: Cold suppresses inflammation, which you actually want for collagen stimulation

Over-massage or apply prolonged pressure with ice: Can worsen bruising.

Chapter 72: Why your Injector can't Advertise- TGA Restrictions

One of the most common questions clients ask is:

"Why won't clinics just say exactly what they use?"

You may already know the names of treatments and products from social media, overseas clinics, or friends. So when an Australian clinic uses more general terms, it can feel confusing — even frustrating.

But there is a clear reason for this.

The Legal Framework

In Australia, many injectable treatments — including wrinkle relaxers and certain dermal fillers — are classified as **prescription-only medications**.

They are regulated by organisations such as AHPRA and the Therapeutic Goods Administration (TGA).

Under these regulations:

- Prescription medications **cannot be advertised directly to the public**
- Clinics **cannot promote specific product names** in marketing
- Language must remain **general, factual, and non-promotional**
- Advertising must not create unrealistic expectations or influence decision-making

This is why you will see wording like:

- "wrinkle reduction treatment"
- "volume restoration"
- "lip enhancement"

These are not vague descriptions — they are **legally compliant terms**.

Advertising vs Consultation

The most important distinction to understand is this:

Advertising is public. Consultation is medical.

In advertising — websites, social media, brochures — practitioners must:

- follow strict guidelines
- avoid naming prescription products
- keep messageing broad and compliant

However, in a **clinical consultation**, the environment is completely different.

Once you are in a private setting with a qualified practitioner:

- your medical history can be reviewed
- your facial anatomy can be assessed
- your goals and concerns can be explored

At this point:

- **specific product options can be discussed**
- **treatment plans can be explained in detail**
- **risks, benefits, and alternatives can be clearly outlined**

This is where personalised, transparent information is appropriately given.

Why the Rules Exist

The intention behind these regulations is to:

- prevent misleading or exaggerated claims
- reduce pressure-based or impulsive decisions
- ensure treatments are recommended based on **clinical need**, not marketing
- protect vulnerable individuals from unrealistic expectations

It shifts the focus away from promotion and toward **professional assessment**.

The Reality of Social Media

The challenge is that the internet is global —but regulations are local.

Australian consumers are exposed daily to:

- overseas clinics openly naming products
- influencers sharing treatment experiences
- before-and-after transformations without context
- simplified or commercialised messageing

This content does not follow Australian regulations.

So while Australian practitioners must communicate carefully, clients are often arriving with detailed — and sometimes inaccurate — expectations.

Why It Can Feel Confusing

This difference between what you see online and what you hear in clinic can create uncertainty.

You might feel:

- information is being withheld
- answers are too general
- your injector is not being direct

In reality, your injector is:

- complying with legal requirements
- protecting their professional registration
- ensuring information is given in the **right setting**

What Happens in the Consultation

The consultation is where everything becomes clear.

This is where your injector can:

- explain exactly what they are recommending
- discuss why a particular product or approach suits you
- tailor treatment to your individual anatomy and goals
- answer all of your questions openly

It is a **medical conversation**, not a marketing message.

What You Should Expect as a Client

A reputable injector will:

- use compliant, general language in public
- provide detailed, personalised information in private
- prioritise your safety over promotion
- guide you based on experience — not trends

If anything, these regulations reinforce the importance of choosing a practitioner who:

- takes time to consult properly
- educates you thoroughly
- and treats you as an individual, not a transaction

Understanding the Bigger Picture

We are living in a time where information is easily accessible, but not always reliable.

Australian regulations aim to ensure that when it comes to medical treatments:

- decisions are made thoughtfully
- information is given responsibly
- and care is delivered safely

The role of your injector is not simply to provide a treatment —it is to help you navigate everything you have seen, heard, and read, and translate it into something appropriate for you.

PART 6- HOLISTIC AGEING, WELLNESS & LONGEVITY

Chapter 73: Health Is Wealth

I am a great advocate for integrative medicine, recognizing that our internal health is reflected in our external appearance. The way we eat, drink, sleep, and manage stress directly influences how we look. Many aesthetic concerns are symptoms of underlying health issues, and addressing the root cause leads to lasting beauty and rejuvenation.

How Health Affects Appearance

1. Lifestyle Factors and Their Visible Impact

Alcohol Causes bloating, puffy eyes, and ruddy (red, inflamed) skin due to dehydration and liver stress.

Cigarettes Leads to poor circulation, smoker's lines, and wrinkled, grey-toned skin from oxygen deprivation.

Dehydration Results in dry, crepey skin and increased fine lines due to lack of hydration at the cellular level.

Obesity Can contribute to fuller facial features, double chins, and increased facial fat deposits, sometimes making ageing signs more prominent.

2. Hormonal Health and Its Aesthetic Impact

Thyroid Issues : Hypothyroidism can cause hair loss, weight gain, and dry, flaky skin, while hyperthyroidism may lead to thin, fragile skin and excessive hair shedding.

Perimenopause & Postmenopause :The loss of oestrogen leads to skin thinning, dryness, fine lines, and loss of elasticity.

Testosterone Imbalance : Can contribute to excessive facial hair in women or hair loss on the scalp.

3. Mental Health and the Face

Depression, Anxiety & Insomnia :Poor sleep causes dark circles, fine lines, dull skin, and increased facial tension (frown lines, clenched jaw).

Anorexia & Malnutrition :Leads to severe facial fat loss, hollow cheeks, thinning hair, and dull skin due to lack of essential nutrients.

Grief and Sadness: Emotionally, sadness can be seen in the droop of the corners of the mouth, tension in the forehead, and a general loss of facial vibrancy.

4. The Role of Vitamins & Minerals in Skin Health

Vitamin C Deficiency: Causes weakened gums, dull skin, and slower collagen production.

Vitamin D Deficiency :Can lead to dull, dry skin and increased skin ageing due to its role in cell turnover.

B Vitamins & the MTHFR Gene Mutation: Many people have undiagnosed MTHFR gene mutations, affecting their ability to process B vitamins, impacting oestrogen metabolism and skin quality.

Lack of Minerals (Zinc, Magnesium, Selenium, etc.) Affects immune function, skin hydration, and overall skin integrity.

5. Chronic Health Conditions and Aesthetic Changes

Stress & Cortisol Overload :Leads to premature ageing, breakouts, dull skin, and deepened facial lines.

Diabetes : Can cause poor wound healing, dark patches (acanthosis nigricans), and overall dull skin tone.

Fibromyalgia: Often linked to chronic fatigue, pale skin, and premature ageing signs due to persistent pain and stress.

Cosmetic Procedures & Medical Conditions

Many medical conditions affect when and how cosmetic treatments can be performed. Here are a few key considerations:

Cancer & Chemotherapy :Skin becomes fragile, and immune function is compromised. When is it safe to start cosmetic procedures post-treatment? It's usually recommended to wait at least 6-12 months post-chemo and only proceed under medical guidance.

Acne & Roaccutane (Isotretinoin): Patients on Roaccutane should avoid laser treatments and deep peels as the skin is highly sensitive and prone to scarring. Treatments should resume 6 months post-medication.

Herpes Simplex (Cold Sores) : Cosmetic treatments like lip fillers or microneedling can trigger outbreaks. Pre-treatment antiviral medication (e.g., Valacyclovir) is recommended to prevent post-procedure flare-ups.

Final Thoughts: A Holistic Approach to Beauty

True rejuvenation is not just about injectables and skin treatments it's about nourishing the body, balancing hormones, manageing stress, and understanding the deep connection between health and beauty.

Rather than masking symptoms, I believe in addressing the root cause, helping individuals heal from within so their outer beauty naturally radiates vitality and wellness. Because at the end of the day, health truly is wealth.

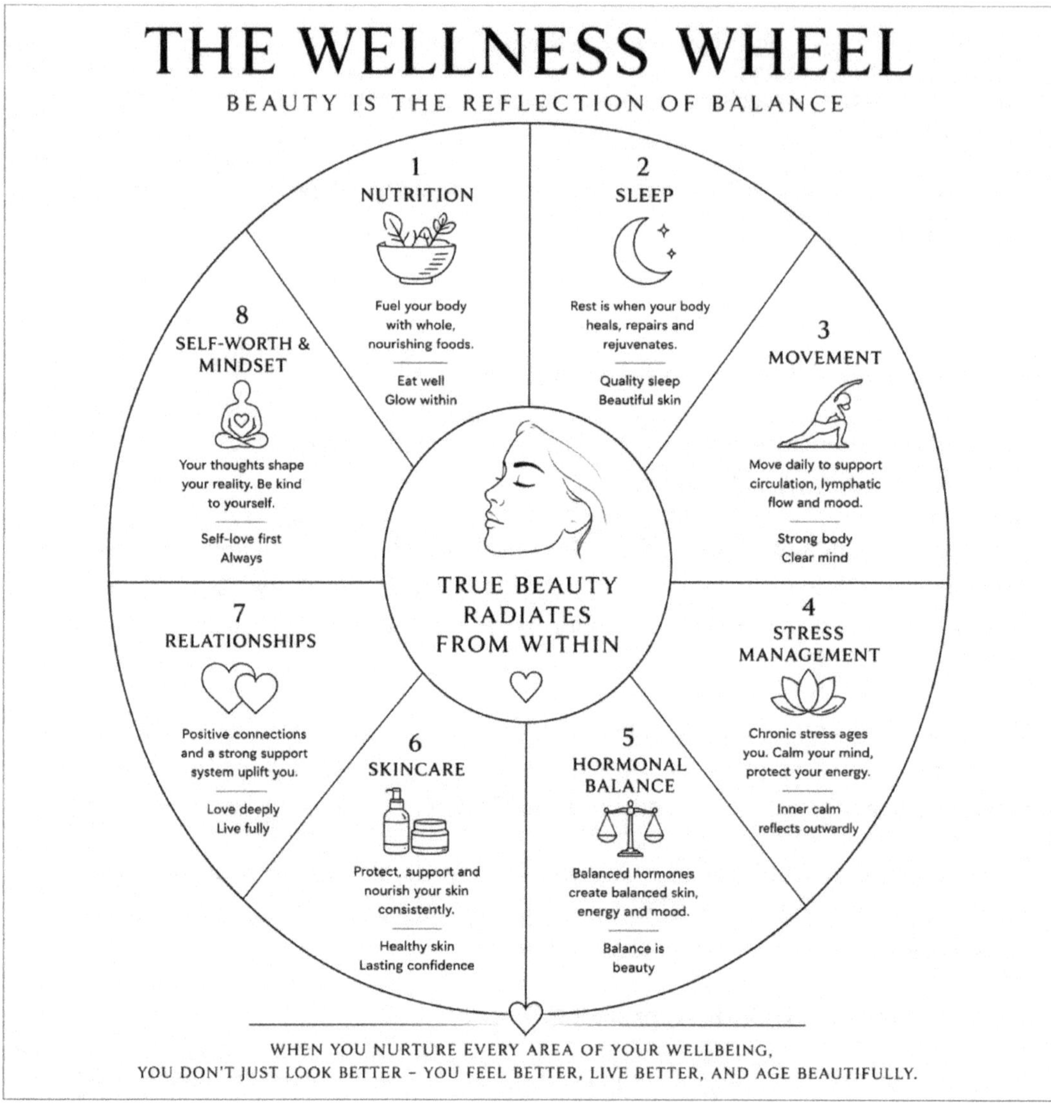
THE WELLNESS WHEEL
BEAUTY IS THE REFLECTION OF BALANCE
1
NUTRITION
Fuel your body with whole, nourishing foods.
Eat well
Glow within
2
SLEEP
Rest is when your body heals, repairs and rejuvenates.
Quality sleep
Beautiful skin
3
MOVEMENT
Move daily to support circulation, lymphatic flow and mood.
Strong body
Clear mind
4
STRESS MANAGEMENT
Chronic stress ages you. Calm your mind, protect your energy.
Inner calm
reflects outwardly
5
HORMONAL BALANCE
Balanced hormones create balanced skin, energy and mood.
Balance is
beauty
6
SKINCARE
Protect, support and nourish your skin consistently.
Healthy skin
Lasting confidence
7
RELATIONSHIPS
Positive connections and a strong support system uplift you.
Love deeply
Live fully
8
SELF-WORTH & MINDSET
Your thoughts shape your reality. Be kind to yourself.
Self-love first
Always
TRUE BEAUTY RADIATES FROM WITHIN
WHEN YOU NURTURE EVERY AREA OF YOUR WELLBEING,
YOU DON'T JUST LOOK BETTER - YOU FEEL BETTER, LIVE BETTER, AND AGE BEAUTIFULLY.

Chapter 74: Beauty Starts in the Gut

They say beauty comes from within, and in many ways, that starts with the gut. The health of our gut microbiome directly impacts our skin, hair, energy levels, and overall well-being. Many people focus on external beauty treatments without realizing that poor gut health can manifest as skin issues, inflammation, and premature ageing.

How Today's Diet Harms the Gut

Our modern lifestyle has disrupted gut health, leading to an imbalance in the gut microbiome (dysbiosis). Some of the biggest offenders include:

Antibiotics in Food: Wipe out both good and bad bacteria, leading to an unhealthy microbiome.

Too Much Gluten: Can trigger gut inflammation and leaky gut syndrome, especially in sensitive individuals.

Excess Sugar: Feeds bad bacteria and yeast (candida), contributing to acne, dull skin, and bloating.

Too Much Lactose (Dairy Products) Dairy intolerance can cause skin breakouts, puffiness, and digestive discomfort.

Gut Imbalance & Beauty Problems

When the gut microbiome is imbalanced, it can show up in various beauty concerns:

Acne: Overgrowth of bad bacteria and candida can cause hormonal imbalances, inflammation, and breakouts.

Eczema & Rosacea: Linked to leaky gut and inflammation.

Dull, Dry Skin: Poor gut health reduces nutrient absorption, leading to lacklustre skin.

Dark Circles & Puffiness: Toxins from gut imbalances burden the liver and kidneys, causing fluid retention and dark under-eye circles.

Thinning Hair: Nutrient deficiencies from poor digestion impact hair growth and scalp health.

How to Repair Leaky Gut

A damaged gut lining (leaky gut) allows toxins and undigested food particles to enter the bloodstream, triggering inflammation, autoimmune reactions, and skin conditions. Here's how to heal it:

1. Nutrients & Supplements for Gut Repair

Butyric Acid: A short-chain fatty acid that helps heal the gut lining and reduce inflammation.

Glutathione: A powerful antioxidant that supports liver detoxification and gut barrier integrity.

Berberine: A natural antibacterial that reduces bad bacteria overgrowth and improves insulin sensitivity.

Oregano Oil: Helps eliminate harmful bacteria, parasites, and candida overgrowth.

Slippery Elm: Soothes and coats the gut lining, reducing inflammation.

Triphala: An Ayurvedic herbal blend that supports digestion and detoxification.

Water: Hydration is essential for flushing out toxins and supporting digestive function.

2. Reduce Foods That Trigger Inflammation

To heal the gut, it is essential to remove inflammatory foods, including:

Refined Sugar (feeds bad bacteria and candida).

Processed Foods & Artificial Additives (disrupt microbiome balance).

Excessive Gluten & Dairy (can trigger inflammation in sensitive individuals).

3. Support Digestion & Reduce Bloating

Many people lack digestive enzymes, leading to poor breakdown of foods like red meat and lectins (found in legumes, grains, and nightshades). When undigested food sits in the small intestine, it can cause bacterial overgrowth, bloating, gas, and puffiness.

Digestive Enzymes: Help break down food properly, preventing gut irritation.

Probiotics & Prebiotics: Balance good bacteria for better digestion and skin health.

Fermented Foods: (Kimchi, sauerkraut, kefir) naturally restore gut microbiome balance.

Testing for Gut Health

For those experiencing chronic skin issues, bloating, fatigue, or food intolerances, it is beneficial to see an integrative doctor to analyse stool samples for gut bacteria levels, yeast overgrowth, and markers of inflammation.

The Effects of Candida Overgrowth on Skin & Beauty

Candida (a type of yeast) is naturally present in the body, but excess sugar, antibiotics, and stress can cause it to overgrow. When candida takes over, it can wreak havoc on the skin.

Common Symptoms of Candida Overgrowth:

Persistent acne, rashes, or fungal skin infections.

White coating on the tongue (oral thrush).

Digestive issues like bloating, gas, and sugar cravings.

Chronic fatigue and brain fog.

How to Treat Candida Naturally:

Cut out sugar & refined carbs (which feed candida).

Increase probiotics to restore gut balance.

Use natural antifungals like oregano oil, berberine, and caprylic acid.

Aloe Vera: A Superfood for Gut & Skin

Aloe vera isn't just for soothing sunburns it is a powerful gut healer!

Aloe Vera Benefits for the Gut:

Soothes and repairs the gut lining.

Supports healthy digestion and reduces bloating.

Helps balance gut bacteria.

Aloe Vera Benefits for Skin:

Hydrates and calms inflammation.

Contains vitamins and antioxidants that boost collagen production.

Supports wound healing and reduces acne scars.

Drinking aloe vera juice (with no added sugar) can be a great way to support gut and skin health simultaneously.

Final Thoughts: Gut Health is the Foundation of Beauty

The gut-skin connection is undeniable. Many common skin issues are rooted in poor digestion, microbiome imbalances, and leaky gut.

By healing the gut with the right foods, supplements, and lifestyle changes, we can achieve clearer skin, stronger hair, reduced inflammation, and a more radiant complexion true beauty from the inside out.

Chapter 75: Thyroid Health and Its Impact on Facial Appearance

When discussing beauty and rejuvenation, it's essential to start with the foundations of health. One of the most overlooked contributors to facial puffiness, tired appearance, and skin texture changes is thyroid dysfunction—specifically hypothyroidism. The thyroid gland plays a crucial role in regulating metabolism, energy production, and cellular repair. When the thyroid is underactive (hypothyroidism), the entire body slows down, and the face often provides early visual clues that something is not functioning optimally.

Common Symptoms of Hypothyroidism

Persistent fatigue

Weight gain, even with unchanged diet and exercise habits

Dry skin, Feeling cold easily

Depression or low mood, Constipation

Hair thinning, particularly the outer third of the eyebrows

Puffy face and eyelids

Hoarseness of voice, Slowed heart rate

From an aesthetic viewpoint, two signs are particularly notable:

Puffiness of the face, especially around the eyes and jawline.

Thinning of the lateral (outer) third of the eyebrows, a classic feature often missed unless specifically looked for.

These subtle changes can make a face appear older, tired, or heavier, even if no other signs of ageing are present.

Thyroid Testing and the T3 / Reverse T3 Trap

Routine thyroid tests often measure TSH (thyroid-stimulating hormone) and T4 (thyroxine). In many cases, these results may come back as "normal," leading patients to be told that their thyroid is functioning properly.

However, many symptoms can still persist despite "normal" blood tests.

This can happen when the active form of thyroid hormone, T3 (triiodothyronine), is not adequately available at the cellular level.

Even if T4 levels are normal, if the body is converting T4 into an inactive form called Reverse T3 (rT3) rather than into active T3, the cells are essentially starved of functional thyroid hormone.

This is why patients may continue to experience hypothyroid symptoms despite being prescribed thyroxine (T4 replacement therapy).

One crucial factor in this conversion process is iodine. Adequate iodine levels are needed to ensure that T4 is properly converted into bioavailable T3 rather than rT3.

What to Do if Symptoms Persist

If you or your clients are noticing ongoing symptoms of hypothyroidism — puffiness, facial swelling, thinning of the brows, or sluggishness — despite being on thyroid medication, it's important to:

See a doctor knowledgeable about full thyroid panels An integrative medicine Dr.

Request testing for Reverse T3 (rT3) and Free T3 levels

Assess iodine status if appropriate

Addressing these imbalances can significantly improve not only energy, mood, and overall health but also enhance the appearance of the face—reducing puffiness and helping to restore natural vibrancy.

Beauty Begins with Health

True aesthetic rejuvenation begins from within.

No injectable, filler, or laser can mask the signs of an underlying health issue like hypothyroidism.

As aesthetic practitioners, it's important to recognize these signs and, where appropriate, suggest medical evaluation to ensure the best long-term outcomes for clients.

A healthy thyroid often means a brighter, less puffy, more youthful appearance—naturally.

Chapter 76: Menopause

Menopause is a profound transition, not just internally but visibly on the skin and body. The hormonal shifts that occur—primarily the decline in oestrogen and progesterone—directly impact collagen levels, fat distribution, and skin hydration. This chapter explores the biological, aesthetic, and medical approaches to addressing these changes, ensuring a smoother transition into the next phase of life with confidence and vitality.

1. The Biological Impact of Menopause on the Face & Body

Hormonal Decline & Its Effect on the Skin

• **Loss of Collagen & Elasticity** → Sagging, fine lines, deeper wrinkles

• **Reduction in Skin Hydration** → Dryness, crepey texture

• **Thinning of the Epidermis** → Increased sensitivity and slower healing

• **Fat Redistribution** → Loss of facial volume, while fat accumulates in the midsection

Fat Distribution & Body Shape Changes

• **Midriff Weight Gain** → Due to declining oestrogen levels, fat shifts from hips and thighs to the abdomen

• **Loss of Muscle Mass** → Slower metabolism, contributing to stubborn fat deposits

2. Medical & Hormonal Treatments

Hormone Blood Tests & Bioidentical Hormone Therapy (BHRT)

• **Blood Tests** to assess levels of oestrogen, progesterone, testosterone, and DHEA

• **Bioidentical Hormones** (BHRT) can restore lost oestrogen, improving skin texture, hydration, and overall well-being

• **Testosterone & DHEA**: Can support muscle tone, skin thickness, and libido

Oestrogen for the Skin

• **Topical Oestrogen Creams**: Improve hydration, elasticity, and overall radiance

• **Oral or Patch Oestrogen Therapy**: Helps with systemic symptoms (hot flashes, bone density, mood) while supporting skin structure

• **Collagen Stimulation via Hormone Support**: Oestrogen encourages fibroblasts to produce more collagen, slowing down the ageing process

3. Aesthetic Treatments for Menopausal Skin

Facial Treatments: Rejuvenation & Volume Restoration

Collagen Biostimulators – Sculptra, Radiesse, and PRP (Platelet-Rich Plasma) help rebuild lost collagen

Hyaluronic Acid Fillers – Restore volume loss in the mid-face, lips, and temples

Skin Boosters & Hydration Fillers – Profhilo, Juvederm Volite, or Teosyal Redensity to deeply hydrate the skin

Neuromodulators (Botox, Dysport) – Soften expression lines and prevent further deepening of wrinkles

Radiofrequency (RF) & Ultrasound Treatments (Ultherapy, Morpheus8) – Tighten sagging skin non-surgically

Chemical Peels & Laser Resurfacing – Improve skin texture, pigmentation, and elasticity

Daily Skincare Routine for Menopausal Skin

• **Retinol or Prescription Tretinoin** – Stimulates skin renewal

• **Vitamin C & Antioxidants** – Brighten skin and combat oxidative stress

• **Hyaluronic Acid & Peptides** – Maintain hydration and plumpness

• **SPF 50+ Sunscreen** – Prevents further collagen degradation

4. Addressing the Body: Fat Redistribution & Contouring

Stubborn Midriff Fat: Aesthetic & Surgical Solutions

As menopause causes fat accumulation around the midsection, diet and exercise may not be enough. The following treatments help contour the body:

Liposculpture & Liposuction

• Targets stubborn fat in the abdomen, waist, and back

• Can be combined with fat transfer to restore lost volume in the face or hands

Non-Surgical Fat Reduction

• **Cryolipolysis (CoolSculpting)** – Freezes fat cells, gradually eliminating them

• **Radiofrequency (Vanquish, TruSculpt, Exilis)** – Uses heat to shrink fat and tighten skin

Skin Tightening for the Body

• **RF Microneedling (Morpheus8 Body, Renuvion)** – Tightens loose skin and improves texture

• **HIFU (High-Intensity Focused Ultrasound)** – Non-invasive lifting for areas like the arms, abdomen, and thighs

5. Lifestyle, Nutrition & Supplement Support

Key Nutrients for Menopausal Skin & Body

• **Collagen Peptides** – Maintain skin elasticity and firmness

• **Omega-3 Fatty Acids** – Combat inflammation and dryness

• **Magnesium & Vitamin D** – Support muscle function and mood

• **Phytoestrogens (Soy, Flaxseed)** – May help balance declining oestrogen

Exercise & Body Composition

• **Strength Training** – Helps counteract muscle loss and reshape the body

• **Pilates & Yoga** – Improves posture, flexibility, and stress levels

• **Cardio Workouts** – Helps manage weight and support heart health

Conclusion: Embracing Menopause with Confidence

Menopause doesn't mean surrendering to ageing—it's an opportunity to take charge of your health, appearance, and well-being. With hormonal support, aesthetic treatments, and lifestyle adjustments, you can age beautifully, naturally, and vibrantly.

THE MENOPAUSE FACIAL AGEING TIMELINE

HOW HORMONAL CHANGES IMPACT YOUR SKIN, VOLUME & STRUCTURE OVER TIME

Every woman is unique. This timeline shows common changes that can occur.

PERIMENOPAUSE
(LATE 30s – EARLY 40s)

HORMONES FLUCTUATE

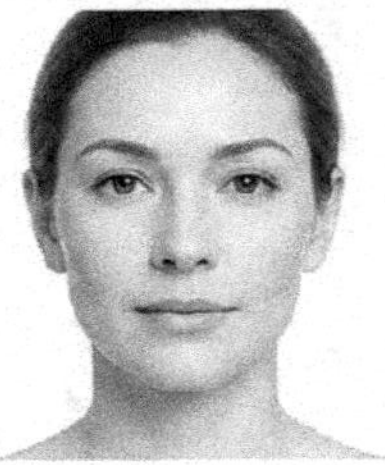

WHAT YOU MAY NOTICE

- Subtle skin sensitivity
- Occasional breakouts or inflammation
- Slight puffiness
- Dullness & dehydration
- Fine lines beginning to appear

EARLY MENOPAUSE
(40s)

ESTROGEN DECLINES

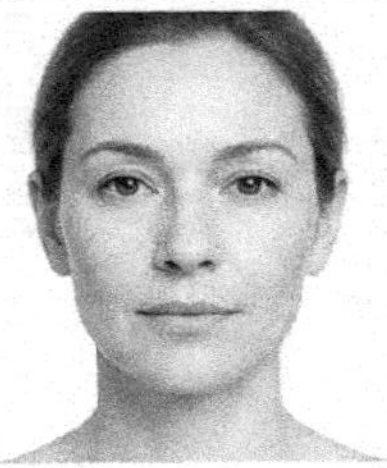

WHAT YOU MAY NOTICE

- Skin becomes drier
- Fine lines increase (especially around eyes & mouth)
- Loss of radiance
- Early volume loss in cheeks
- Skin may feel thinner

MID MENOPAUSE
(EARLY–MID 50s)

ESTROGEN LOW

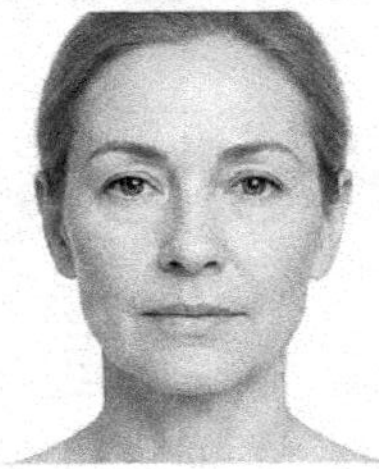

WHAT YOU MAY NOTICE

- Noticeable volume loss in cheeks & temples
- Deeper nasolabial lines
- More pronounced marionette lines
- Loss of jawline definition
- Crepey texture begins

LATE MENOPAUSE
(LATE 50s – 60s)

COLLAGEN & ELASTIN LOSS ACCELERATES

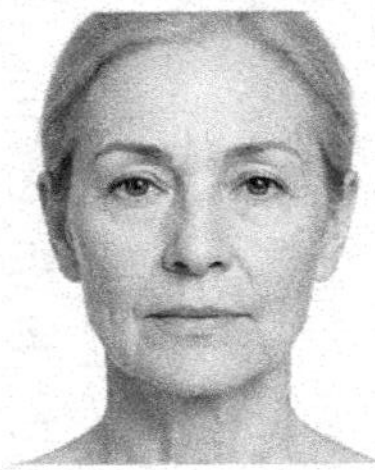

WHAT YOU MAY NOTICE

- Significant volume loss (midface, temples, under eyes)
- Deeper wrinkles & folds
- Sagging around jawline and jowls
- Thinner, crepier skin
- Uneven tone & pigmentation

POST MENOPAUSE
(60s+)

STRUCTURAL AGEING ADVANCES

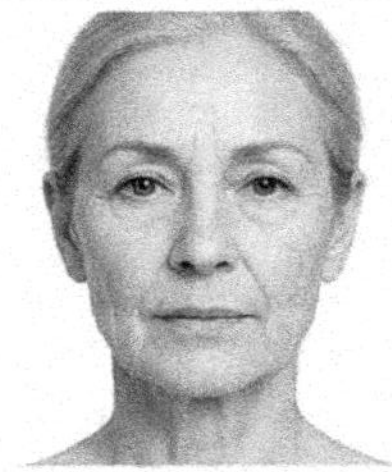

WHAT YOU MAY NOTICE

- Advanced volume loss
- Deep facial folds
- Pronounced sagging
- Very thin, fragile skin
- Loss of facial fat pads
- Dryness & dullness

THE BIOLOGICAL DRIVERS BEHIND FACIAL AGEING IN MENOPAUSE

ESTROGEN DECLINE
Leads to reduced collagen production, thinning skin and loss of elasticity.

COLLAGEN LOSS
Up to 30% loss in the first 5 years of menopause, continues over time.

VOLUME LOSS
Fat pads shrink and shift, especially in cheeks, temples and under eyes.

ELASTIN BREAKDOWN
Skin becomes less firm, more lax and prone to wrinkling and sagging.

DEHYDRATION
Skin barrier weakens, leading tnd dryness, dullness and sensitivity.

BONE RESORPTION
Facial bone loss reduces structural support, affecting contours.

SUPPORT, PROTECT, REJUVENATE

A holistic approach can help slow visible ageing and support skin health through menopause.

HORMONES • NUTRITION • SLEEP
STRESS MANAGEMENT
SKINCARE • MOVEMENT

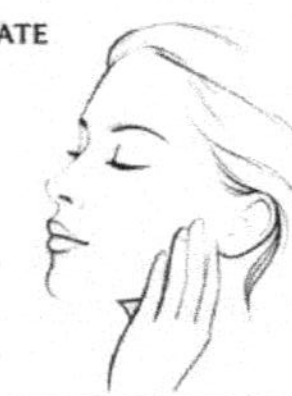

Chapter 77: Sugar: The Enemy!

In the pursuit of youthful, radiant skin, one of the most insidious adversaries is sugar. While its sweet allure is hard to resist, excessive sugar consumption wreaks havoc not only on our internal health but also on our external appearance.

The Hidden Dangers of Excess Sugar

1. Hidden Sugars in Processed Foods

Modern diets are laden with hidden sugars, often concealed under names like high fructose corn syrup, sucrose, dextrose, and more. These sugars are prevalent in processed foods, making it easy to consume excessive amounts unknowingly.

2. The Addictive Nature of Sugar

Sugar triggers the release of dopamine in the brain, creating feelings of pleasure and reward. This response can lead to cravings and overconsumption, similar to addictive substances.

Sugar's Impact on Skin Health

1. Glycation: The Silent Skin Agitator

Glycation is a natural process where excess sugar molecules bind to proteins like collagen and elastin, forming harmful compounds known as Advanced Glycation End Products (AGEs). This process compromises the integrity of these proteins, leading to:

Loss of Skin Elasticity: Skin becomes less firm and more prone to sagging.

Formation of Wrinkles: The structural damage accelerates the appearance of fine lines and wrinkles.

Dullness and Discoloration: AGEs can cause the skin to appear dull and uneven in tone.

Elevated blood sugar directly catalyzes glycation, leading to the formation of AGEs that compromise skin structure.

2. Overgrowth of Candida

Excessive sugar intake can promote the overgrowth of Candida, a type of yeast that naturally resides in the body. When Candida proliferates beyond normal levels, it can lead to:

Skin Issues: Such as fungal infections, rashes, and exacerbation of conditions like eczema.

Digestive Problems: Including bloating, gas, and discomfort.

Fatigue and Brain Fog: General feelings of tiredness and cognitive difficulties.

3. Weight Gain and Empty Calories

Sugary foods are often high in calories but low in essential nutrients, leading to weight gain and nutritional deficiencies. This not only affects overall health but also contributes to:

Increased Fat Deposits: Particularly in areas like the face and neck, affecting facial contours.

Inflammation: Which can exacerbate skin conditions like acne and rosacea.

Combating Glycation: Skin Treatments and Lifestyle Changes

While preventing glycation is ideal, certain treatments can help mitigate its effects:

1. Chemical Peels

Chemical peels involve applying a solution to the skin that exfoliates the top layers, promoting the growth of new, healthier skin. This process can improve skin texture, tone, and reduce the appearance of fine lines.

2. Laser Treatments

Laser therapies, such as fractional laser resurfacing, target deeper skin layers to stimulate collagen production and break down AGEs. This can lead to firmer, more youthful-looking skin.

3. Cosmeceuticals

Topical products containing ingredients like retinoids, antioxidants (e.g., vitamin C), and peptides can help repair and protect the skin from glycation damage. These ingredients promote collagen synthesis and neutralize free radicals.

Preventive Measures

To minimize glycation and its detrimental effects on the skin:

Limit Sugar Intake: Be mindful of both obvious and hidden sugars in your diet.

Maintain a Balanced Diet: Focus on whole foods rich in antioxidants, which combat oxidative stress and support skin health.

Stay Hydrated: Adequate water intake helps flush out toxins and supports overall skin vitality.

Sun Protection: UV exposure can exacerbate glycation; using sunscreen daily can help protect your skin.

By understanding the profound impact of sugar on our skin and overall health, we can make informed choices to preserve our natural beauty and well-being.

Chapter 78: The Most Important Beauty Treatment is Free!

Water: The Ultimate Beauty Secret

In my opinion, the most essential beauty treatment doesn't cost a cent it Is water! Hydration is the foundation of good skin, internal health, and overall well-being. While people chase the latest skincare trends and cosmetic treatments, many overlook the simplest, most powerful anti-ageing tool is proper hydration.

What Does Water Do for Your Skin and Body?

1. Water & The Skin

Hydrated skin appears plumper, smoother, and more radiant.

Dehydrated skin looks dull, wrinkled, and tired, often with more pronounced fine lines.

Reduces dryness and flakiness, improving skin texture, Flushes toxins that contribute to breakouts and inflammation, Helps prevent premature ageing by maintaining skin elasticity.

2. Water & The Liver

The liver is the body's natural detoxifier. Water helps flush out toxins, preventing congestion that can lead to dull skin, acne, and inflammation.

Proper hydration reduces dark circles and puffiness, which are often signs of liver stress and poor circulation.

3. Water & The Bowels

Hydration is key to regular bowel movements. When we are dehydrated, our digestive system slows down, leading to constipation and bloating.

Regular bowel movements prevent toxin buildup, which can contribute to skin congestion and breakouts.

My Morning Hydration Ritual

Every morning, before coffee or tea, I drink an entire litre of water is a non-negotiable part of my beauty routine.

Why? We lose water while we sleep, leading to morning dehydration.

Drinking water first thing helps flush toxins, rehydrate the body, and wake up the digestive system.

It gets the bowels moving, ensuring regular elimination, It prevents headaches most headaches are due to dehydration!

It hydrates the brain, helping with mental clarity and focus.
Coffee and tea are diuretics, which means they can contribute to dehydration if consumed first thing.

Hydrated Skin vs. Dehydrated Skin: The Visible Difference

Hydrated Skin:

Glows naturally, Looks plump and youthful, Has fewer visible fine lines, Feels smooth and supple

Dehydrated Skin:

Looks dull and tired, Shows fine lines and wrinkles more prominently, Appears rough and flaky, Can look puffy yet dry at the same time

Water & The Kidneys: Say Goodbye to Dark Circles

Dark circles aren't t always from lack of sleep they can also be a sign of dehydration and poor kidney function. Drinking enough water helps flush the kidneys, reducing the appearance of dark circles and under-eye puffiness.

Hydrogen Water- The latest wellness trend

Hydrogen water has become one of the newest trends in the wellness, longevity and biohacking world. But what exactly is it?

Hydrogen water is simply water infused with extra molecular hydrogen gas (H_2). The theory is that these tiny hydrogen molecules may help reduce oxidative stress and inflammation within the body.

Regular water is H_2O. Hydrogen water still remains H_2O — but with additional dissolved hydrogen gas added into it.

How Do Hydrogen Water Bottles Work?

Most hydrogen water bottles use a process called electrolysis.

Inside the bottle are metal plates, usually titanium coated with platinum. When activated, an electrical current passes through the water and splits the water molecules into hydrogen and oxygen gases.

Electrolysis process

The hydrogen gas dissolves back into the water while the oxygen is separated or released.

This creates tiny hydrogen bubbles suspended within the water. Some premium bottles claim to create "nano-bubbles," which may allow the hydrogen to remain dissolved for longer.

Because hydrogen is the smallest molecule in existence, it escapes very quickly. This is why freshly generated hydrogen water is considered most effective.

How Do Hydrogen Tablets Work?

Hydrogen tablets create hydrogen through a chemical reaction once dropped into water. Most contain magnesium compounds and organic acids. When the tablet dissolves, hydrogen gas is released into the water, creating the fizzing bubbles you see.

Magnesium reaction

Because hydrogen gas escapes rapidly, the water should ideally be consumed soon after the tablet dissolves.

Claimed Benefits of Hydrogen Water

Research into molecular hydrogen is still evolving, but potential benefits being studied include:

- Reduction of oxidative stress, Anti-inflammatory effects, Improved hydration recovery after exercise
- Mitochondrial support and energy production, Reduction in muscle fatigue
- Possible cognitive and healthy ageing support

Some researchers believe hydrogen acts as a "selective antioxidant," meaning it may neutralise harmful free radicals without interfering with beneficial cellular signalling.

However, while early studies are promising, the science is still emerging and many claims are ahead of the evidence.

My Thoughts

Hydrogen water is probably not a miracle cure — but it may have some supportive wellness benefits.

In my opinion, the basics still matter most: good hydration, quality sleep, movement, stress reduction, whole foods, reducing inflammation overall

Hydrogen water may simply become one extra tool in the wellness toolbox rather than the magic answer to ageing or health. As with many trends in the wellness industry, balance and realistic expectations are important.

Final Thoughts: The Simplest Beauty Hack

Before you spend hundreds on skincare and treatments, ask yourself-are you drinking enough water? Good hydration is the most overlooked yet powerful beauty treatment. It benefits your skin, digestion, energy, and overall health and best of all, it is completely free.

Start your day with water. Drink 2-3 litres a day and your body and skin will thank you.

Chapter 79: Beauty Sleep: The most underrated Anti-Ageing Treatment

You can spend thousands on skincare, injectables, lasers, and collagen stimulators — but if you are chronically sleep deprived, your body struggles to repair itself properly.

Sleep is not a luxury. It is biological repair.

During deep sleep, your body switches into restoration mode:

- Growth hormone is released
- Collagen repair increases, Inflammation reduces
- Cortisol drops, Skin hydration improves
- Cellular repair accelerates, The brain detoxifies waste products
- Muscles and connective tissue recover

Poor sleep accelerates ageing both internally and externally.

Dark circles, puffiness, dull skin, fluid retention, increased cortisol, sugar cravings, poor healing, inflammation, and even faster collagen breakdown can all be linked to poor-quality sleep.

How Much Sleep Do We Need?

Most adults need approximately:

- **7–9 hours** per night, Consistent sleep and wake times
- Deep uninterrupted sleep cycles

The body works in approximately **90-minute sleep cycles**, moving through light sleep, deep sleep, and REM sleep.

Many sleep specialists also refer to repair rhythms occurring roughly every **4 hours**, where the body alternates through deeper hormonal and neurological restoration phases overnight.

Missing these deeper cycles repeatedly can affect:

- Mood, Memory, Hormones, Weight
- Skin quality, Immune function, Nervous system regulation

Why Stress Keeps People Awake

Many people believe they "just can't sleep."

Often the real issue is:

Their nervous system no longer feels safe enough to switch off.

The body can become stuck in:

- **Fight or flight mode** (hyper-alert, anxious, wired)
- Or a frozen stress response sometimes referred to as a limbic "freeze" state

When the nervous system perceives danger — even emotional danger, chronic stress, financial worry, trauma, relationship stress, overwork, or overstimulation — the brain keeps producing stress hormones.

Your body thinks:

"Stay alert. Don't fully relax."

So even when exhausted, the brain remains "on."

Many people are tired but wired.

Resetting the Nervous System for Better Sleep

Good sleep is not just about being tired.

It is about teaching the body that it is safe to relax again.

Simple Ways to Calm the Nervous System

Reduce Evening Stimulation

At night:

- Avoid doom scrolling, Reduce blue light exposure
- Dim lights where possible, Avoid stressful conversations
- Reduce caffeine late in the day, Limit alcohol close to bedtime

Blue light from phones and screens suppresses natural melatonin production — the hormone that helps regulate sleep.

Breathwork to Calm the Vagus Nerve

One of the quickest ways to shift the body out of stress mode is controlled breathing.

Try this:

- Breathe in for 4
- Hold for 6
- Slowly exhale for 8

Repeat several times.

Longer exhalations help activate the **parasympathetic nervous system** — often called the "rest and repair" state.

This also helps soothe the **vagus nerve**, which plays a major role in calming the heart rate, digestion, breathing, and stress response.

The Backwards Counting Trick

A simple but surprisingly effective technique:

- Count backwards slowly from 50
- If your mind wanders, gently restart

This works because it interrupts repetitive anxious thinking and gives the brain a neutral focus until it gradually powers down.

My Favourite Japanese Pressure Point for Sleep

One of my favourite natural sleep techniques comes from traditional acupressure.

How to Find It

- Place 3 fingers below the wrist crease on the inner arm
- Locate the tender spot between the two central tendons
- Press firmly with your thumb for about 1 minute
- Repeat on the other wrist

This point is commonly known in acupuncture as the **Pericardium 6 point (P6 or Nei Guan)**.

Why Might It Work?

Stimulating this point may help:

- Calm the nervous system, Reduce anxiety, Ease nausea
- Relax chest tension
- Activate parasympathetic pathways

Some research suggests acupressure may influence nerve signalling pathways connected to relaxation and vagal regulation.

Many people find it surprisingly calming.

Supplements Sometimes Used for Stress and Sleep

Ashwagandha

Ashwagandha is an adaptogenic herb traditionally used to help the body cope with stress.

Some people find it helpful for:

- Anxiety, Stress resilience, Sleep quality
- Cortisol regulation

However, supplements can interact with medications and are not suitable for everyone.

Melatonin

Melatonin is a hormone naturally produced by the brain in darkness.

It helps regulate:

- Sleep timing, Circadian rhythm, Jet lag recovery

Supplemental melatonin may sometimes help:

- Shift workers, Jet lag
- Temporary sleep disruption, Older adults with reduced natural melatonin production

But more is not always better.

Timing and dosage matter.

When to See Your Doctor

If sleep problems persist:

- Constant waking, Severe anxiety
- Loud snoring, Sleep apnoea symptoms
- Ongoing insomnia, Depression, Exhaustion

…it is important to speak with your doctor.

Sometimes a short medical intervention may help interrupt the cycle of chronic sleep deprivation and nervous system overload.

In some cases, doctors may prescribe a short course of medications such as Diazepam for temporary relief, although these medications can cause dependence and are generally not intended for long-term use.

Beauty Sleep Is Real

The face often reflects the state of the nervous system.

A calm body heals better. A rested brain repairs better.A regulated nervous system ages better.

Sometimes the most powerful anti-ageing treatment is not another injectable.

It is teaching the body how to feel safe enough to rest.

Part 7 - Future Trends

Chapter 80: Anti-Ageing Trends

Ageing gracefully is no longer just about skincare and injectables scientific advancements in longevity and regenerative medicine are revolutionizing the way we approach ageing. From IV infusions to peptide therapy, cutting-edge treatments are emerging that focus on cellular health, hormone balance, and mitochondrial function.

Here are some of the latest anti-ageing trends that are shaping the future of longevity.

1. IV Infusions: Replenishing from the Inside Out

Intravenous (IV) therapy delivers vitamins, minerals, antioxidants, and hydration directly into the bloodstream, bypassing the digestive system for maximum absorption.

Popular IV infusions for anti-ageing include:

Glutathione: A powerful antioxidant that brightens skin, detoxifies the liver, and reduces oxidative stress.

Vitamin C: Boosts collagen production and immunity.

B Vitamins: Essential for energy, metabolism, and brain function.

NAD+ (Nicotinamide Adenine Dinucleotide): A game-changer in longevity science.

2. NAD+ Therapy: Cellular Energy & DNA Repair

NAD+ is a coenzyme found in every cell that plays a critical role in energy production and DNA repair. As we age, NAD+ levels decline, leading to fatigue, inflammation, and slower cellular repair.

NAD+ infusions or supplements (like NMN and NR) help to:

Improve mitochondrial function (the powerhouse of cells), Increase energy and cognitive function, Slow down ageing at the cellular level.

NMN (Nicotinamide Mononucleotide) & NR (Nicotinamide Riboside):

These precursors to NAD+ boost cellular metabolism and longevity.

Studies suggest they may delay age-related diseases and improve skin health.

3. Low Dose Naltrexone (LDN): Inflammation & Immune Support

LDN, originally used to treat opioid addiction, is now being studied for its ability to regulate the immune system and reduce chronic inflammation a key driver of ageing.

Potential anti-ageing benefits of LDN:

Reduces chronic inflammation, which contributes to ageing and disease, May help with autoimmune conditions, fibromyalgia, and chronic pain, Can improve sleep and mood, essential for longevity.

4. Transdermal Hormones: Balancing the Ageing Body

Hormonal imbalances contribute to skin ageing, weight gain, fatigue, and cognitive decline. Instead of oral hormone replacement, transdermal (topical) hormone therapy is gaining popularity due to its better absorption and lower risk of liver stress.

Key anti-ageing hormones include:

Oestrogen (Bioidentical HRT) Maintains skin elasticity, prevents bone loss, and supports cognitive function.

Testosterone:(for men and women) Preserves muscle mass, libido, and mental clarity.

Progesterone: Regulates mood, sleep, and inflammation.

DHEA & Pregnenolone: Anti-ageing hormones that support energy, cognition, and immune function.

5. RED LED light Therapy

Red LED light therapy is a non-invasive treatment that stimulates cellular energy (ATP), enhancing the skin's natural repair and regeneration processes. It promotes collagen and elastin production, helping to improve skin firmness and reduce the appearance of fine lines and wrinkles. Red light also decreases inflammation, accelerates tissue healing, and supports recovery following aesthetic procedures.

6. PEMF Mats: Electromagnetic Healing

Pulsed Electromagnetic Field (PEMF) therapy uses low-frequency electromagnetic waves to stimulate cellular repair, reduce inflammation, and enhance circulation.

Anti-ageing benefits of PEMF therapy:

Improves sleep and cellular regeneration, Reduces pain and inflammation, Supports bone density and joint health, Enhances mitochondrial function, slowing cellular ageing.

7. Amino Acids for Muscle Preservation & Longevity

Muscle loss (sarcopenia) is a major concern with ageing, affecting metabolism, strength, and skin integrity. Amino acids play a crucial role in muscle maintenance, collagen production, and energy metabolism.

Key amino acids for anti-ageing:

L-Glutamine: Supports gut health, muscle recovery, and immune function.

L-Carnitine: Aids in fat metabolism and energy production.

Collagen Peptides: Boost skin elasticity, hair health, and joint function.

BCAAs (Branched-Chain Amino Acids): Preserve muscle mass and improve endurance.

8. Other Cutting-Edge Anti-Ageing Trends

Peptides & Growth Factors

GHK-Cu (Copper Peptide): Known for its skin regeneration and wound healing properties.

Epitalon: A longevity peptide that may extend lifespan by regulating telomere length.

Thymosin Beta-4: Promotes tissue repair and reduces inflammation.

Cold Therapy (Cryotherapy & Ice Baths)

Reduces inflammation and oxidative stress, Enhances circulation and fat metabolism, Increases endorphins and energy levels.

Red Light Therapy (Photobiomodulation)

Stimulates collagen production and improves skin texture, Enhances cellular energy (ATP production), Helps with wound healing, hair growth, and pain relief.

Fasting & Autophagy

Intermittent fasting and prolonged fasting trigger autophagy, the body's natural process of removing damaged cells and regenerating new ones. Fasting is linked to increased longevity, reduced inflammation, and improved metabolic health.

9. Peptides: What They Are and Why Everyone Is Talking About Them

A peptide is a short chain of amino acids (the building blocks of protein). You can think of peptides as biological "messengers". In the body, different peptides signal different actions — such as inflammation control, tissue repair, pigmentation, growth hormone signalling, immune modulation, or sleep–wake rhythm regulation.

In aesthetics and longevity medicine, peptides are popular because they're marketed as "targeted" and "natural," with claims around skin quality, healing, fat loss, energy, sleep, and healthy ageing. However, the science and regulation are mixed: some peptides are legitimate medicines, while others are experimental or unapproved.

The Anti-Ageing Peptide Trend

Peptides sit at the intersection of three booming trends:

Longevity medicine (optimising sleep, recovery, inflammation, metabolic health)
Regenerative aesthetics (skin quality, collagen support, wound healing)
Biohacking culture (self-experimentation, online peptide "stacks")
This has created a fast-moving market where marketing often runs ahead of evidence.
A key message for consumers is this:

Not all peptides are equal. Some have solid medical uses. Others have early research only. Some sold online are poor quality, incorrectly dosed, or not what they claim.

Common Peptides People Ask About (and What They're Promoted For)

Skin and collagen support GHK-Cu (Copper peptide)

Most commonly used topically in skincare
Promoted for skin repair and collagen support
Topical cosmetic products are widely available; injectable forms raise bigger safety and regulatory issues

Longevity and sleep rhythm Epithalon (Epitalon / Epithalamin)

A short synthetic peptide linked to the pineal gland and circadian rhythm research
Promoted for sleep quality, "longevity," and cellular ageing support
Evidence is limited and it is not a mainstream approved medicine in Australia.

Healing and tissue repair (popular online, high caution) BPC-157 and TB-500 / Thymosin beta fragments

Promoted for tendon, ligament, gut repair, and injury recovery
Much of the hype is based on preclinical or early research and heavy online marketing
This is one of the most common areas where people buy unsafe "research peptides" online

Immune and inflammation support (medical-adjacent use) Thymosin Alpha-1 (TA1)

Studied for immune modulation
In some countries used in specific medical contexts
Access and appropriateness depend entirely on medical oversight and local regulation

Pigmentation (not "anti-ageing," but common in aesthetics circles) Melanotan

Promoted for tanning and sometimes appetite/sexual effects
Higher risk profile, commonly sourced illegally, and not something I recommend
Important note for readers: many peptide claims are off-label or not proven, and results vary widely.

Where to Get Peptides Safely (Australia)

In Australia, many peptides discussed online are not on the ARTG (not approved/registered for general supply). When a product is "unapproved," legal access may still be possible through the correct medical pathways.

1) Through a registered medical practitioner using TGA pathways

The TGA allows access to unapproved therapeutic goods via the Special Access Scheme (SAS) and other pathways, where a practitioner applies or notifies for a specific patient and clinical need.

2) Via legitimate pharmacy compounding (prescription only)

Some medicines can be compounded for an individual patient when clinically appropriate. Compounding is governed by professional standards and quality expectations, and it is not meant to be "mass produced" or casually supplied.

3) Clinical trials

For emerging therapies, clinical trials are often the safest and most transparent access route.

The big red flag

If someone is selling peptides directly to the public online, especially labelled "research use only," that is a major safety risk. Purity, sterility, and dosing accuracy can be unreliable.

Rapamycin — The Emerging Longevity Drug?

One of the latest and most controversial trends in the anti-ageing and biohacking world is Rapamycin, also known as sirolimus.

Originally developed as an immunosuppressive medication for organ transplant patients, Rapamycin is now attracting enormous interest in longevity medicine because of its potential effects on cellular ageing pathways.

What Is Rapamycin?

Rapamycin was first discovered in bacteria found in the soil of Easter Island (Rapa Nui), which is where its name originated.

In medicine, it has traditionally been used: to prevent organ rejection after transplantation, in some cancer therapies, in certain rare diseases involving abnormal cell growth

However, scientists later discovered something fascinating:

Rapamycin appeared to extend lifespan in multiple animal studies.

This sparked a wave of research into its possible role in slowing biological ageing.

How Does It Work?

Rapamycin works by influencing an important cellular signalling pathway called mTOR (Mammalian Target of Rapamycin).

mTOR pathway

Think of mTOR as the body's nutrient and growth sensor. It regulates cell growth, protein synthesis, metabolism and ageing. When mTOR is constantly activated—often by excess calories, sugar and continuous growth signals—cells focus on growth rather than repair, which may contribute to accelerated ageing.

Low-dose Rapamycin partially inhibits mTOR, shifting the body's focus from growth to cellular maintenance and repair.

Researchers believe this may:

Enhance cellular repair, Activate autophagy (the body's natural cellular clean-up process), Remove damaged proteins and worn-out cell components, Reduce chronic inflammation, Improve the resilience and function of ageing cells

Autophagy — The Cellular Clean-Up Process

One of the most discussed anti-ageing mechanisms linked to Rapamycin is autophagy.

Autophagy concept

Autophagy is one of the most promising mechanisms linked to healthy ageing. Often described as the body's internal recycling system, it removes damaged proteins, dysfunctional cell parts and cellular waste, recycling them into new building blocks. By keeping cells cleaner and functioning more efficiently, autophagy may help support healthier ageing and reduce the accumulation of age-related cellular damage.

Although research into Rapamycin and longevity is encouraging, its use for anti-ageing remains investigational and is still being actively studied.

Why Is Low-Dose Rapamycin Trending?

In the longevity community, some doctors are now prescribing intermittent low-dose Rapamycin protocols "off-label" for potential healthy ageing support.

Unlike transplant medicine where daily high doses suppress the immune system, longevity enthusiasts often use: much lower doses, less frequent dosing schedules

The goal is not immune suppression, but gentle modulation of ageing pathways.

Potential areas being researched include: healthy lifespan extension, brain ageing, inflammation reduction, immune system resilience, cardiovascular ageing, skin ageing and tissue repair

What Does the Research Show?

Animal studies have been impressive. Rapamycin has extended lifespan in: mice, yeast, worms, flies. Even when started later in life.

Human data, however, is still limited.

At present:

- there is no definitive proof Rapamycin extends human lifespan
- long-term safety data for healthy individuals is lacking
- much of the excitement comes from animal and mechanistic research

Potential Risks and Side Effects

Because Rapamycin affects major growth and immune pathways, it is not a harmless supplement.

Possible side effects include: mouth ulcers, elevated cholesterol, impaired wound healing, immune suppression, increased infection risk, insulin resistance in some individuals

This is why medical supervision is essential.

My Thoughts

Rapamycin is one of the most fascinating developments in longevity science because it targets ageing pathways at a cellular level rather than simply masking symptoms of ageing.

It represents a shift away from superficial anti-ageing toward attempting to influence the biology of ageing itself.

However, while the science is exciting, we are still early in understanding: who benefits, optimal dosing, long-term safety, potential risks

At this stage, Rapamycin remains an emerging and experimental area of longevity medicine rather than a proven anti-ageing miracle.

As always, the foundations of healthy ageing still remain: nutrition, movement, sleep, stress management, muscle maintenance, social connection, purpose and emotional wellbeing

No longevity drug replaces those fundamentals.

Final Thoughts: The Future of Anti-Ageing

We are entering an exciting era of longevity science, where the focus is shifting from just treating ageing signs externally to optimizing health at a cellular level. While injectables and skincare remain valuable tools, true anti-ageing goes far beyond aesthetics "it is about extending vitality, cognitive function, and overall quality of life.

From IV infusions and NAD+ therapy to hormonal balance, peptides, and biohacking, the future of ageing gracefully is about integrative, regenerative, and preventive medicine.

The goal? Not just to look younger but to feel stronger, sharper, and healthier for years to come.

Chapter 81: Secretomes – The Healing Messages of Regenerative Medicine

One of the most exciting developments in aesthetic medicine is the move away from simply filling lines and wrinkles and towards treatments that encourage the body to repair and regenerate itself.

For years, the focus was on replacing what had been lost. We added volume with fillers, relaxed muscles with Botox, and resurfaced the skin with lasers and peels. While these treatments remain valuable, a new category of regenerative therapies has emerged that aims to improve the quality of the skin itself.

One of these therapies is the **secretome**.

Although relatively new to many patients, secretomes are becoming an increasingly discussed topic in regenerative aesthetics, skin rejuvenation, hair restoration, and tissue repair.

What Is a Secretome?

A secretome is the collection of biological substances naturally released by a living cell. Cells are constantly communicating with each other. They do this by releasing chemical messengers that tell neighbouring cells what to do.

These messages may encourage cells to:

- Produce collagen, Produce elastin, Reduce inflammation
- Repair damaged tissue, Improve blood supply, Accelerate healing, Improve skin quality

The complete collection of these healing signals is known as the secretome.

Think of it as the cell's communication package.

Rather than being one single ingredient, a secretome contains hundreds of naturally occurring biological messengers working together.

What Does a Secretome Contain?

The exact contents vary depending on the manufacturing process, but may include:

- Growth factors, Cytokines, Peptides, Proteins, Amino acids, Extracellular vesicles, Exosomes, Anti-inflammatory mediators, Regenerative signalling molecules

A useful way to understand it is that exosomes are one part of a secretome.

The secretome is the entire orchestra.

Exosomes are one of the instruments.

Where Do Secretomes Come From?

Most commercially available secretomes are derived from laboratory-cultured stem cells.

These may include:

- Mesenchymal stem cells, Adipose-derived stem cells
- Umbilical cord-derived stem cells, Placental-derived stem cells

Importantly, the final product usually contains no living stem cells.

Instead, scientists culture the cells and collect the beneficial substances they release.

The cells themselves are removed.

What remains is the secretome — the collection of regenerative molecules produced by those cells.

Because no living cells remain, many manufacturers consider secretomes safer and easier to handle than cellular therapies.

How Are Secretomes Used?

Secretomes are commonly applied following procedures that create temporary channels within the skin.

These include:

- Microneedling, Radiofrequency microneedling, Fractional laser resurfacing, Chemical peels, Skin needling, Hair restoration procedures

The treatment creates pathways that allow the secretome to penetrate the skin more effectively.

In some countries and jurisdictions, secretomes may also be administered through mesotherapy-style techniques.

Regulations vary significantly around the world, and practitioners should always follow local guidelines.

What Do Secretomes Do?

Secretomes are designed to enhance the body's natural healing processes.

Their primary role is communication.

They do not fill. They do not freeze muscles. They do not create volume.

Instead, they send biological signals encouraging cells to function more efficiently.

Potential effects include:

Improved Collagen Production Fibroblasts may be stimulated to produce new collagen, improving firmness and elasticity.

Improved Skin Texture Many patients report smoother skin and improved overall texture.

Improved Hydration Healthier skin often retains moisture more effectively.

Reduced Inflammation Some components of secretomes possess anti-inflammatory properties that may help calm irritated skin.

Enhanced Healing Recovery following microneedling, laser treatments, and other procedures may be accelerated.

Hair Growth Support Secretomes are increasingly being used alongside hair restoration treatments to support follicular health.

What Results Can Patients Expect?

Results vary depending on the individual and the treatment protocol used.

Most patients are not looking at immediate dramatic changes.

Secretomes are regenerative treatments.

They work gradually.

Patients may notice:

- Improved skin glow, Improved hydration, Smoother skin texture, Reduced redness, Improved skin resilience, Better recovery after procedures, Gradual improvement in fine lines

Results typically develop over weeks to months as the skin undergoes its natural repair processes.

Secretomes Versus Exosomes

This is where confusion often occurs.

Many people mistakenly believe secretomes and exosomes are the same thing.

They are not.

Exosomes

Exosomes are tiny extracellular vesicles released by cells.

They act as biological courier packages, carrying information from one cell to another.

Their job is communication.

Secretomes

A secretome includes exosomes but also contains many other regenerative substances.

If exosomes are the letters, the secretome is the entire post office.

Secretomes provide a broader range of signalling molecules than exosomes alone.

Secretomes	Exosomes
Broad collection of regenerative factors	Specific extracellular vesicles
Contains exosomes	One component only
Multiple signalling pathways	Primarily cellular messaging
More comprehensive biological mixture	More targeted communication system

Secretomes Versus PRP

Platelet-Rich Plasma (PRP) remains one of the most established regenerative treatments in aesthetic medicine.

However, PRP works differently.

PRP

PRP is produced from the patient's own blood. Blood is collected and centrifuged to concentrate platelets.

These platelets release growth factors that stimulate healing.

Secretomes

Secretomes are manufactured products derived from cultured cells rather than the patient's blood.

No blood collection is required.

Advantages of PRP

- Autologous (comes from the patient), Long history of use, Excellent safety profile, Natural treatment, Widely accepted

Advantages of Secretomes

- Consistent manufacturing, No blood draw required, Higher concentration of signalling molecules, Broad regenerative profile, Easy to use

Why Would Someone Choose Secretomes?

The answer depends on treatment goals.

Patients who dislike blood collection may prefer secretomes.

Practitioners seeking a highly concentrated regenerative product may favour secretomes.

Others prefer PRP because it comes directly from the patient's own body.

Some clinics combine regenerative approaches to maximise outcomes.

As research continues, we will gain a clearer understanding of which patients benefit most from each treatment.

The Future of Regenerative Aesthetics

The future of aesthetics is unlikely to be about creating larger cheeks or bigger lips.

Increasingly, patients are asking for something different.

They want healthier skin. They want stronger skin.

They want skin that looks refreshed rather than altered.

Secretomes represent part of this shift.

Rather than replacing tissue, they aim to encourage the body to repair itself.

Whether used alongside microneedling, lasers, PRP, or other regenerative treatments, secretomes are helping move aesthetic medicine into an exciting new era—one where regeneration, rather than replacement, becomes the primary goal.

Chapter 82: Professional Skin Resurfacing and Rejuvenation Treatments

One of the most common questions patients ask is:

"What treatment will make my skin look brighter, smoother, and healthier?"

The answer depends on the condition of the skin, your age, your concerns, and your long-term goals.

Today, aesthetic medicine offers a wide range of treatments designed to improve skin quality. Some treatments exfoliate the surface, some hydrate, some stimulate collagen production, and others encourage regeneration and repair.

Understanding how each treatment works can help you make informed decisions about your skin journey.

Microdermabrasion

Microdermabrasion is one of the oldest and most established forms of skin resurfacing.

The treatment works by gently removing the outer layer of dead skin cells from the stratum corneum using either a diamond-tipped wand or fine crystals combined with suction.

Think of it as polishing the skin.

Microdermabrasion can improve:

- Dull skin, Rough texture, Mild pigmentation
- Congested pores, Superficial fine lines

Most patients notice an immediate improvement in smoothness and brightness. Because the treatment is relatively gentle, there is usually little to no downtime.

While microdermabrasion improves the skin's surface appearance, it does not significantly stimulate collagen production deeper within the skin.

Dermasound

Dermasound is a professional ultrasonic treatment that exfoliates, hydrates, and enhances the penetration of active skincare ingredients.

Unlike microdermabrasion, which physically abrades the skin, Dermasound uses low-frequency ultrasound waves.

The treatment generally consists of three phases.

First, ultrasonic exfoliation loosens and removes dead skin cells.

Second, sonophoresis temporarily increases the skin's permeability, allowing treatment serums to penetrate more effectively.

Third, gentle microcurrent stimulation may enhance circulation and cellular activity.

Dermasound is widely used by GlyMed Plus practitioners because it can significantly improve the absorption of professional skincare products.

Benefits may include:

- Increased hydration, Improved skin texture, Enhanced product penetration, Brighter complexion
- Reduced congestion, Improved circulation

Because it is so gentle, Dermasound is suitable for even sensitive skin types.

Dermapen Microneedling

Dermapen represents a different category of skin rejuvenation.

Rather than exfoliating the surface, Dermapen creates thousands of tiny controlled micro-injuries within the skin using sterile needles.

These micro-injuries trigger the body's natural wound-healing response.

As the skin repairs itself, it produces:

- New collagen, New elastin, Improved blood supply, Stronger skin structure

This process is known as collagen induction therapy.

Dermapen treatments may improve:

- Fine lines and wrinkles, Acne scars, Surgical scars
- Enlarged pores, Stretch marks, Skin laxity, Overall skin texture

Unlike microdermabrasion, which works primarily on the surface, microneedling creates changes deeper within the dermis where collagen is produced.

Many practitioners combine microneedling with Platelet-Rich Plasma (PRP), polynucleotides, secretomes, exosomes, and skin boosters to enhance regenerative outcomes.

Understanding the Skin Rejuvenation Toolbox

Patients are often overwhelmed by the number of treatments available today.

The truth is that each treatment has a different purpose.

Some remove dead skin cells. Some stimulate collagen. Some improve hydration.

Others encourage cellular repair and regeneration.

The best treatment is not necessarily the newest treatment.

The best treatment is the one that addresses your particular skin concerns and forms part of a long-term treatment plan.

Treatment	What It Does	Best For
Home Skincare	Maintains skin health and protects collagen	Everyone
Microdermabrasion	Mechanical exfoliation and brightening	Dull skin and congestion
Dermasound	Ultrasonic exfoliation and product infusion	Sensitive, dehydrated and ageing skin
Enzyme Treatments	Dissolve dead skin cells naturally	Sensitive skin maintenance
Chemical Peels	Accelerate skin renewal	Pigmentation, acne and sun damage
Dermapen Microneedling	Stimulates collagen and elastin	Scars, wrinkles and enlarged pores
PRP	Uses your own growth factors to stimulate healing	Skin rejuvenation and hair restoration
Secretomes	Deliver regenerative signalling molecules	Skin quality and repair
Exosomes	Cellular messengers that support regeneration	Ageing skin and hair restoration
Skin Boosters	Improve hydration and skin quality	Dehydrated or crepey skin
Polynucleotides	Tissue repair and skin rejuvenation	Eyes, neck and thin skin
Biofillers	Natural volume and regeneration	Mild volume loss
Radiofrequency Microneedling	Combines collagen stimulation with skin tightening	Acne scars and laxity
IPL	Treats pigmentation and redness	Sun damage and rosacea
Fractional Laser	Resurfaces and remodels skin	Wrinkles and scarring
HIFU	Ultrasound skin tightening	Mild to moderate sagging
Biostimulators	Stimulate collagen production	Volume loss and ageing
Dermal Fillers	Replace lost volume	Lips, cheeks, folds and jawline
Botox	Relaxes muscles causing expression lines	Forehead, frown and crow's feet

My Philosophy

After more than thirty years in aesthetic medicine, I have learned that beautiful skin is rarely the result of a single treatment.

Healthy skin comes from a combination of good skincare, sun protection, healthy lifestyle habits, and carefully selected professional treatments.

Think of your skin like a garden.

You cannot throw down one bag of fertiliser and expect it to flourish forever.

It requires nourishment, maintenance, protection, and care.

The same is true for your skin. The goal should never be perfection.

The goal should be healthy, vibrant skin that reflects the very best version of you.

Chapter 83: Understanding Skin Peels- From Glow to Regeneration

Skin peels have been used for decades to improve the appearance, texture and quality of the skin. Modern peels are no longer just about "peeling skin off." Today they range from superficial glow peels with no downtime to deeper medical peels that stimulate collagen and improve pigmentation, acne and ageing.

A peel works by applying acids or active solutions to the skin to accelerate exfoliation, stimulate cellular turnover and encourage regeneration.

Different peels work at different depths within the skin.

What Can Skin Peels Improve?

Depending on the type and strength, peels may help improve:

- dull skin, uneven texture, pigmentation, acne
- congestion, enlarged pores, fine lines, sun damage, melasma
- post inflammatory pigmentation, rough skin, superficial scarring

The Different Depths of Peels

Superficial Peels

- work mainly in the epidermis, minimal downtime, often called "lunchtime peels", suitable for maintenance and glow

Medium Depth Peels

- reach deeper into the epidermis and superficial dermis, more peeling and downtime, target pigmentation and ageing more aggressively

Deep Peels

- penetrate into the deeper dermis, significant downtime, stronger collagen stimulation, require experienced medical supervision

AHA Peels — Alpha Hydroxy Acids

AHAs are water-soluble acids that work mainly on the surface layers of the skin. They help dissolve the "glue" between dead skin cells.

They are excellent for: dull skin, fine lines, dehydration, superficial pigmentation, skin texture

Glycolic Acid Peel

Derived from sugar cane.

Because glycolic acid molecules are very small, they penetrate deeply and quickly.

Indications: pigmentation, dullness, fine lines, uneven texture, acne scarring

Downtime: redness for 1–3 days, light flaking possible, mild sensitivity

Aftercare: strict sunscreen, avoid active skincare for several days, moisturise well, avoid heat and sweating initially

Lactic Acid Peel

Derived from milk sugars.

Lactic acid is gentler and more hydrating than glycolic acid.

Indications: sensitive skin, dry skin, mild pigmentation, dullness, early ageing

Downtime: minimal, mild pinkness or flaking

Benefits: hydrates while exfoliating, often suitable for mature or reactive skins

Mandelic Acid Peel

Derived from bitter almonds.

Mandelic acid has a larger molecular size so it penetrates more slowly and gently.

Indications: acne, oily skin, rosacea-prone skin, pigmentation in darker skin types

Downtime: very minimal, occasional mild dryness

BHA Peels — Beta Hydroxy Acids

BHAs are oil-soluble acids that penetrate into pores and sebaceous glands.

Salicylic Acid Peel

One of the most popular acne peels.

Indications: acne, blackheads, congestion, oily skin, enlarged pores

How It Works

Salicylic acid dissolves oil and debris within pores while also reducing inflammation.

Downtime: dryness, peeling around acne areas, temporary purging possible

Aftercare: avoid over-drying products, moisturise, sunscreen essential

Combination Peels

Modern peels often combine several acids for synergistic effects.

These may include:

- glycolic + salicylic, lactic + mandelic

- TCA combinations, retinol combinations

Combination peels allow practitioners to target: pigmentation, acne, texture, ageing, simultaneously.

Examples of Combination Peels

Jessner Peel

A classic combination peel containing: salicylic acid, lactic acid, resorcinol

Indications: acne, pigmentation, sun damage, oily skin

Downtime: visible peeling for 5–7 days, redness, dryness

Retinol Peels

Retinol peels stimulate rapid cell turnover and collagen stimulation.

Indications: ageing, acne, pigmentation, rough texture

Downtime: peeling for several days, temporary dryness and sensitivity

TCA Peels — Trichloroacetic Acid

TCA is a medium-to-deep peel depending on concentration.

It penetrates deeper than superficial AHAs.

Indications: deeper pigmentation, acne scarring, sun damage, wrinkles, skin laxity

Downtime: frosting during treatment, peeling 5–10 days, redness may persist for weeks

Important

TCA peels should be performed carefully, especially in darker skin types, due to risk of post-inflammatory hyperpigmentation.

Deep Phenol Peels

Phenol peels are among the deepest peels available.

They create dramatic resurfacing but with substantial downtime and risk.

Indications: severe sun damage, deep wrinkles, advanced ageing

Downtime: weeks of recovery, significant redness, strict aftercare

These are now less common due to newer technologies such as lasers and regenerative treatments.

PRX — The "Non-Peeling Peel"

PRX-T33 has become extremely popular because it stimulates the skin without visible peeling.

It combines: TCA, hydrogen peroxide, kojic acid

The hydrogen peroxide modifies the action of the TCA, allowing stimulation beneath the surface without aggressive exfoliation.

Why People Love PRX

- little to no visible peeling
- no major downtime, glow and tightening effect
- suitable before events, stimulates collagen

Indications: skin laxity, dull skin, crepey skin, pigmentation, ageing skin, neck and décolletage rejuvenation

Downtime: mild redness possible, occasional dryness, usually minimal interruption to daily life

Important Peel Aftercare

After any peel:

- sunscreen is essential, avoid heat, saunas and sweating initially
- avoid picking peeling skin, avoid retinoids and strong actives temporarily
- hydrate the skin barrier, follow practitioner instructions carefully

The deeper the peel, the more critical aftercare becomes.

My Thoughts

Not every peel needs to produce dramatic visible peeling to be effective.

Modern skin rejuvenation is moving toward:

- controlled stimulation, collagen regeneration, improving skin quality gradually, less downtime

The key is choosing the right peel for: skin type, skin colour, lifestyle, concerns, tolerance for downtime

A good practitioner understands not only acids, but skin biology, inflammation and healing pathways.

Sometimes the best results come not from the strongest peel — but from the right peel, repeated consistently over time.

Chapter 84: Your Homecare Skincare Routine

The Foundation of Healthy Skin

One of the most common questions I am asked is:

"What is the best skincare routine?"

After more than 30 years in aesthetics, my answer is surprisingly simple.

The best skincare routine is the one you will actually do every day.

You don't need twenty products. You don't need a bathroom cabinet full of expensive creams. You need consistency and a basic understanding of what your skin requires.

Most healthy skincare routines follow three simple steps:

Morning

- Cleanse, Treat, Protect

Evening

- Cleanse, Treat, Repair

The products may vary depending on your skin type, but the principles remain the same.

Why Vitamin A and Vitamin C Matter

If I could choose only two ingredients for healthy ageing, they would be Vitamin A and Vitamin C.

Vitamin A (Retinol or Retinoic Acid)

Vitamin A is often called the gold standard of skincare.

It helps:

- Increase cell turnover, Stimulate collagen production, Improve fine lines
- Reduce pigmentation, Improve acne, Smooth skin texture, Support healthy skin renewal

Vitamin A works best at night because sunlight can reduce its effectiveness.

Think of Vitamin A as your skin's personal trainer. It encourages skin cells to behave like younger, healthier versions of themselves.

Vitamin C

Vitamin C is one of the most powerful antioxidants available.

It helps:

- Brighten dull skin, Protect against environmental damage
- Support collagen production, Reduce pigmentation
- Improve skin radiance, Enhance sunscreen protection

Vitamin C is best applied in the morning underneath sunscreen.

Think of Vitamin C as your skin's bodyguard.

Normal Skin

If your skin is generally balanced, not overly oily or dry, your goal is maintenance and prevention.

Morning

Cleanse with a gentle cleanser.

Apply: Vitamin C serum, Lightweight moisturiser, SPF 30–50 sunscreen

Evening

Cleanse thoroughly.

Apply: Vitamin A serum or retinol, Moisturiser

Simple and effective.

Oily and Acne-Prone Skin

Acne is not simply a teenage problem. Many adults, particularly women around menopause, experience persistent breakouts.

The goals are to: Reduce excess oil, Minimise congestion, Control inflammation, Support healthy cell turnover

Morning

Cleanse with a salicylic acid cleanser.

Apply: Vitamin C, Niacinamide serum, Oil-free moisturiser, SPF 50

Evening

Cleanse.

Apply: Vitamin A, Salicylic acid or acne treatment if needed, Lightweight moisturiser

Avoid over-cleansing. Stripping the skin often causes it to produce even more oil.

Pigmented Skin

Pigmentation can result from sun exposure, hormones, inflammation, ageing, or previous acne.

The treatment goals are: Reduce melanin production, Protect against UV damage, Encourage cell turnover

Morning

Cleanse.

Apply: Vitamin C, Tyrosinase inhibitors, SPF 50 every day

Tyrosinase inhibitors may include: Kojic acid, Arbutin, Liquorice extract, Tranexamic acid

Evening

Cleanse.

Apply: Prescription hydroquinone compound if prescribed, Retinoic acid (Vitamin A), Moisturiser

This is one of the most effective combinations for stubborn pigmentation.

As I often tell patients: *"Pigmentation is easy to create and difficult to remove."*

Daily sunscreen is non-negotiable.

Menopausal Skin

Menopause causes a rapid decline in collagen, elastin and natural hydration.

Many women notice: Dryness, Sensitivity, Crepey skin, Loss of glow, Increased pigmentation

Morning

Cleanse gently.

Apply: Vitamin C, Hyaluronic acid serum, Ceramide moisturiser, SPF 50

Evening

Cleanse.

Apply: Vitamin A, Peptide serum, Rich moisturiser

Menopausal skin needs nourishment, not aggression.

Mature Ageing Skin

As we age, skin cell turnover slows dramatically.

The focus shifts towards: Collagen stimulation, Hydration, Protection, Repair

Morning

Cleanse.

Apply: Vitamin C, Growth factors or peptides, Moisturiser, SPF 50

Evening

Cleanse.

Apply: Vitamin A, Peptides, Moisturiser

Remember, healthy skin at seventy can often look better than neglected skin at forty.

Thin Anglo-Saxon Skin

Many fair-skinned Australians have naturally thin skin with significant sun damage.

Common concerns include: Broken capillaries, Fine lines, Fragility, Easy bruising

Morning

Gentle cleanser.

Apply: Vitamin C, Peptide serum, SPF 50

Evening

Cleanse.

Apply: Low-strength Vitamin A, Moisturiser rich in ceramides

Avoid excessive exfoliation.

Thin skin needs strengthening.

Mediterranean and European Skin

Mediterranean skin often has: More natural oil, Better collagen density, Greater pigmentation risk

Morning

Cleanse.

Apply: Vitamin C, Antioxidant serum, SPF 50

Evening

Cleanse.

Apply: Vitamin A, Moisturiser

Focus on preventing pigmentation and maintaining collagen.

Fitzpatrick IV–VI Skin

(Indian, Middle Eastern, Asian, African and darker skin tones)

These skin types generally age well due to increased melanin and collagen density.

However they are more prone to: Hyperpigmentation, Melasma, Post-inflammatory pigmentation

Morning

Cleanse.

Apply: Vitamin C, Pigment inhibitors, SPF 50

Evening

Cleanse.

Apply: Vitamin A, Pigment-control serum, Moisturiser

Avoid aggressive treatments that create unnecessary inflammation.

In darker skin types, inflammation often leaves pigment behind.

The Importance of Exfoliation

Healthy skin naturally renews itself approximately every 28 days when we are young.

By our fifties and sixties, this process can take 45 to 60 days or longer.

Exfoliation helps remove dead skin cells and allows active ingredients to penetrate more effectively.

Options include: Lactic acid, Glycolic acid, Mandelic acid, Enzyme exfoliants, Professional peels

Even Cleopatra reportedly bathed in sour milk, unknowingly benefiting from lactic acid — one of the gentlest and most effective exfoliants still used today.

My Simple Rule

If you remember nothing else from this chapter, remember this:

Morning: Vitamin C and sunscreen.

Night: Vitamin A and moisturiser.

Everything else is simply tailoring the routine to your particular skin type.

Beautiful skin is rarely the result of one miracle treatment.

It is usually the result of thousands of small decisions made consistently over many years.

The best skincare routine is not the most expensive. It is the one you do every single day.

Chapter 85: Fitzpatrick Skin Classification

Why Skin Type Is Not Just About Colour

Understanding the Fitzpatrick Skin Classification is foundational in aesthetic medicine—but it is often misunderstood, oversimplified, or underestimated. Skin tone alone does not determine risk. Genetics, inflammatory response, melanocyte activity, and cultural skin behaviours all play a critical role in how skin reacts to injectables, energy devices, and chemical peels.

This chapter is essential reading for anyone treating skin of colour, mixed-ethnicity patients, or those with a history of pigmentation—even when the skin appears fair.

The Fitzpatrick Skin Types (I–VI)

The Fitzpatrick scale classifies skin based on melanin response to UV exposure, not ethnicity alone.

- Type I – Very fair, always burns, never tans
- Type II – Fair, usually burns, minimal tan
- Type III – Light–medium, sometimes burns, gradually tans
- Type IV – Medium–olive, rarely burns, tans easily
- Type V – Brown skin, very rarely burns
- Type VI – Dark brown to black skin, never burns

Key Clinical Truth

A patient may look Fitzpatrick II or III yet genetically behave like a IV or V when injured or inflamed.

This is where many pigmentation complications occur.

Genetics: Why Fair Skin Can Still Hyperpigment

Skin response is inherited—not just skin colour.

A fair-skinned patient with:

Mediterranean, Middle Eastern,

Asian, Latin, Indigenous or mixed heritage

may carry highly active melanocytes, predisposing them to:

- Post-inflammatory hyperpigmentation (PIH), Melasma reactivation, Prolonged erythema → pigmentation shift

This is why asking about family background matters, even when the skin appears light.. Pigmentation risk is about melanocyte behaviour, not how pale the skin looks on the day of treatment.

Sculptra and Pigmentation Risk (Especially Fitzpatrick IV–VI)

Sculptra is a biostimulatory injectable. It works by creating a controlled inflammatory cascade that stimulates collagen production over time.

Why This Matters for Fitzpatrick V–VI

- Inflammation = melanocyte activation, Deep or superficial placement errors increase risk, Nodules or prolonged inflammation raise the likelihood of PIH

Hyperpigmentation after Sculptra is not common, but when it occurs, it is more likely in:

- Fitzpatrick V and VI
- Patients with previous PIH or melisma, Areas of thin skin or previous trauma

Clinical Pearls

- Use conservative dilution, Avoid superficial placement, Meticulous technique and massage education are essential, Pre-condition high-risk skin when appropriate

The Critical Importance of Fitzpatrick in Chemical Peels

Chemical peels are one of the highest-risk treatments for pigmentation when Fitzpatrick type is ignored.

Higher Fitzpatrick = Higher PIH Risk

Especially with:

- Medium to deep peels, Overlapping passes, Inadequate priming, Poor post-treatment sun avoidance

Safer Peel Strategies for Skin of Colour

- Start low and slow, Prefer superficial, progressive treatments
- Extend intervals between sessions, Avoid aggressive endpoints (frosting ≠ success in darker skin)

Pre-treatment skin preparation is non-negotiable for Fitzpatrick IV–VI.

Injectables and Skin of Colour: Specific Considerations

When treating skin of colour, injectors must adapt—not avoid.

Key Differences

- Thicker dermis in many ethnic skins, Increased fibroblast and melanocyte activity, Greater risk of visible pigment change after inflammation

Best Practice Principles

- Minimise trauma: fewer entry points, gentle technique
- Avoid unnecessary inflammation, Respect vascular and anatomical variations, Avoid treating through active inflammation or acne

Skin of colour does beautifully with injectables—but only when treated intelligently and respectfully.

Post-Inflammatory Hyperpigmentation (PIH)

What Is PIH?

PIH is excess melanin production following:

- Injection trauma, Heat (energy devices), Chemical irritation, Infection or inflammation

It may appear as:

- Brown, grey, or slate discoloration, Patchy or localised marks, Delayed onset (weeks after treatment)

How to Treat PIH (Clinical Overview)

Treatment must be calm, patient, and layered.

Core Principles

- Reduce inflammation, Suppress melanocyte overactivity, Support barrier repair, Protect from UV and heat

Treatment Strategies

- Strict sun protection (daily, non-negotiable)
- Topical pigment regulators (non-irritating), Barrier-repair skincare, Avoid aggressive treatments until pigment stabilises

The worst mistake is "chasing" pigment with more inflammation.
In Fitzpatrick V–VI, patience is not optional—it is the treatment.

Fitzpatrick Is a Safety Tool, Not a Label
The Fitzpatrick classification is not about putting people into boxes—it is about preventing harm.

When respected, it:

- Improves outcomes, Reduces complications, Builds trust with patients, Elevates your clinical skill

FITZPATRICK SKIN TYPES – ALL TYPES

Black and White Portraits – Examples

TYPE I	TYPE II	TYPE III	TYPE IV	TYPE V	TYPE VI
Very fair	Fair	Medium	Olive	Brown	Deeply Pigmented
Always burns, never tans	Usually burns, tans minimally	Sometimes mild burn, tans gradually	Rarely burns, tans easily	Very rarely burns, tans very easily	Never burns, deeply pigmented

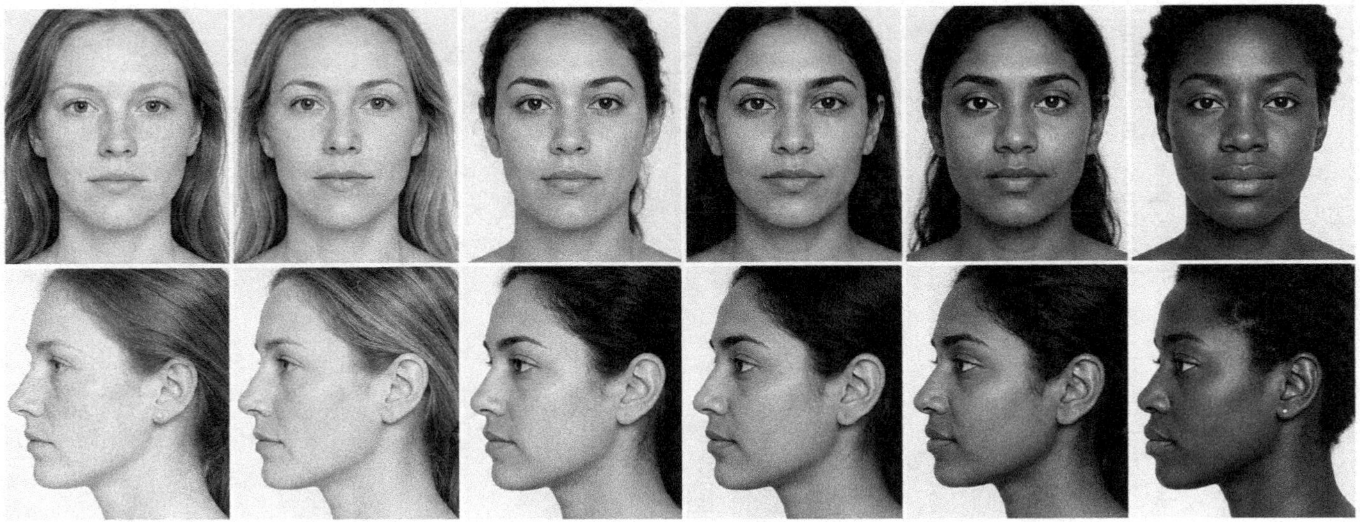

TYPE I	TYPE II	TYPE III	TYPE IV	TYPE V	TYPE VI
Pale white skin	Fair white skin	Light olive to beige skin	Olive or moderate brown skin	Brown skin	Deep brown to black skin
Freckles common	Sometimes freckles	Sometimes freckles	Rarely freckles	Very rarely freckles	Never freckles
Red or blonde hair	Blonde or light brown hair	Brown hair	Dark brown hair	Dark brown to black hair	Black hair
Blue or green eyes	Blue, green, or hazel eyes	Hazel or brown eyes	Brown eyes	Dark brown eyes	Dark brown eyes

Chapter 86: Beauty Across Borders – Treating Faces from Around the World

Understanding Cultural Aesthetics, Ethnic Anatomy, and Global Trends in Cosmetic Injectables

In our increasingly globalized world, aesthetic practitioners must recognize and respect the rich diversity of facial structures, skin types, and cultural ideals of beauty. The "one-size-fits-all" approach is outdated—true artistry lies in enhancing unique features, not erasing them. This chapter explores how different nationalities and ethnic groups perceive beauty and how we can treat their features with skill, cultural sensitivity, and precision.

1. East and Southeast Asians (Chinese, Japanese, Korean, Vietnamese, etc.)

Facial Features:

• Flatter midface

• Wider, shorter nose with a lower nasal bridge

• Smaller eyes with epicanthic folds

• Wider buccal region (cheeks)

• Often smooth and thick dermis with lower pore visibility

Beauty Ideals:

• V-shaped jawline

• High nasal bridge

• Larger eyes with "double eyelids"

• Smooth, clear skin

Popular Treatments:

• Receding Chin Filler and jawline (masseters) thinning with Botox

• Nose bridge augmentation (filler)

• Cheek contouring

• Lip hydration, not volume

• Under-eye filler to address tear troughs

• Eyebrow shaping to lift and widen the eye appearance

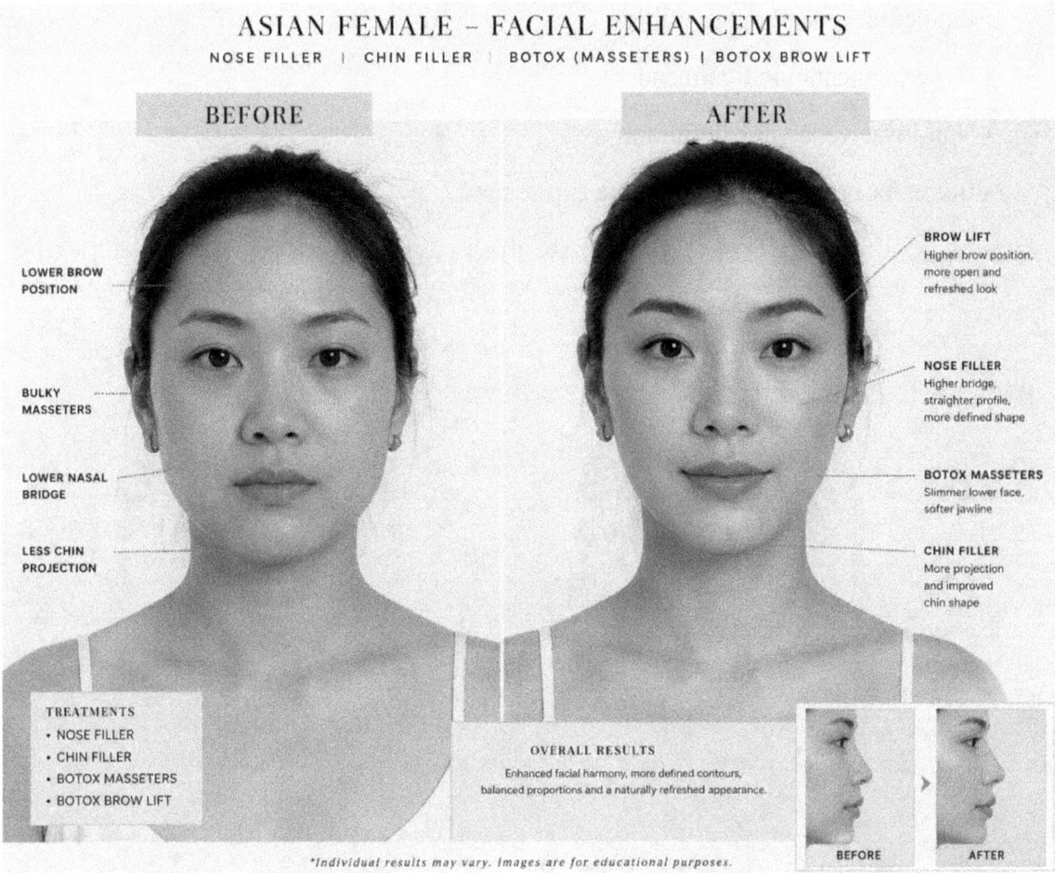

2. African and African-American Clients

Facial Features:

• Strong bone structure

• Fuller lips

• Wider nasal base

• Thicker dermis, more melanin (slower ageing, but keloid risk)

Beauty Ideals:

• Enhanced, natural cheekbones

• Lip contouring, not reduction

• Skin glow and tone

• Defined jawline

Popular Treatments:

• Sculptra or Radiesse for natural contour

• Lip definition without overfilling

• Hyperpigmentation treatments

• Non-invasive jawline definition

• Botox for brow lift, not flattening expression

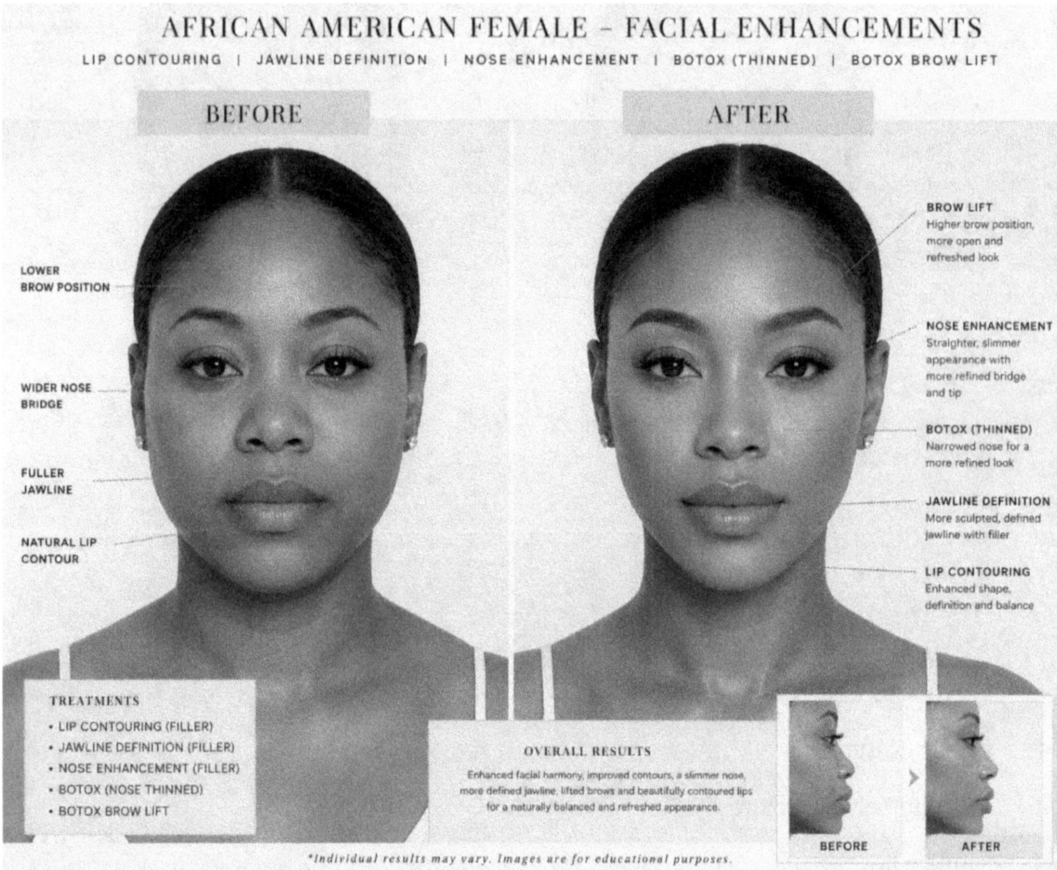

3. South Americans (Brazilian, Colombian, Argentinian, etc.)

Facial Features:

• Mixed heritage: Indigenous, European, African

• Strong, diverse bone structure

• Lush lips and expressive features

Beauty Ideals:

• Youthful fullness, High cheekbones

• Defined lips and sculpted nose

• Glowy, tanned skin

Popular Treatments:

- Cheek enhancement (Voluma, Radiesse)
- Lip filler with a balance of volume and shape
- Botox for smooth skin and brow lift
- PRP or skin boosters for luminosity

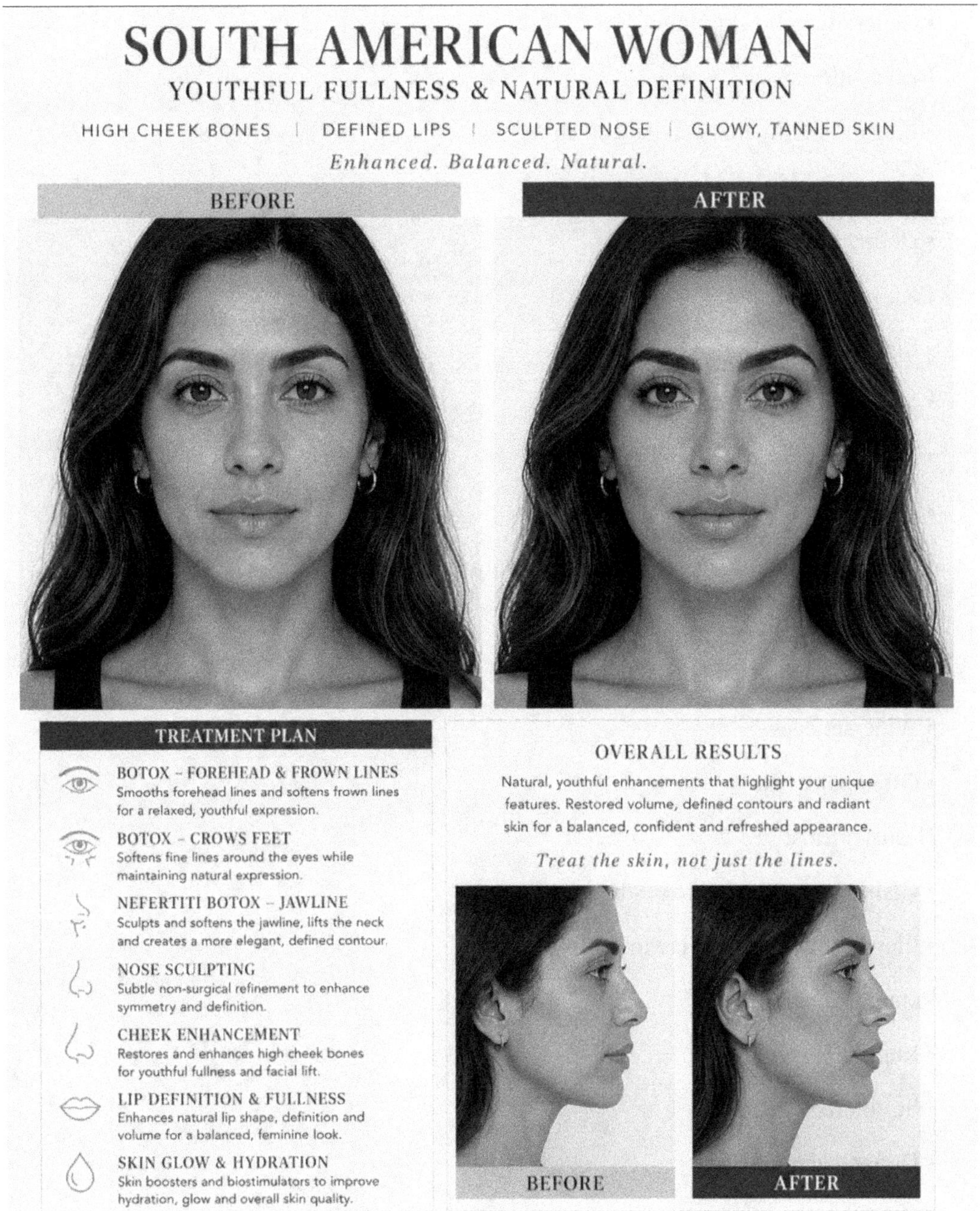

4. Western Europeans (French, Spanish, Italian, etc.)

Facial Features:

- Balanced proportions
- Prominent noses (often Roman-style)
- Thinner lips in some regions
- Generally good skin tone

Beauty Ideals:

- Elegant, minimalistic enhancements
- Natural-looking lips
- Defined but soft features

Popular Treatments:

- Lip refinement
- Micro Botox or baby Botox
- Mid-face volume restoration
- Skin tightening without bulk

5. Eastern Europeans (Russian, Ukrainian, Polish, etc.)

Facial Features:

- High cheekbones, Sharp chin
- Wide-set eyes
- Often paler skin

Beauty Ideals:

- Glamorous, model-like aesthetics
- Plump lips, Snatched jawline, Bold cheeks

Popular Treatments:

- Russian lip technique
- Structured cheek filler
- Defined chin and jaw
- Full-face contour packages

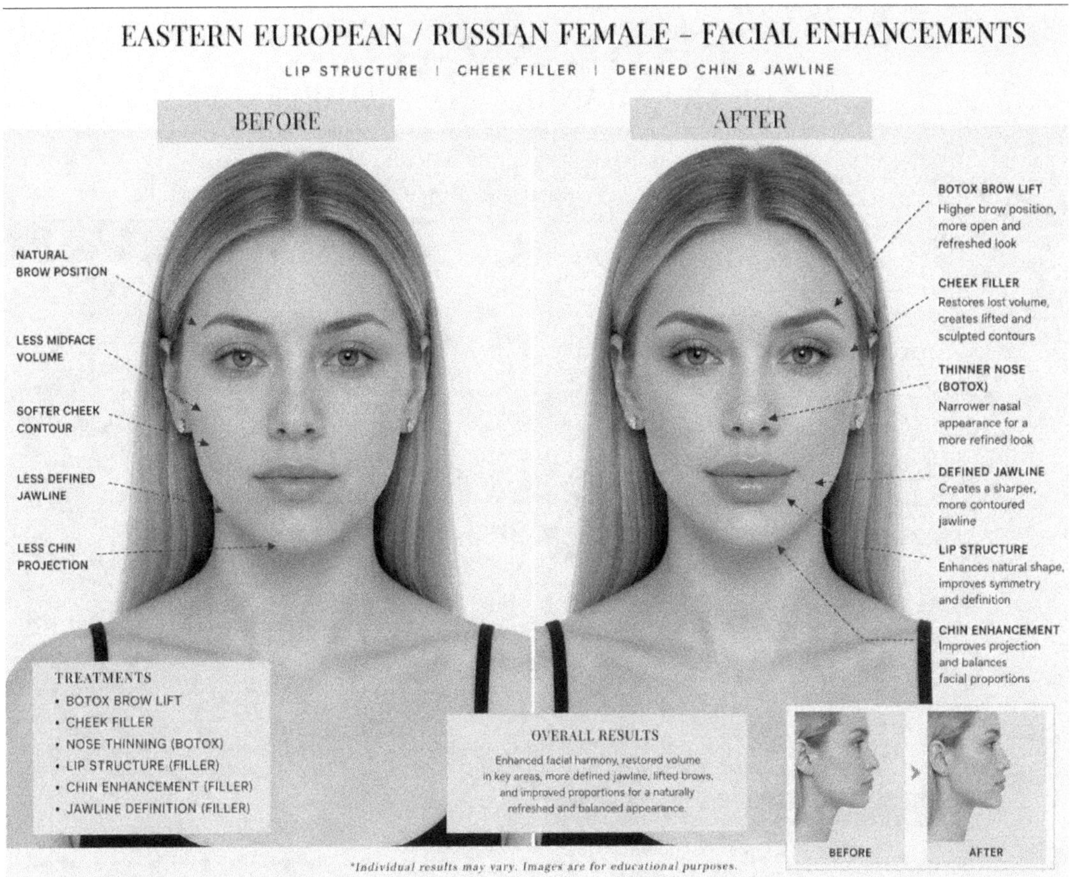

6. English (British Isles)

Facial Features:

• Fair skin, prone to redness

• Thin to medium lips

• Lower facial volume in ageing

Beauty Ideals:

• Natural enhancement

• Subtle freshness

• Soft lips and eyes

Popular Treatments:

• Baby Botox, Tear trough filler

• Gentle lip filler

• PRP for skin clarity

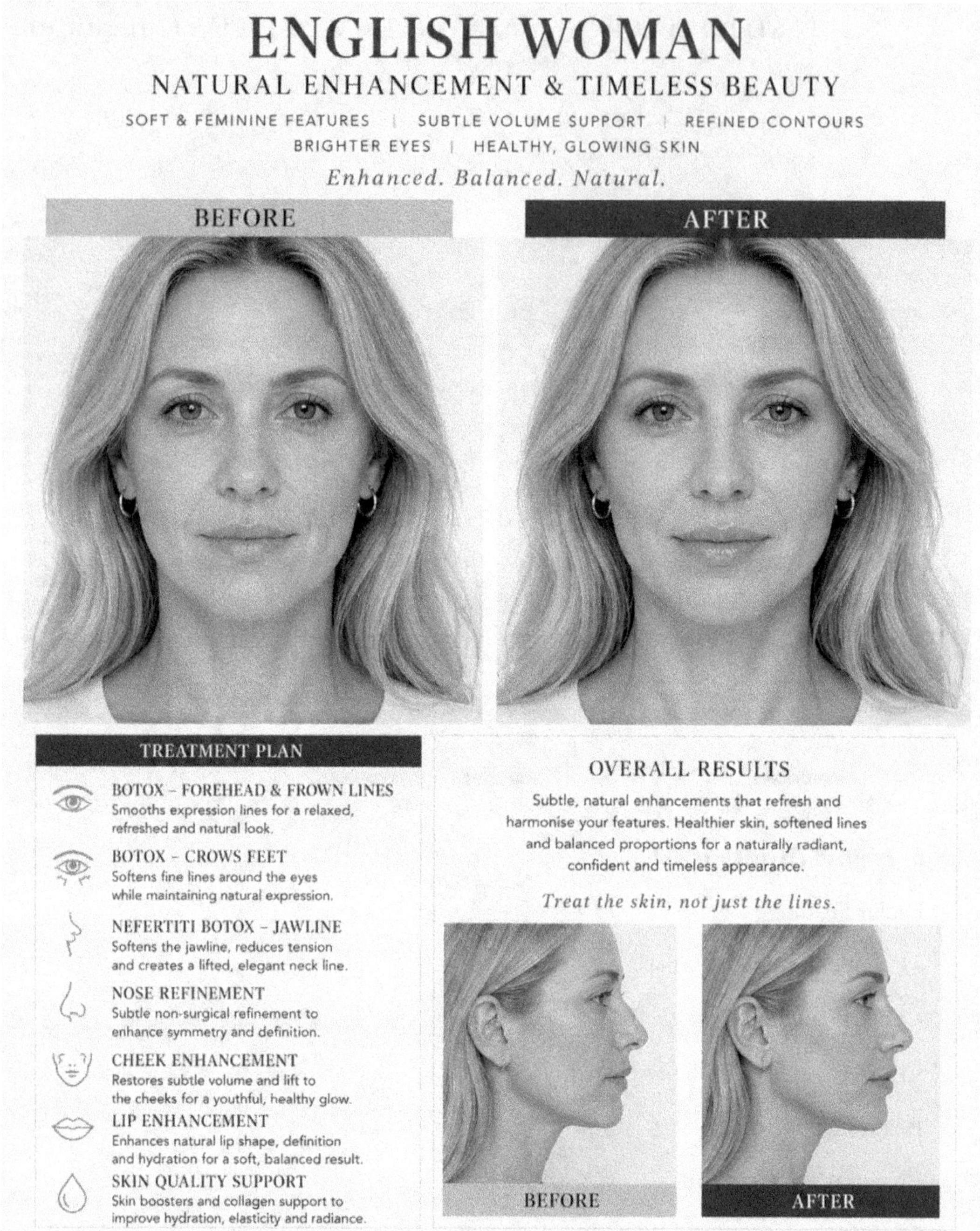

ENGLISH WOMAN
NATURAL ENHANCEMENT & TIMELESS BEAUTY
SOFT & FEMININE FEATURES | SUBTLE VOLUME SUPPORT | REFINED CONTOURS
BRIGHTER EYES | HEALTHY, GLOWING SKIN
Enhanced. Balanced. Natural.
BEFORE
AFTER
TREATMENT PLAN
BOTOX – FOREHEAD & FROWN LINES
Smooths expression lines for a relaxed, refreshed and natural look.
BOTOX – CROWS FEET
Softens fine lines around the eyes while maintaining natural expression.
NEFERTITI BOTOX – JAWLINE
Softens the jawline, reduces tension and creates a lifted, elegant neck line.
NOSE REFINEMENT
Subtle non-surgical refinement to enhance symmetry and definition.
CHEEK ENHANCEMENT
Restores subtle volume and lift to the cheeks for a youthful, healthy glow.
LIP ENHANCEMENT
Enhances natural lip shape, definition and hydration for a soft, balanced result.
SKIN QUALITY SUPPORT
Skin boosters and collagen support to improve hydration, elasticity and radiance.
OVERALL RESULTS
Subtle, natural enhancements that refresh and harmonise your features. Healthier skin, softened lines and balanced proportions for a naturally radiant, confident and timeless appearance.
Treat the skin, not just the lines.
BEFORE
AFTER

7. Americans (USA)

Facial Features:

• Highly diverse (melting pot of ethnicities)

• Media-driven beauty ideals

Beauty Ideals:

• Youthful glow

• Symmetry and proportion

• Plump lips, smooth foreheads

Popular Treatments:

• Full facial rejuvenation (packages)

• Lip filler, cheek and jaw contour

• Skin resurfacing, Preventative Botox

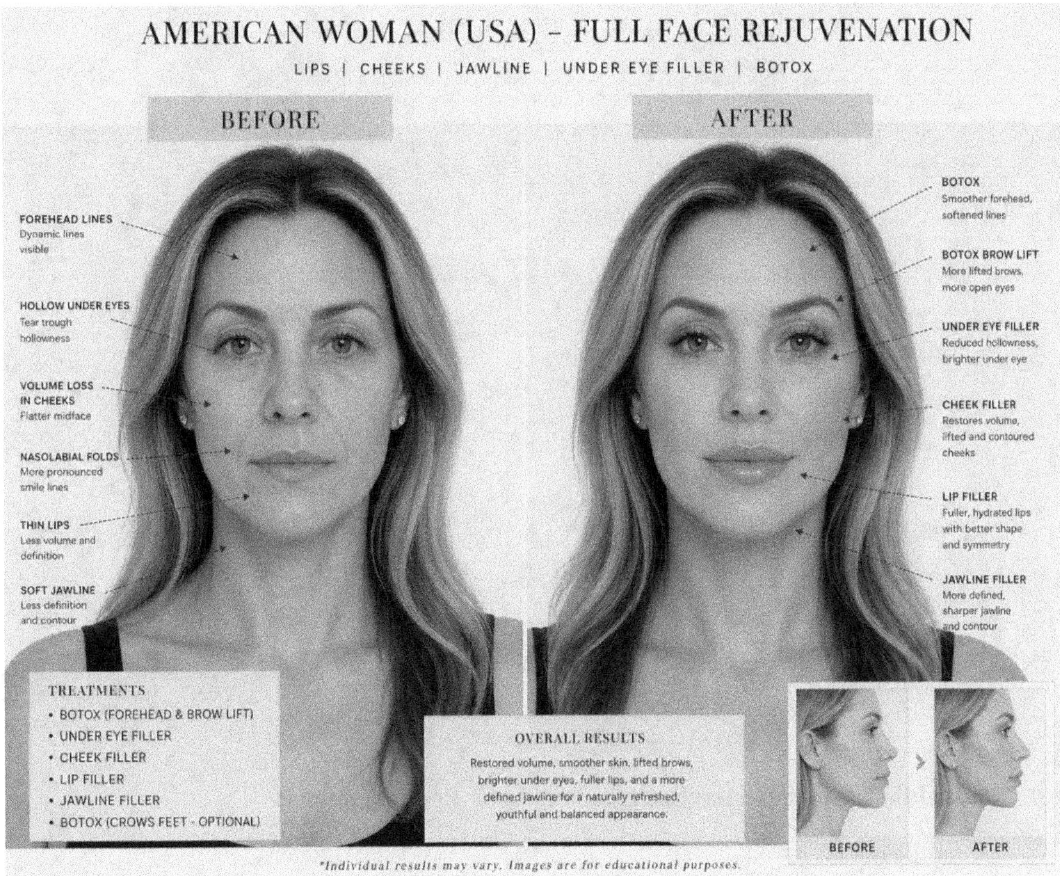

8. Australians

Facial Features:

• Also diverse—Anglo-Celtic majority but with large Asian, Indigenous, and Mediterranean influences

• Often sun-damaged skin

Beauty Ideals:

• Natural and fresh look, Subtle tweaks

• Healthy skin focus

Popular Treatments:

• Skin boosters, PRP and collagen biostimulators

• Lip hydration

• Anti-wrinkle for crow's feet and frown

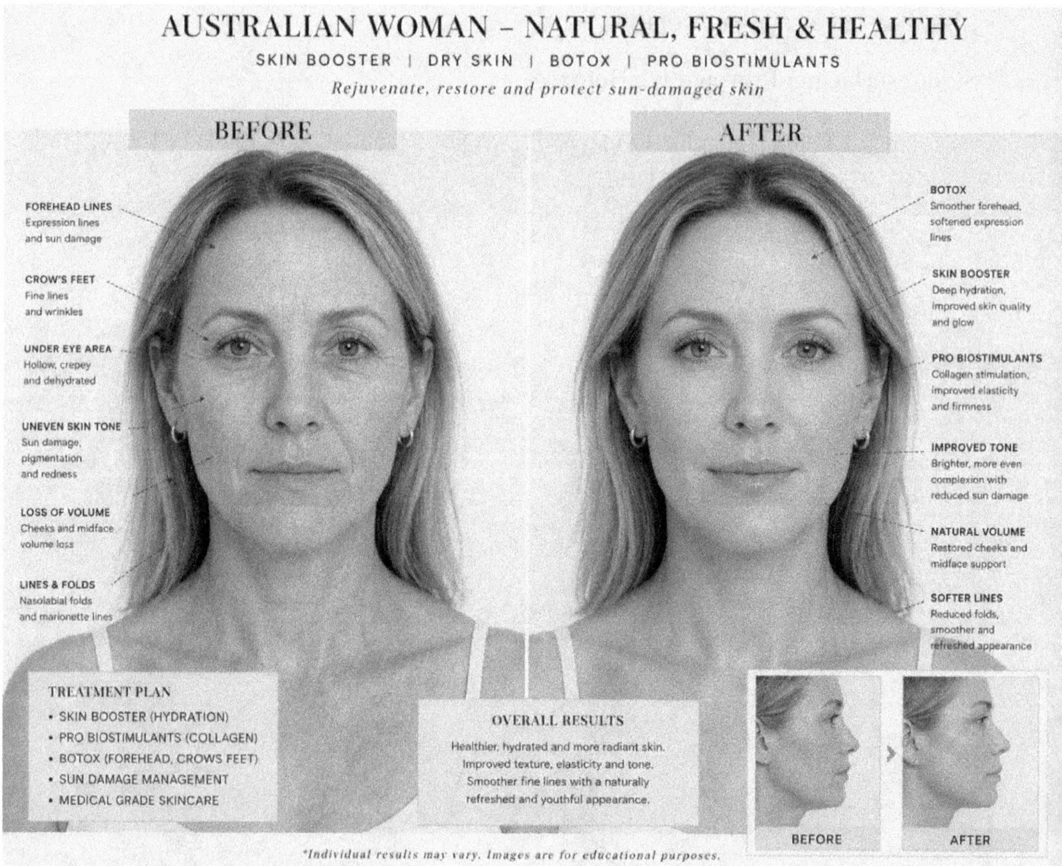

9. Middle Eastern (Lebanese, Iranian, Arab Peninsula, etc.)

Facial Features:

• Strong nose profile, Deep-set eyes, Full lips

• Olive skin tone

Beauty Ideals:

• Sculpted features, Defined cheeks

• Perfect nose profile

• Sharp brows

Popular Treatments:

- Non-surgical rhinoplasty, Lip shaping
- Brow lift with threads or Botox
- Cheek contouring

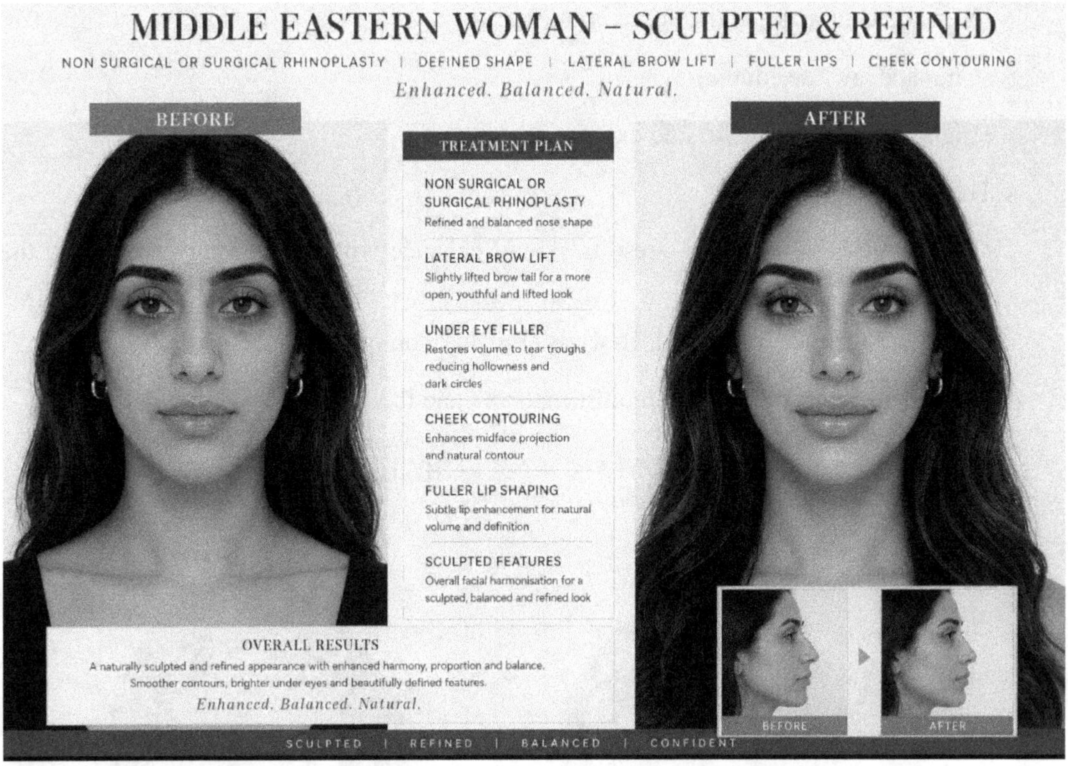

10. India (South Asian Aesthetics)

Facial Features:

- Medium to full lips, Strong jawline and chin
- Wider midface with well-defined bone structure
- Often high cheekbones and almond-shaped eyes
- Medium to deep skin tones with melanin-rich dermis (slower ageing but prone to pigmentation)

Beauty Ideals:

- Smooth, radiant skin
- Symmetrical and softly contoured features
- Refined nose and balanced lips
- Defined jawline and softly lifted cheeks

• Natural expressions with minimal wrinkle lines

Popular Treatments:

• Skin texture and pigmentation improvement (PRP, skin boosters, light peels)

• Subtle lip enhancement—balance and hydrate, not overfill

• Midface volumization to restore youthfulness

• Chin and jawline contouring

• Light Botox for brow lift and expression softening

Trends:

• Natural glam is preferred—results should enhance without drawing attention to the "work"

• Bridal aesthetic is influential: flawless skin, harmonious features

• Increasing interest in collagen biostimulators and thread lifts

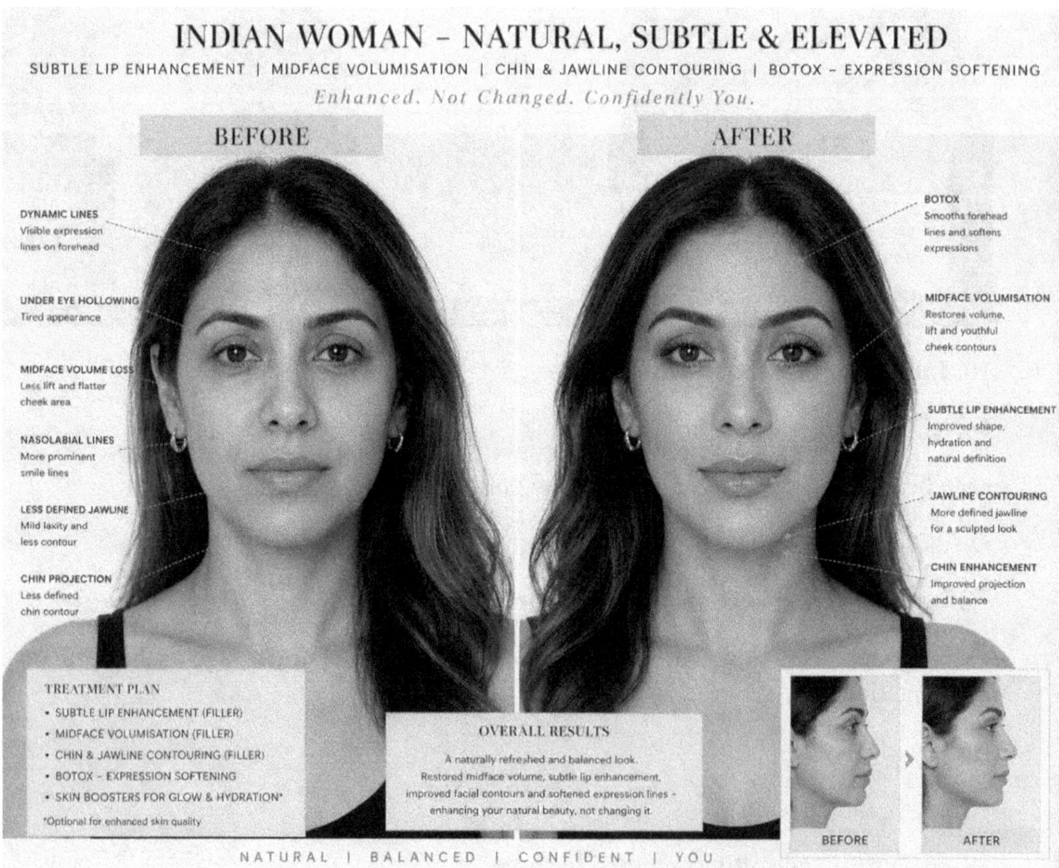

Lip Characteristics

Ethnicity/Region	Natural Lip Characteristics	Aesthetic Preferences & Trends	Treatment Approach
English	Thin to medium lips; more definition in the upper lip	Desire for subtle plumpness, symmetry, and hydration	Soft filler for shape and hydration; avoid overfilling
Western European	Moderate fullness; often well-defined shape (e.g., French/Italian)	Favor natural enhancement, soft volume, and proportion	Minimalist techniques with light filler in vermilion border
Eastern European	Naturally fuller lips, particularly lower lip	Bold, structured look; Russian lip technique is popular	Use firm filler, vertical columns for lift and height (e.g., Russian lips)
USA	Highly varied; trend-driven; media influence	Full lips are fashionable; Cupid's bow definition is often emphasized	Contour + volume combo; "Instagram" lips trend with keyhole pout
Asian (East/Southeast)	Evenly proportioned lips; smaller, with less projection	Hydration and shape enhancement, not volume	Use soft filler; focus on cupid's bow and vermilion border
Indian (South Asian)	Medium to full lips; often with good definition and melanin-rich tone	Smoother texture, mild enhancement, and lip symmetry	Focus on lip symmetry, subtle volumizing; balance pigmentation with gloss or hydration
Australia	Diverse population (Anglo, Mediterranean, Asian mix); sun exposure affects texture	Trend toward natural, hydrated lips with mild volume	Balance and blend approach; skin boosters often used alongside filler

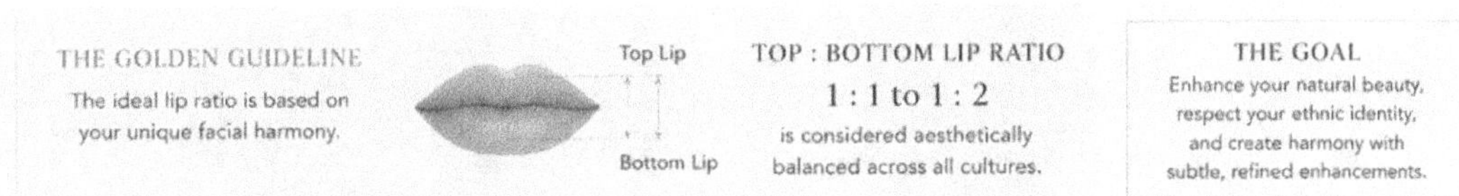

LIP IDEALS AROUND THE WORLD

FAVOURED TOP & BOTTOM LIP RATIO

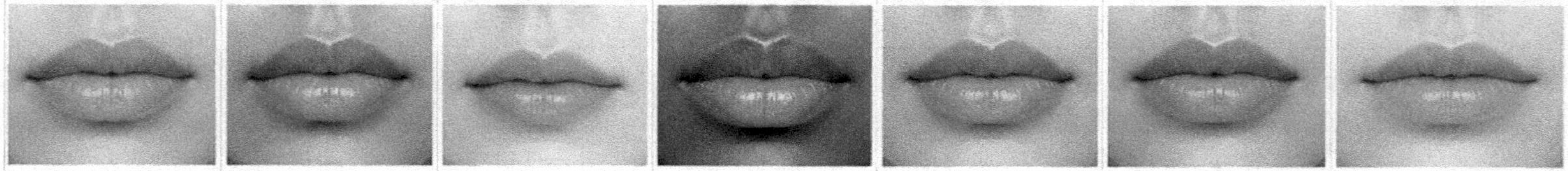

AUSTRALIAN WOMAN	INDIAN WOMAN	EAST ASIAN WOMAN	AFRICAN / AFRO CARIBBEAN WOMAN	MIDDLE EASTERN WOMAN	MEDITERRANEAN WOMAN	NORTHERN EUROPEAN / SCANDINAVIAN WOMAN
1 : 1.3 to 1 : 1.5	1 : 1.5 to 1 : 1.7	1 : 1 to 1 : 1.2	1 : 1.6 to 1 : 2	1 : 1.3 to 1 : 1.6	1 : 1.3 to 1 : 1.6	1 : 1 to 1 : 1.2
Slightly fuller bottom lip	Noticeably fuller bottom lip	Balanced or subtle bottom lip fullness	Fuller bottom lip	Slightly fuller bottom lip	Slightly fuller bottom lip	Balanced or subtle bottom lip fullness
• Soft, natural fullness • Balanced proportions • Soft cupid's bow • Effortless, healthy look	• Full, well-defined lips • Soft cupid's bow • Good volume • Harmonious balance	• Soft, subtle fullness • Low to medium volume • Gentle cupid's bow • Refined, delicate look	• Full, voluminous lips • Soft or less defined cupid's bow • Bold, natural shape • Hydrated, healthy look	• Sculpted, defined lips • Pronounced cupid's bow • Balanced volume • Elegant, symmetrical look	• Full, natural-looking lips • Defined cupid's bow • Balanced proportions • Warm, sensual look	• Soft, subtle lips • Low to medium volume • Gentle cupid's bow • Natural, understated look

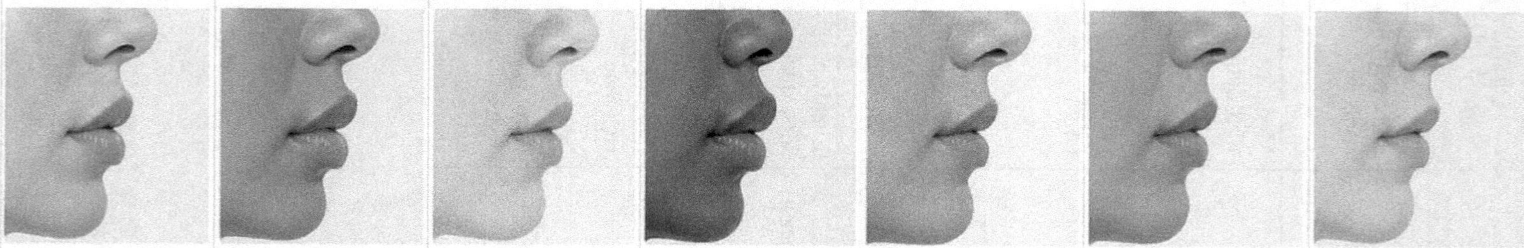

AUSTRALIAN WOMAN	INDIAN WOMAN	EAST ASIAN WOMAN	AFRICAN / AFRO CARIBBEAN WOMAN	MIDDLE EASTERN WOMAN	MEDITERRANEAN WOMAN	NORTHERN EUROPEAN / SCANDINAVIAN WOMAN
Natural projection Mild pout Balanced profile	Good projection Softly rounded Balanced profile	Natural projection Soft contour Refined profile	Strong projection Full pout Beautifully defined profile	Defined projection Sculpted shape Balanced profile	Balanced projection Softly defined Harmonious profile	Subtle projection Soft contour Natural profile

International Trends

Trends by Region

Region	Injecting Trends
East Asia	Chin and jaw slimming with Botox; subtle filler in nose bridge and under-eye areas.
Africa/African-Am.	Cheek sculpting with biostimulators; lip contouring without added volume.
South America	Full facial harmonization; structured filler for cheeks and lips.
Western Europe	Micro-Botox; minimal lip filler; subtle midface rejuvenation.
Eastern Europe	Russian lips; high cheek filler; defined chin and jawline.
UK	Baby Botox; tear trough filler; soft, natural lip enhancement.
USA	Full-face packages; preventative Botox; HD contouring across cheeks and jawline.
Australia	Skin boosters; PRP; conservative filler use to maintain a natural look.
Middle East	Non-surgical rhinoplasty; defined cheekbones; bold lips and brows.
India	Skin texture improvement; subtle lip and midface filler; jawline refinement.

Beauty trends around the world are fascinating because they reflect far more than fashion.
Climate, culture, beauty ideals, social media, and even economic trends all shape what each country considers attractive.

Here's an expanded global look at the beauty aesthetics different countries have become famous for — and how these trends have influenced the cosmetic industry worldwide.

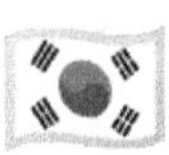

South Korea — Glass Skin & Advanced Aesthetic Culture

South Korea has transformed global beauty more than almost any other nation in the past decade.
K-beauty focuses on luminous "glass skin" — skin that appears poreless, hydrated, translucent, and reflective like glass. Multi-step skincare routines including essences, ampoules, sheet masks, and SPF have become mainstream worldwide.

Korean beauty also popularized:

- Gradient lips, Straight brows
- "Aegyo-sal" under-eye fullness for a youthful look
- Skin boosters and regenerative treatments
- Subtle jawline contouring, Preventative aesthetic treatments at a younger age

The philosophy is prevention, hydration, and refinement rather than dramatic transformation.

Japan — Mochi Skin & Soft Feminine Beauty

Japan embraces "mochi skin" — soft, smooth, pillowy skin resembling Japanese rice cake.
Japanese beauty trends favor delicacy, elegance, and youthful femininity rather than overt glamour.

Iconic Japanese trends include:

- Under-eye blush ("Igari makeup"), Doll-like lashes
- Circle lenses for enlarged eyes, Lightweight skincare layering
- Soft matte or satin skin, Minimal contouring

Japanese beauty philosophy centers around ritual, simplicity, and skin harmony.

France — Effortless Chic & Natural Ageing

France is synonymous with understated sophistication.
French women are famous for the "less is more" approach — glowing skin, brushed brows, healthy hair, and makeup that appears almost invisible.

French beauty trends include:

- "No makeup" makeup, Pharmacy skincare
- Minimal injectables, Strobing instead of heavy contour
- Acceptance of natural ageing, Red lips paired with otherwise minimal makeup

French beauty celebrates individuality and confidence over perfection.

Brazil — Body Confidence & Sensual Beauty

Brazil has long been associated with athletic, sun-kissed beauty and body confidence.
Brazilian beauty culture strongly emphasizes the body alongside facial aesthetics.

Known trends include:

- Glowing bronzed skin, Body contouring
- Lymphatic drainage massage, Curves and fitness culture
- Hair smoothing treatments, Beach-inspired effortless beauty

Brazil is also one of the world's largest consumers of cosmetic surgery and aesthetic procedures.

India — Ayurvedic Beauty & Expressive Eyes

India blends ancient Ayurvedic traditions with modern beauty innovation.
Beauty rituals often include turmeric, sandalwood, rose water, neem, oils, and herbal preparations passed down through generations.

Indian beauty is famous for:

- Kohl-lined expressive eyes
- Thick glossy hair, Bridal glamour
- Gold-toned makeup, Holistic wellness practices
- Scalp oiling and massage rituals

There is a strong connection between beauty, spirituality, and wellness in Indian culture.

Scandinavia — Minimalism & Skin Health

Scandinavia beauty reflects simplicity, wellness, and sustainability.
Rather than dramatic makeup, Scandinavian beauty focuses on healthy skin, clean aesthetics, and understated elegance.

Typical Scandi beauty features:

- Minimal makeup, Grey-toned nude lips
- Skin barrier health, Natural brows
- Sustainable skincare
- "Quiet luxury" beauty

The aesthetic is polished without looking overly done.

China — High-Tech Beauty & Porcelain Skin

China combines traditional herbal medicine with cutting-edge beauty technology.
Chinese beauty trends increasingly focus on precision skincare, anti-pollution formulas, and high-tech devices.

Popular ideals include:

- Porcelain skin
- Brightening skincare, V-shaped jawlines
- Delicate facial proportions, Herbal ingredients like ginseng and green tea
- Advanced beauty tech devices

China is also rapidly influencing global beauty commerce through livestream shopping and social media beauty culture.

Russia — Glamour, Volume & Russian Lips

Russia is known for glamorous, high-maintenance beauty aesthetics with an emphasis on dramatic femininity.

Russian beauty trends include:

- Bold lashes and layered mascara, Sculpted cheekbones
- Full glamorous hair, Matte flawless skin
- Defined brows, Statement lips

One of the most influential trends to emerge from Russia is the "Russian Lip" technique in aesthetic medicine.

The Russian Lip Trend

Russian Lips use vertical filler placement techniques designed to:

- Create a flatter heart-shaped lip
- Increase lip height rather than forward projection
- Define the cupid's bow
- Produce a doll-like lifted appearance

While highly popular on social media, the technique requires careful anatomical understanding to avoid vascular compromise, migration, or an overfilled appearance.

Russia has strongly influenced global trends toward dramatic lip shaping and facial contouring aesthetics.

Italy — Mediterranean Glamour

Italy celebrates sensuality, confidence, and timeless glamour.
Italian beauty emphasizes:

- Olive skin, Voluminous hair
- Strong brows, Bronze tones
- Elegant femininity, Expressive eyes

Italian beauty often feels luxurious and effortlessly sexy without appearing excessive.

Middle East & Arab Beauty — Intensity & Luxury

Middle East beauty culture is known for glamour, precision, and long-lasting makeup designed for hot climates.

Signature elements include:

- Dramatic eye makeup
- Oud-based fragrances, Full brows and lashes
- High-pigment cosmetics
- Matte flawless skin, Advanced aesthetic procedures

The region has also heavily influenced trends in:

- Full lips, Sharp contouring
- Fox-eye aesthetics, Luxury fragrance culture

Germany — Clean Beauty & Functional Wellness

Germany approaches beauty with practicality and wellness in mind.
German beauty trends prioritize:

- Eco-conscious products
- Functional skincare, Clean ingredients
- Gender-neutral aesthetics
- Fitness and health, Minimal cosmetic excess

German consumers tend to value science-backed formulations and sustainability over trend-driven beauty.

The Globalisation of Beauty

Social media has blurred international beauty boundaries.
Today, someone in Sydney may ask for:

- Korean glass skin, Russian lips
- Brazilian body contouring, French minimalism
- Scandinavian skin wellness

all in the same consultation.

The challenge for aesthetic practitioners is balancing trends with anatomy, individuality, and natural outcomes.

Because ultimately, the most beautiful results are the ones that still allow a person to look like themselves — just fresher, healthier, and more confident.

Part 8- 30 Years of Lessons & Final Thoughts

Chapter 87: What 30 Years has Taught me

Never stop learning. Never stop refining.

From the moment I decided to go into aesthetics, something in me shifted.

My mind was curious.
My heart was invested.
And I developed a hunger to learn that has never left me.

Over the years, I have completed hundreds of courses and certificates — from functional and nutritional medicine, to advanced injectable training, to international conferences. I have trained with companies, with doctors, with peers, and I have always remained open to learning something new.

Thirty years later, I am still learning.

Because the moment you think you know it all in this industry is the moment you stop growing

Education never ends

Aesthetics is not a static field.

It evolves:

New products, New techniques, New understanding of anatomy and ageing

What we believed ten years ago is not always what we believe today

And that is a good thing because it means we are improving refining becoming safer and more effective

For me, education has never been about collecting certificates

It has been about **refining my ability to deliver better outcomes**

I have witnessed the evolution

When I first started, the choices were simple

We had: Botox, Collagen injections

That was it

Then came Sculptra
A very different way of thinking — not filling, but stimulating

And then came hyaluronic acid fillers
Starting with early products like Restylane

From that point, everything changed

The HA world expanded rapidly:

Different technologies, Different consistencies, Different uses

We moved from basic filling to **sculpting, layering, and refining**

And now, we are entering another phase:

Biostimulants, Skin boosters, Regenerative treatments

The industry has evolved from:
filling → shaping → regenerating

The industry has changed — and so have the patients

When I first began, aesthetic treatments were less common
and often more conservative

Now:

Treatments are mainstream, Patients are more informed, Expectations are higher

And with that has come:

More opportunity, But also more responsibility

Because not everything that is possible is appropriate

I have learnt the importance of restraint

One of the biggest lessons over time has been this:

Just because you can do something does not mean you should

Early in the industry, the focus was often on:

Filling lines

Adding volume

Now, with experience, I understand:

Less can achieve more, Balance is more important than correction, Natural results last

Restraint is not about doing less
It is about doing what is **right**

I have seen what works — and what doesn't

Trends come and go, Lip shapes change, Cheek projection changes

Techniques evolve

But what remains consistent is this:

Natural results never go out of style

Overfilled faces, Overtreated features, Aggressive trends

They may look current for a moment but they rarely age well

I have learnt to treat the whole person

Aesthetics is not just about the face

It is about:

Health, Hormones, Lifestyle, Emotional wellbeing

Over time, I have expanded my knowledge into:

Functional medicine, Nutrition, Hormonal balance

Because the skin reflects what is happening internally

And when you address boththe results are far more powerful

Ageing has changed

We are now seeing something quite remarkable

Patients in their 60s looking like they are in their 40s

And in my own case, now in my 70s, I can say this honestly

I still feel: Energetic, Engaged, Spiritually younger than my age

And I do believe that my work, my knowledge, and my approach to aesthetics has contributed to that

Because aesthetics is not just about looking good

It is about:
feeling good in your own skin

Aesthetics is about more than appearance

When a patient feels better about how they look it affects how they move through the world

Their confidence
Their energy
Their presence

There is a lightness that returns

A joy

The French call it joie de vivre
— the joy of living

And that, to me, is what good aesthetic work supports

I am still learning

Even after 30 years

I still: Attend courses, Listen to new ideas, Refine my techniques

Because this industry demands it

But more importantly my patients deserve it

A final thought

Thirty years has taught me this:

It is not about doing more, It is about understanding more

It is not about following trends, It is about recognising what lasts

And it is not about changing faces, It is about supporting people to feel like themselves again

Treat the skin, respect the face, and never stop learning

Chapter 88: Cosmetic Treatments Myths

Separating Fact from Fiction

Over the past 30 years in aesthetic medicine, I have heard just about every myth imaginable.

Some have been around for decades. Others have spread through social media, celebrity gossip, and online forums. Unfortunately, misinformation often travels faster than facts.

Many patients arrive at their consultation feeling confused. They have heard horror stories from a friend, read something alarming online, or seen an overfilled celebrity and assumed all cosmetic treatments produce the same result.

The truth usually lies somewhere in the middle.

Let's look at some of the most common cosmetic treatment myths and separate fact from fiction.

Myth 1: Botox Is a Poison

This is probably the most common concern I hear.

Technically, botulinum toxin is derived from a bacterium. However, so are many medications used safely in modern medicine.

The important thing to understand is that cosmetic treatments use extremely small, purified, carefully measured doses.

Botulinum toxin has been used medically for decades to treat conditions such as muscle spasms, migraines, excessive sweating, and eye disorders long before it became popular for wrinkles.

When administered by a trained practitioner, it has an excellent safety profile.

The dose used cosmetically is tiny compared with doses used in many medical treatments.

Myth 2: Botox Will Make Me Look Frozen

Botox does not create a frozen appearance.
Poorly performed Botox creates a frozen appearance.

When injected appropriately, Botox simply relaxes selected muscles that create unwanted wrinkles. The goal is to soften expression lines while allowing natural facial movement to remain.
Most people should look refreshed, rested, and less tired—not expressionless.
A good treatment should never be obvious.

Myth 3: Fillers Stretch the Skin

Many people believe that once fillers are used, the skin becomes permanently stretched.
This is largely untrue.
Hyaluronic acid fillers gradually break down over time. As they dissolve, the skin generally returns to its previous state.

In fact, hyaluronic acid attracts water and may improve hydration and skin quality during its lifespan.
Problems occur when excessive amounts of filler are repeatedly placed over many years without adequate assessment or when migration occurs.

The issue is usually over-treatment, not stretching.

Myth 4: Once You Start, You Can Never Stop

This is one of the biggest misconceptions in aesthetics.

If you stop having Botox, your muscles simply regain their normal movement over time.
If you stop having fillers, the product gradually dissolves.
If you stop having skin treatments, your skin simply continues to age naturally.
You do not suddenly look worse than before.

In fact, many patients have enjoyed years of improved appearance and collagen stimulation from previous treatments.
There is no cosmetic treatment addiction built into the products themselves.
The choice to continue is entirely yours.

Myth 5: More Filler Equals Better Results

In aesthetic medicine, more is not always better.
Some of the most beautiful outcomes come from using less product, placed strategically.

An overfilled face often loses natural contours, facial movement, and balance.
The goal should never be to chase volume, The goal should be harmony.

As I often tell patients:
"Looking like yourself on a really good day is the ideal result."

Myth 6: Cosmetic Treatments Are Only for Vanity

This is one of the most unfair myths.

Many patients seek treatment because they feel their face no longer reflects how they feel inside.

A teacher may look permanently angry because of frown lines.
A nurse working night shifts may appear exhausted due to hollow eyes.
A woman going through menopause may feel she has aged rapidly in a short period of time.
Most patients are not trying to become someone else.
They simply want their appearance to better reflect their energy, confidence, and wellbeing.

Myth 7: Natural Products Are Always Safer

The word "natural" is often misunderstood.

Many natural substances can be harmful, while many scientifically developed medical products have undergone years of testing and research.

Safety depends on:
The product, The patient, The practitioner, The technique

Not whether something is marketed as natural.

Myth 8: Fillers Always Migrate

Migration can occur, but it is not inevitable.

Migration is influenced by: Product choice, Injection technique, Placement depth, Volume used, Individual anatomy, Repeated over-treatment

When fillers are selected carefully and injected appropriately, many remain stable and perform exactly as intended.

Myth 9: Cosmetic Treatments Prevent Ageing Forever

I wish this one were true. No treatment stops ageing.

Ageing is a natural biological process influenced by genetics, hormones, sun exposure, lifestyle, nutrition, sleep, and time.

Cosmetic treatments can slow visible signs of ageing, restore lost volume, improve skin quality, and help patients look refreshed.

They cannot stop the clock completely.
The goal is not to avoid ageing, The goal is to age well.

Myth 10: Everyone Needs Cosmetic Treatments

Absolutely not.
Some people choose cosmetic treatments, Others do not.
Both choices are valid.

Good skin care, sun protection, healthy nutrition, exercise, quality sleep, meaningful relationships, and a sense of purpose contribute enormously to how we look and feel.
Cosmetic treatments are simply one tool among many.
They should never define a person's worth or self-esteem.

The Biggest Myth of All

Perhaps the biggest myth is that beauty equals perfection.

After treating thousands of patients, I have learned that the most attractive people are rarely the most perfect.

They are the people who look healthy, authentic, expressive, and comfortable in their own skin.

A wrinkle from laughter, A dimple, A crooked smile.
A feature inherited from a beloved parent.

These are often the very things that make a face memorable.
Cosmetic treatments work best when they enhance individuality rather than erase it.
The goal is not perfection, The goal is confidence.
And confidence will always be more beautiful than perfection.

.

Chapter 89: When to Consider a Facelift

A facelift is not about trying to look 25 again. A good facelift is about restoring structure, lifting descended tissues, softening heaviness, and helping the outside reflect how you still feel inside.

One of the biggest misconceptions is believing ageing is only about loose skin. It isn't. Ageing is a combination of:

- bone resorption, fat pad descent
- ligament laxity, collagen and elastin loss
- muscle changes, skin thinning, volume depletion.

This is why many people who simply "pull the skin tight" still look aged or become disappointed with their results. The skin is only the outer wrapping. If the deeper structures are not addressed, the heaviness, marionette lines, jowls, and hollowing often remain.

I personally had a skin-only facelift years ago and was disappointed. Although the skin was tightened initially, I still had marionette lines and ongoing sagging because the underlying structures had not truly been repositioned. Over time, when skin alone is repeatedly pulled, the collagen weakens and stretches again, allowing the face to descend

In my opinion, if someone is considering surgery, it is worth understanding the difference between procedures and investing in a proper lift rather than simply tightening loose skin.

Signs You May Be Ready for a Facelift

A facelift may be worth considering when:

- fillers no longer give a natural result
- the lower face feels heavy, jowls become prominent
- marionette lines deepen, neck laxity develops
- cheeks flatten and descend, makeup sits poorly due to skin laxity
- you constantly feel you need more filler just to "hold things up."

Usually this occurs somewhere from the late 40s onward, although genetics, weight loss, smoking, sun damage, stress, and menopause all influence facial ageing.

Different Types of Facelifts

Skin-Only Facelift

This older technique focuses mainly on tightening and removing excess skin.

Advantages: shorter surgery, lower cost, quicker recovery.

Disadvantages:

- does not address deeper facial structures
- results often shorter lived, skin can stretch again
- may create a pulled look, marionette lines and jowls may persist.

This is why many modern surgeons now favour deeper structural lifting techniques.

SMAS Facelift

The SMAS (Superficial Musculoaponeurotic System) is a deeper fibromuscular layer beneath the skin.

Instead of pulling only skin, the surgeon lifts and repositions the SMAS layer.

Advantages: more natural result, better jawline definition, longer lasting, less tension on skin, improved lower face support.

This became a major advancement over skin-only facelifts.

Deep Plane Facelift

The deep plane facelift is considered by many surgeons to be the gold standard for advanced facial rejuvenation.

Rather than separating skin from deeper tissues extensively, the deeper facial structures are released and repositioned together as one unit.

Advantages:

- natural movement, less "pulled" appearance, stronger midface lift, softens nasolabial folds, improves marionette lines, longer lasting results.

This technique addresses facial descent at its true anatomical level.

However, it is technically demanding and should only be performed by highly experienced facial surgeons.

Ponytail Lift

Popularised as a more subtle and often younger-looking lift.

The ponytail lift uses hidden incisions around the hairline to create an upward and lateral elevation of the face.

Advantages: minimal visible scars, fresher appearance, less invasive, good for early ageing.

Disadvantages:

- not ideal for severe laxity, less dramatic neck improvement
- may not adequately treat heavier lower faces.

Vertical Facelift

A vertical lift repositions the face upward rather than sideways.

This often creates a more natural restoration because facial ageing tends to descend downward over time.

Advantages: natural rejuvenation, less stretched appearance, improved cheek support, softer lower face.

Many modern surgeons incorporate vertical vector lifting principles into deep plane surgery.

Keyhole or Minimal Access Facelift

Also called short scar or mini facelifts.

These involve smaller incisions and are often suited for mild ageing.

Advantages: quicker recovery, less invasive, subtle improvement.

Disadvantages: limited longevity, less effective for neck laxity or heavier jowls.

Facelifts and Volume Loss

A facelift lifts tissue, but it does not fully replace lost facial volume.

This is why many patients still require: fat transfer, biostimulants, skin treatments, carefully placed filler, regenerative treatments.

Ageing is not only sagging — it is also deflation.

A beautifully lifted face can still appear tired if the temples, cheeks, or around the mouth remain hollow.

This is where facial balancing becomes important.

Fat Transfer vs Fillers After Facelift

Many surgeons prefer fat transfer after facelift surgery because it uses the patient's own tissue and can create softer, more natural restoration.

Fat transfer may help: temples, cheeks, under eyes, around the mouth, jawline transitions.

Some patients still choose small amounts of filler for refinement, particularly: lips, fine marionette correction, chin shaping, hydration treatments.

The best results usually come from combining surgery with conservative regenerative aesthetic treatments rather than overfilling.

The Debate Around Sculptra and Facelifts

Sculptra stimulates collagen formation and can be wonderful for restoring facial support and skin quality.

However, some surgeons are cautious about operating on patients who have had large amounts of Sculptra because:

- it stimulates collagen and fibrosis, tissue planes may become thicker
- surgical dissection can become more difficult, anatomy may feel less predictable during surgery.

This does not mean Sculptra is "bad." It simply means the surgeon should know your injectable history.

As a general guide, many surgeons prefer patients not to have Sculptra close to surgery. Often waiting 12–24 months after significant Sculptra treatment is considered safer, although this varies depending on:

- amount injected, areas treated, surgeon preference, individual tissue response.

Always disclose: fillers, threads, biostimulants, fat transfer history, before facial surgery.

Maintaining Facelift Results

A facelift cannot stop ageing. Maintenance matters.

Lymphatic Drainage

Good lymphatic flow may help reduce: puffiness, post-surgical swelling, fluid stagnation.

Helpful tools include:

- gua sha, gentle facial massage, ice rollers, manual lymphatic drainage, sleeping slightly elevated, reducing inflammation.

Facial Muscle Strengthening

Facial muscles weaken with age just like the body.

Gentle facial muscle activation may help support circulation and tone. Examples include:

- facial yoga, resistance exercises, microcurrent devices, good posture, jaw and neck strengthening.

However, excessive repetitive movement can also deepen expression lines, so balance is important.

Skin Quality Maintenance

To maintain results:

- SPF daily, avoid smoking, maintain stable weight
- support hormones where appropriate, collagen-supportive treatments, regenerative therapies, healthy sleep and nutrition.

Treatments commonly used after facelift healing may include: PRP, skin needling, LED, exosomes, gentle lasers, biostimulants, conservative injectables.

The best facelift is the one that still looks like you — just fresher, healthier, and less tired.

Chapter 90: My Treatment Planning Roadmap

Creating a plan, not just a treatment

Every face is different. Every patient is different.

There is no single formula.

What I create instead is a roadmap—a treatment plan that is personalised, realistic, and designed to achieve natural results over time.

The best outcomes do not come from isolated treatments. They come from a thoughtful, long-term strategy.

I Work With the Person, Not the Procedure

Before I think about treatment, I consider:

* What concerns the patient, What they hope to achieve, Their lifestyle, Their budget, Their comfort level

* Sometimes, what is not being said

Often, what a patient asks for is not the full story.

A treatment plan is not something I impose. It is something we create together.

I guide. I educate. I explain what is possible.

Most importantly, the patient must feel comfortable, informed, and in control of their decisions.

This is a partnership.

Timing Matters

One of the first questions I ask is:

"Do you have an event coming up?"

A wedding., A holiday. A milestone celebration.

Because timing matters.

Many treatments need time to settle. Others need to be staged. Some improve gradually over weeks or months.

This is where I begin to build a timeline.

Mapping the Journey

Once I understand the patient's goals, I create a plan that includes:

* What to do first, What to introduce later, How long to wait between treatments, What results to expect along the way

The plan is then explained clearly and often written down for the patient.

Clarity creates confidence.

Starting Gently

For many patients, especially those new to aesthetics, I prefer to start with something simple.

Often, this may be anti-wrinkle treatment in the frown area.

Why?

Because it allows the patient to:

* Experience treatment in a gentle way

* Build trust in the process

* See a result without dramatic change

* Understand how treatment feels

* Learn how their face responds

Building Confidence Before Deeper Treatments

Once a patient feels comfortable, we can progress.

This may include: Dermal fillers, Biostimulators, Skin rejuvenation treatments, Regenerative procedures

Starting gently is important for two reasons.

First, it prepares the patient for future treatments.

Second, it allows them to gain confidence before moving into more advanced correction.

This staged approach often creates: Better outcomes, Less anxiety, More natural progression, Greater patient satisfaction

Treat the Cause, Not Just the Concern

A key part of treatment planning is understanding where the problem is actually coming from.

A concern may be:

Thin lips, Lines around the mouth, Under-eye hollowing, Jowls, Loss of definition

However, treating the visible concern is not always treating the cause.

For example, a patient may present with deep nasolabial folds, yet the real issue may be mid-face volume loss.

Another patient may complain about jowls when the underlying problem is structural support loss higher in the face.

Treating only what is visible can lead to overcorrection and disappointing outcomes.

My goal is to identify what will make the biggest difference and create a plan that addresses the cause, not just the symptom.

Every Patient Is Different

Every patient arrives with unique circumstances.

Some have limited budgets.

Some have unrealistic expectations.

Some are nervous.

Others have had previous treatments that influence what is possible.

A successful plan works within the patient's reality.

Consistency Matters

One of the most important parts of achieving optimal outcomes is consistency.

Moving from practitioner to practitioner, or constantly changing treatment plans, can make it difficult to achieve a cohesive result.

A long-term treatment plan works best when it is followed, reviewed, and adjusted over time.

Education Is Empowering

At every stage, I explain:

* What we are doing, Why we are doing it, What to expect next

Patients should never feel rushed or surprised by a treatment.

Education builds trust, confidence, and better decision-making.

My Mindset When a Patient Sits in Front of Me

When I assess a patient, my thinking is simple:

“What can I improve?”

More importantly:

“How can I enhance this person’s appearance in a way that remains natural, balanced, and authentic?”

I am not trying to change who they are.

I am asking:

* How can I achieve the desired result without overfilling?

* How can I maintain harmony and facial balance?

* How can I guide this patient safely throughout their journey?

Aesthetic Medicine Is a Journey

Aesthetic treatment is not a one-time event.

It evolves as the face changes, treatments settle, and goals shift over time.

That is why a roadmap matters.

It provides direction. It builds trust. It creates results that last.

Final Thoughts

The best outcomes rarely come from doing everything at once.

They come from thoughtful planning, staged treatments, clear communication, and a shared understanding of where you are going.

Treat the cause, not just the concern.

Chapter 91: Final Thoughts- Where Aesthetics Meets the Soul

Ageing well is more than appearance

As I reflect on my journey in aesthetics, I realise it has never been just about treatments.

It has been about people

About connection, About helping someone feel better in themselves

And somewhere along the way, this work became something deeper

Aesthetic medicine and personal growth began to meet and I found myself on a parallel journey — one of **spiritual evolution**

More than skin deep

Over the years, I have come to understand that what we do is not just physical

When a patient looks in the mirror and feels: Softer, Brighter, More like themselves

Something shifts

Their confidence lifts, Their energy changes, They carry themselves differently

That is not vanity, That is **self-connection**

A moment that stayed with me

At one point in my life, I was told by a highly regarded spiritual teacher that she had a vision of me as a priestess of Hathor in Dendera, Egypt

Hathor, the goddess of beauty, love, and healing

Now, I am not someone who lives in past lives or needs to define myself by them

But what stayed with me was not the story It was the meaning

Because throughout my life, I have always felt drawn to: Healing, Beauty, Helping others reconnect with themselves And in many ways, that is exactly what this work has allowed me to do

Finding purpose

This has never felt like just a career, It has felt like a calling

A way of expressing: Care, Skill, Understanding

Through something that touches both the outside and the inside

I have had the privilege of:

- Supporting people through change, Restoring confidence
- Witnessing transformation

Not just in how someone looks but in how they feel about themselves

Ageing with grace

Ageing is not something to fight

It is something to understand, to support, to move through with awareness

We are not here to become someone else

We are here to remain ourselves with a little more softness, a little more balance

And perhaps a little more kindness toward what we see in the mirror

Gratitude

I feel deeply grateful

To every patient who has trusted me, To every teacher who has guided me, To every experience that has shaped me

This journey has given me more than a profession

It has given me: Purpose, Growth, A deeper understanding of people

Who I have become

After all these years, I can say this with honesty

This work has shaped me as much as I have shaped it

I am not just someone who performs treatments

I am someone who sees, who listens, who understands

Sovereign in my choices, grounded in my values

A final reflection

Life is a journey, Not just through time but through understanding

And aesthetics, when done with care and intention, can be part of that journey

Not to change who you are, but to support how you feel within yourself

Thank you for allowing me to share this with you

— Nita

All You NEEDLE to Know

Facial Anatomy, Ageing and Structural Support

References 1–13
Primary Sections Supported: Facial anatomy, Facial ageing, Facial fat compartments, Retaining ligaments, SMAS, Midface anatomy, Tear troughs, Facial support structures, Temple anatomy, Structural treatment planning
1. Coleman SR, Grover R. The Anatomy of the Aging Face: Volume Loss and Changes in Three-Dimensional Topography. Aesthetic Surgery Journal. 2006;26(Suppl):S4–S9.
Referenced for: Facial ageing, volume loss, structural changes. Pages: S4–S9.
2. Rohrich RJ, Pessa JE. The Fat Compartments of the Face: Anatomy and Clinical Implications for Cosmetic Surgery. Plastic and Reconstructive Surgery. 2007;119:2219–2227.
Referenced for: Deep and superficial fat compartments. Pages: 2219–2227.
3. Haddock NT, Saadeh PB, Boutros S, Thorne CH. The Tear Trough and Lid/Cheek Junction: Anatomy and Implications for Surgical Correction. Plastic and Reconstructive Surgery. 2009;123:1332–1340.
Referenced for: Tear trough anatomy and correction. Pages: 1332–1340.
4. Hirmand H. Anatomy and Nonsurgical Correction of the Tear Trough Deformity.
Plastic and Reconstructive Surgery. 2010. Referenced for: Tear trough assessment and classification.
5. Lambros V. Observations on Periorbital and Midface Aging.
Plastic and Reconstructive Surgery. 2007. Referenced for: Facial ageing patterns.
6. Mendelson BC, Wong CH. Surgical Anatomy of the Midcheek and Midface: Facial Layers, Spaces and Midcheek Segments.
Referenced for: Midface anatomy, facial layers and spaces.
7. Özdemir R, Kiliçing H, Ünlü RE, Uysal AC, Sensöz Ö, Baran CN. Anatomicohistologic Study of the Retaining Ligaments of the Face and Use in Face Lift Surgery.
Plastic and Reconstructive Surgery. 2002. Referenced for: Retaining ligaments and SMAS support.
8. Furnas DW. The Retaining Ligaments of the Cheek. Plastic and Reconstructive Surgery.
Referenced for: Cheek retaining ligaments.
9. Alghoul M, Codner MA. Retaining Ligaments of the Face: Review of Anatomy and Clinical Applications. Referenced for: Facial support structures.
10. Stuzin JM, Baker TJ, Gordon HL. The Relationship of the Superficial and Deep Facial Fascias: Relevance to Rhytidectomy and Aging.
Plastic and Reconstructive Surgery. Referenced for: SMAS and fascial anatomy.
11. Knize DM. The Forehead and Temporal Fusions: Applied Anatomy and Surgical Relevance.
Referenced for: Temple and forehead anatomy.
12. Mendelson BC. Facial Retaining Ligaments and Facial Aging.
Referenced for: Facial support structures and ageing.
13. Mendelson BC, Muzaffar AR, Adams WP Jr. Surgical Anatomy of the Midcheek and Malar Fat Pad.
Referenced for: Midface and malar anatomy.

Botulinum Toxin

References 14–16
Primary Sections Supported: Botulinum toxin, Facial musculature, Treatment planning, Dosing principles, Combination therapies
14. Carruthers J, Fagien S, Matarasso SL, et al. Consensus Recommendations on the Use of Botulinum Toxin Type A in Facial Aesthetics. Plastic and Reconstructive Surgery. 2004;114(Suppl):1S–22S.
Referenced for: Assessment, treatment planning and dosing. Pages: 1S–22S.
15. Carruthers JDA, Glogau RG, Blitzer A, et al. Advances in Facial Rejuvenation: Botulinum Toxin Type A, Hyaluronic Acid Dermal Fillers and Combination Therapies. Plastic and Reconstructive Surgery. 2008;121(Suppl 5):5S–30S. Referenced for: Combination treatments. Pages: 5S–30S.

16. Bulam H, Ayhan S, Sezgin B, et al. The Inhibitory Effect of Platelet-Rich Plasma on Botulinum Toxin Type A. Aesthetic Plastic Surgery. 2015;39:134–140. Referenced for: PRP and toxin interaction. Pages: 134–140.

Hyaluronic Acid Fillers

References 17–22
Primary Sections Supported: HA fillers, Lip enhancement, Cheek enhancement, Chin and jawline, Rheology, Adverse events
17. Monheit GD, Coleman KM. Hyaluronic Acid Fillers. Dermatologic Therapy. 2006;19:141–150. Referenced for: HA filler science. Pages: 141–150.
18. Rohrich RJ, Ghavami A, Crosby MA. The Role of Hyaluronic Acid Fillers in Facial Cosmetic Surgery.
Plastic and Reconstructive Surgery. 2007;120(Suppl):41S–54S. Referenced for: Facial rejuvenation with HA fillers. Pages: 41S–54S.
19. Pinsky MA, Thomas JA, Murphy DK, Walker PS. Juvéderm Injectable Gel: A Multicenter Study of Safety and Effectiveness.
Aesthetic Surgery Journal. 2008;28:17–23. Referenced for: Product safety and efficacy. Pages: 17–23.
20. Wahl G. European Evaluation of a New Hyaluronic Acid Filler Incorporating Lidocaine.
Journal of Cosmetic Dermatology. Referenced for: HA filler technology.
21. Snozzi P, van Loghem AJJ. Complication Management Following Rejuvenation Procedures with Hyaluronic Acid Fillers. PRS Global Open. 2018;6:e2061. Referenced for: Complication management.
22. Funt D, Pavicic T. Dermal Fillers in Aesthetics: An Overview of Adverse Events and Treatment Approaches. Clinical, Cosmetic and Investigational Dermatology. 2013;6:295–316.
Referenced for: Adverse events and treatment protocols. Pages: 295–316.

Filler Safety and Vascular Complications

References 23–26
Primary Sections Supported: Vascular occlusion, Blindness prevention, Emergency management, Hyaluronidase, Patient safety
23. Goodman GJ, Magnusson MR, Callan P, et al. A Consensus on Minimizing the Risk of Hyaluronic Acid Embolic Visual Loss and Suggestions for Immediate Bedside Management. Aesthetic Plastic Surgery. 2020.
24. DeLorenzi C. Complications of Injectable Fillers Part 1: Prevention. Aesthetic Surgery Journal. 2014.
25. DeLorenzi C. Complications of Injectable Fillers Part 2: Vascular Complications. Aesthetic Surgery Journal. 2014.
26. Beleznay K, Carruthers JDA, Humphrey S, Jones D. Avoiding and Treating Blindness From Fillers: A Review of the World Literature.
Referenced for: Ophthalmic complications and emergency management.

Platelet-Rich Plasma (PRP) and Regenerative Medicine

Platelet-Rich Plasma (PRP), PRF and Regenerative Medicine
References 27–32
Primary Sections Supported: PRP, PRF, Biofiller, Hair restoration, Regenerative aesthetics, Tissue repair
27. Zenker S. Platelet Rich Plasma (PRP) for Facial Rejuvenation.
28. Gondinet A. Tissue Regeneration: Cell Therapies Using Platelet Rich Plasma and Autologous Cellular Regeneration.
29. Ulusal BG. Platelet-Rich Plasma and Hyaluronic Acid: An Efficient Biostimulation Method for Face Rejuvenation. Journal of Cosmetic Dermatology.
30. Borhan R, Gasnier C, Peygrane P. Autologous Platelet Rich Plasma as a Treatment of Male Androgenetic Alopecia. Journal of Clinical and Experimental Dermatology Research. 2015.
31. Marx RE. Platelet-Rich Plasma: Evidence to Support Its Use.
32. Anitua E, Sanchez M, Orive G, Andia I. The Potential Impact of PRP in Regenerative Medicine.

Facial Rejuvenation and Volume Restoration

References 33–37
Primary Sections Supported: Treatment planning, Volume restoration, Fat grafting principles, Structural ageing, Facial assessment
33. Coleman SR. Structural Fat Grafting: More Than a Permanent Filler.
34. Coleman SR. Facial Recontouring With Lipostructure.
35. Rohrich RJ, Pessa JE. Facial Aging and Its Relationship to Facial Fat Compartments.
36. Lambros V. Models of Facial Aging and Implications for Treatment Planning.
37. Mendelson BC, Wong CH. Changes in the Facial Skeleton With Aging and Their Clinical Relevance.

Core Educational Sources and Clinical Training

The content contained within this publication has also been informed by:
* Advanced Cadaver Anatomy Training, King's College London
* FACE Conference, London
* Needle Art Conference, Philadelphia
* Cosmetex Conference, Australia
* The Aesthetic Show, Las Vegas
* Merz Aesthetics Educational Programs
* Allergan Medical Institute Educational Programs
* Galderma Educational Programs
* PRP and Regenerative Medicine Training Programs
* International Anatomy, Facial Rejuvenation and Complication Management Workshops

Author Note

In addition to the published literature listed above, this book draws upon more than 30 years of clinical experience as an aesthetic nurse, trainer, lecturer, author and educator in cosmetic medicine, regenerative aesthetics and facial rejuvenation.

Disclaimer

This publication is intended for educational purposes only and reflects both published scientific literature and the author's clinical experience. It does not replace formal medical training, product-specific education, manufacturer protocols, individual clinical judgement, local regulations or professional standards of practice.

Readers are encouraged to undertake appropriate accredited training, maintain current professional registration requirements and consult product information, regulatory guidance and clinical mentors before performing any procedure described within this publication.

Conclusion

The Artist's Eye: Beyond Points, Protocols, and Perfection

As we reach the end of All You NEEDLE to Know, I invite you to pause—not with your injector's hand, but with your artist's eye.

Because at the heart of everything I've shared in this book—from muscle anatomy to bio-stimulation, from consultation ethics to product science—lies something deeper: the soul of aesthetic medicine is not just knowledge. It is vision.

We begin this journey memorising safe zones and layer depths. We learn where the vessels run, how the ligaments anchor, how light scatters over bone. But the longer we practice, the more we realise: this work is not just technical. It's emotional. It's intuitive. It's human.

You're Not Just an Injector—You're a Storyteller

Every face you treat tells a story. of laughter and grief. of stress and survival. of identity. Your job is not to rewrite that story—it's to honour it.

A cheek isn't just a cheek. It holds memories of joy. A frown line may hold years of resilience. Our goal is never to erase who someone is. It's to illuminate who they are.

Anatomical points give us safety. But artistry gives us grace.

Faces Aren't Templates—They're Landscapes

If there's one lesson I hope stays with you long after the last page, it's this: don't chase dots. Chase balance.

Symmetry is never perfect. Faces are dynamic, expressive, and beautifully unique. One brow lifts a little higher. One eye softens more. One cheek deflates faster than the other. That's real life—and it's your canvas. When we treat a face holistically, rather than compartmentalised into zones or trends, we create results that feel organic, timeless, and restorative.

Our best work doesn't look "done." It looks right.

Blend, Don't Overfill. Enhance, Don't Inflate.

Natural rejuvenation isn't about chasing volume—it's about manageing light and shadow with subtlety. Smooth transitions between planes. Support where there's collapse. Lift where there's heaviness. Glow where skin has dulled.

And above all- restraint.

The injector who knows when to stop is the one who gains trust, loyalty, and long-term success. We are not here to alter faces. We are here to refine them, refresh them, and sometimes—reveal them.

The Future Is Natural. The Future Is You.

There's a rising tide in our industry. A shift back to authenticity. Patients no longer want to look injected—they want to look like the best version of themselves. This is your invitation to evolve with that change. Lead it. Let your consultations be conversations. Let your needle become an extension of your awareness. Let every treatment plan be bespoke—not just to the face in front of you, but to the soul behind it.

Final Words

You now have all you NEEDLE to know—but what you'll come to understand through experience is this:

- It's not just about the tools—it's how you use them.
- It's not just about the knowledge—it's how you apply it.
- And it's not just about the face—it's how you see.

So go forward—not just as a clinician, but as a compassionate artist.

Inject with skill. Treat with heart.

And remember: the most beautiful results come not from perfection, but from presence.

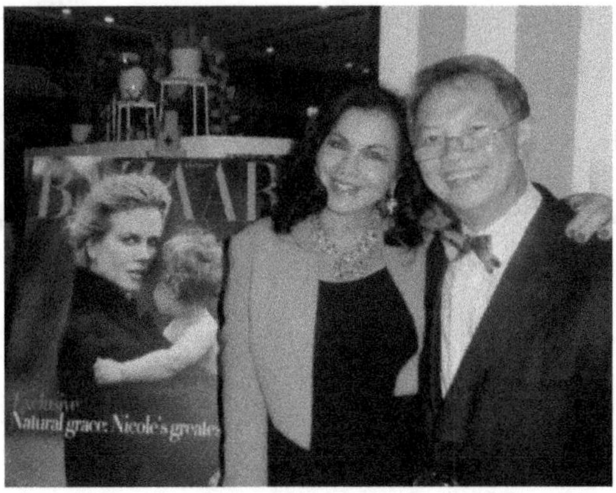

I owe my career to Dr. Soo Keat Lim, his encouragement, support and trust in me has made me forever grateful

Beauty Beyond the Mirror

The Journey to Self-Worth

After more than thirty years in aesthetic medicine, I have come to realise something deeply important:

No injectable, laser, cream, or procedure can ever replace self-worth.

I have seen beautiful women who could not see their beauty.

I have seen handsome men terrified of ageing. I have seen people chasing youth as though growing older were something shameful instead of something sacred.

In the beginning of my career, aesthetics was often about "fixing" lines or replacing volume. But over the years, I began to understand that what many people were truly seeking was not perfection — it was confidence, vitality, and a sense of feeling like themselves again.

There is nothing wrong with wanting to look refreshed. There is nothing wrong with wanting to look well groomed and cared for.

In many ways, looking your best can positively affect how you feel inside. When we feel comfortable in our appearance, it can create confidence, help us present ourselves to the world with pride, and allow our outer appearance to better reflect the energy and spirit we still feel within.

I understand this personally.

As women age, it can sometimes feel confronting when the face in the mirror no longer matches the youthful energy we still carry inside ourselves. For some, aesthetic treatments can gently bridge that gap. Not to become someone else — but to feel more aligned with who they are.

But there is also a delicate line in aesthetics.

Sometimes the pursuit of youth can become endless. A chasing of the tail. One more syringe.

One more treatment.

One more procedure in the hope that external change will finally create internal peace.

Yet true peace never comes from a syringe alone.

Because confidence built only on appearance is fragile.

Eventually time humbles all of us.

What lasts is something much deeper: self-acceptance, self-respect, kindness, wisdom, laughter, experience, resilience, and the ability to love ourselves through every season of life.

The most attractive people I have ever met were not necessarily the youngest or the most flawless. They were the people who radiated warmth, authenticity, humour, compassion, and presence.

Beauty is energy.
Beauty is confidence.
Beauty is how you make people feel.

Aesthetic medicine, when approached with balance and integrity, can be empowering. It can soften insecurities, restore confidence after illness or trauma, and help people feel more comfortable in their own skin. But it should never become a substitute for inner healing.

I believe the goal should never be to look twenty forever.

The goal is to look healthy, vibrant, natural, and harmonious for your age and stage of life.

To age well is not failure.

It is privilege.

There is wisdom in the softened lines around our eyes.

There is character in the faces that have laughed, cried, loved, lost, and survived.

Over the years my own journey has moved from seeking external validation toward something much deeper — self-acceptance. Learning that my worth was never dependent on whether someone chose me, desired me, admired me, or validated me.

True beauty begins when we stop abandoning ourselves.

Today, I still value aesthetics. I still believe in rejuvenation, self-care, and helping people feel confident. But I also believe our spirit, our energy, our health, and our self-love are what truly sustain beauty over a lifetime.

The most beautiful people are not those desperately trying to hold onto youth.

They are the ones who embrace life fully, continue growing, continue learning, continue loving, and allow their outer appearance to evolve naturally alongside their soul.

Because in the end, beauty is not really about looking younger.

Australian Advanced Aesthetics (AAA)

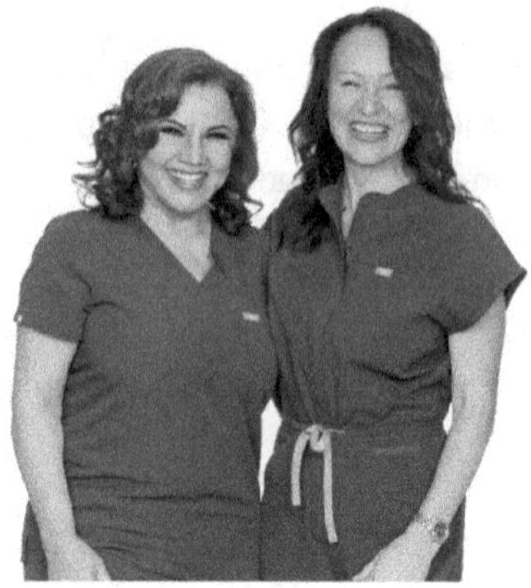

Australian Advanced Aesthetics (AAA) is an educational collective dedicated to advancing excellence, safety, and innovation in cosmetic medicine.

Founded by Dr Bonnie Hawthorne and Registered Nurse Nita McHugh, AAA delivers high-level education through regular hands-on workshops, masterclasses, and immersive aesthetic retreats.

Designed for medical professionals seeking to deepen their clinical knowledge, artistic skill, and confidence, AAA programs focus on evidence-based practice, anatomical precision, patient safety, and ethical aesthetics.

Expressions of interest are welcomed via the official website at www.australianadvancedaesthetics.com.au where upcoming workshops and retreat opportunities are announced.

www.australianadvancedaesthetics.com.au

www.instagram.com/australianadvancedaesthetics

Nita: 0422584682 Dr Bonnie: 0438204009

So you want to become a Cosmetic Nurse

The world of cosmetic nursing often looks glamorous from the outside. Beautiful clinics, glowing skin, social media transformations, luxury brands, and injectors with large followings. What many people do not see behind the scenes is that aesthetics is still nursing. It is medicine. It is anatomy. It is psychology. It is assessment. And above all, it is responsibility.

A syringe may look small in your hand, but the responsibility attached to it is enormous.

Cosmetic nursing is not simply about "doing lips." It is about understanding the ageing process, respecting anatomy, manageing complications, communicating honestly, and helping patients achieve natural, safe outcomes.

The best cosmetic nurses are not just injectors. They are clinicians, educators, artists, counsellors, and lifelong students.

Step One: Become a Registered Nurse

In Australia, the first step is completing a Bachelor of Nursing and becoming registered with Australian Health Practitioner Regulation Agency (AHPRA) under the Nursing and Midwifery Board of Australia.

This usually involves:

- A 3-year Bachelor of Nursing degree
- Clinical placements
- National registration as an RN

Your nursing foundation matters more than many people realise. Nursing teaches:

- Infection control, Patient assessment, Emergency management
- Communication skills, Ethics, Professional boundaries
- Clinical judgement

These skills become invaluable in aesthetics.

Do You Need Hospital Experience First?

Traditionally, cosmetic clinics preferred nurses to complete at least 12 months of hospital experience before entering aesthetics.

Many still do.

Why? Because hospitals teach you how to think critically under pressure. You learn:

- Sterility, Anatomy in real life
- Manageing emergencies, Recognising deteriorating patients
- Professional discipline, Team communication

Areas such as surgical nursing, dermatology, plastics, emergency, ICU, and perioperative nursing can all provide useful experience.

That said, the industry is changing. Some clinics now mentor graduate nurses directly into aesthetics. However, no matter which pathway you take, mentorship is essential.

A weekend course alone does not create an experienced injector.

Cosmetic Training Courses in Australia

After becoming an RN, nurses usually complete foundation cosmetic injectable training courses.

Training commonly includes:

- Anti-wrinkle injections, Dermal fillers, Facial anatomy, Facial ageing
- Consultation skills, Complication management, Cannula techniques
- Infection control, Emergency protocols, Hyalase use, Patient assessment
- Photography and documentation

Australia has many private aesthetic training organisations and academies offering cosmetic education.

Examples include:

- Australian Advanced Aesthetics (AAA)
- Australasian Academy of Cosmetic Dermal Science
- Derma Medical Australia
- Fresh Clinics Education
- Cosmetic Medical Training Australia

Some nurses also pursue:

- Graduate certificates in cosmetic nursing, Cadaver anatomy workshops
- Ultrasound training, Skin and laser education
- Regenerative aesthetics training

The learning never stops.

The Importance of Mentorship

This industry is not mastered quickly.

Social media can create the illusion that aesthetics is easy, but true cosmetic medicine takes years to refine.

A mentor teaches you:

- Patient selection, Conservative treatment planning
- Facial balance, Ethical practice, Complication prevention
- What NOT to inject, How to manage unhappy patients
- How to avoid overfilled faces

A good mentor can shorten years of mistakes.

Continuing Professional Development (CPD)

All registered nurses in Australia are required to complete Continuing Professional Development (CPD).

Currently, nurses must complete:

- Minimum 20 CPD hours yearly

In aesthetics, CPD may include:

- Anatomy training, Conferences, Advanced injectables workshops, Ultrasound education
- Complication management, Emergency vascular occlusion training
- Regenerative medicine education, Skin and laser science
- Business and consultation training

Good injectors remain students forever.

The face is dynamic. Trends change. Products evolve. Techniques improve.

The moment you think you know everything is the moment you become dangerous.

Working With a Prescriber

Cosmetic nurses in Australia cannot independently prescribe Schedule 4 medications such as anti-wrinkle injections.

You must work alongside:

- A prescribing doctor, or
- An authorised nurse practitioner

Current Australian regulations require genuine patient assessment and involvement by the prescriber.

The days of "quick remote scripts" are disappearing as regulations tighten.

Patient safety is becoming the focus — as it should be.

The Reality of Cosmetic Nursing

Aesthetics is rewarding, creative, and exciting. But it is also:

- Highly regulated, Competitive, Emotionally demanding
- Anatomically complex, Constantly evolving

Patients bring more than lines and wrinkles into your clinic.

They bring:

- Insecurities, Trauma
- Relationship breakdowns, Ageing fears, Loss of identity
- Social pressure, Unrealistic expectations

Sometimes they simply want to look less tired. Sometimes they want confidence back after illness, divorce, grief, menopause, or life itself.

This is why consultation skills matter just as much as injecting skills.

The Art of Natural Results

The best cosmetic work should not scream, "What have you had done?"

Patients should look:

- Fresher, Healthier, Less tired, More confident
- Like themselves

Good aesthetics is subtle.

Overfilled faces, distorted anatomy, and trend-driven treatments often happen when injectors chase social media rather than anatomy.

Natural rejuvenation is about restoring structure, support, skin quality, and harmony — not creating clones.

My Advice to Future Cosmetic Nurses

Do not rush.

Learn anatomy deeply, Respect the face., Respect complications.
Find mentors. Keep learning. Treat conservatively.
Underpromise and overdeliver.

And never forget:

Behind every face is a human being trusting you with their confidence, their appearance, and sometimes their self-worth.

That trust should never be taken lightly.

Index

C

D

I

J

K

L

M

O

N

Q

R

P

S

T

U

www.ingramcontent.com/pod-product-compliance
Lightning Source LLC
LaVergne TN
LVHW082018200926
848481LV00010B/2881